A HISTORY OF SCOTTISH MEDICINE

THEMES AND INFLUENCES

Helen M. Dingwall

EDINBURGH UNIVERSITY PRESS

For Dr W. G. Middleton
with gratitude

© Helen Dingwall, 2003
Edinburgh University Press Ltd
22 George Square, Edinburgh

Typeset in Linotype Ehrhardt
by Koinonia Ltd, Bury, and
printed and bound in Great Britain by
The Cromwell Press, Trowbridge, Wilts

A CIP record of this book is available
from the British Library

ISBN 0 7486 0865 6 (paperback)

CONTENTS

ABBREVIATIONS

Bull. Hist. Med.	*Bulletin of the History of Medicine*
Comrie, *History*	Comrie, J. D., *History of Scottish Medicine.* 2 Vols (Oxford, 1932)
EUL	Edinburgh University Library
Hamilton, *Healers*	Hamilton, D., *The Healers. A History of Medicine in Scotland* (Edinburgh, 1981)
Lynch, *History*	Lynch, M., *Scotland. A New History* (London, 1991)
Med. Hist.	*Medical History*
NAS	National Archive of Scotland
NLS	National Library of Scotland
Porter, *Greatest Benefit*	Porter, R., *The Greatest Benefit to Mankind. A Medical History of Humanity from Antiquity to the Present* (London, 1997)
Proc. Roy. Coll. Phys. Ed.	*Proceedings of the Royal College of Physicians of Edinburgh*
Soc. Hist. Med.	*Social History of Medicine*

NOTE ON REFERENCING

In the main text, full references are given for first citation, and a shortened version for subsequent citations. The Further Reading section contains items not referenced within the text, and the Select Bibliography comprises a short list of major works cited in the book.

ACKNOWLEDGEMENTS

This book has been many years in the making. It has changed out of all recognition since the first tentative outline was submitted to Edinburgh University Press; changed, it is to be hoped, for the better. I wish to acknowledge the help and support of many individuals and institutions who have made the work possible. Considerable help has been received from the staff of a number of institutions, including the Royal College of Surgeons of Edinburgh, the Royal College of Physicians of Edinburgh, the National Library of Scotland, the National Archive of Scotland, the Library of the Royal College of Surgeons of Ireland and the Libraries of Stirling, Glasgow and Edinburgh Universities. I am grateful to Sir John Clerk for permission to consult the Clerk of Penicuik papers.

Among the many individuals who must be acknowledged are, first and foremost, the entire staff of the Department of History at the University of Stirling, who have been of considerable help and support, often through rather stormy times in recent years. Dr M. A. Penman, Dr I. G. C. Hutchison, Dr J. L. M. Jenkinson and Dr E. V. Macleod have all made useful comment on sections of the book, and this is much appreciated. I am also grateful to Dr M. Barfoot, Dr M. Dupree, Professor H. J. Cook, Mr D. Hamilton and Professor L. Rosner for helpful advice and criticism. Errors of fact or interpretation that remain are, of course, my own.

This book was in large part conceived and created for, and as a result of, my special subject course on the history of medicine and society in Scotland. The students who took this course regularly provided original and stimulating insights and suggestions, without which the book would have been much the poorer. Their contribution is acknowledged with appreciation.

Holly Roberts and Nicola Carr of Edinburgh University Press remained sanguine throughout many delays and missed deadlines, and their help and encouragement were most welcome, as was the assistance of editors Eddie Clark and Alison Rae.

As most authors will acknowledge, no book can be completed without the help and support of family and friends. I am happy to extend my thanks to my sister Elizabeth, and to Bill, James and Andrew, Robert and Anne, and also to Irene Drummond, Patricia Cripps and Doris Williamson.

Finally, I am indebted, for support and, importantly, friendship and encouragement, to Professor G. C. Peden, Dr R. B. McKean, Professor M. Lynch and Professor C. A. Whatley; and for medical reasons to Mr E. W. J. Cameron, Dr A. J. Jacob, Dr F. C. McRae, Dr N. R. Grubb and, most of all, to Dr W. G. Middleton, to whom this book is dedicated with grateful thanks. There is much that is very good about medicine in Scotland today.

INTRODUCTION

TWO MILLENNIA OF MEDICINE IN SCOTLAND

To write a global history of medicine in Scotland is virtually impossible. How can one modestly-sized volume account with any measure of adequacy for the evolution and increasing complexity of medicine and medical practice in a small, but equally complex and often disproportionately important nation? It is necessary not only to chart the progress of medical and surgical training, professionalisation, institutionalisation, practice and the experiences of the consumers of medical care, but also to assess these developments in terms of a number of complex, interacting forces, including Scottishness, Scotland, Britain and Empire. Medicine in the rural areas and remote highlands and islands of Scotland was, and in some ways still is, very different from lowland urban medicine. The distinctively Scottish influence is perhaps less now than it was three centuries ago, though it may not be insignificant that a fair proportion of the medical personnel who occupy the highest national institutional posts, including the British Medical Association, are Scots. It has been claimed that surveys have shown that doctors with Scottish accents are trusted more than those without. This may be a statistical quirk, or even mildly amusing, but may also be taken more seriously.

The major aim of the book is to account for the progress of Scottish medicine in the context of the evolution and progress of the nation. The Scottishness, it may be claimed, is a false notion. It may be argued that medical practice in Roman-occupied Scotland was influenced by Romans. Traditional medical care in the south-west of Scotland may have had much in common with Irish practices. Could there have been in any sense Scottish medicine before Scotland existed as a geographical entity? Did the strong and well-used European contacts made by Scottish doctors in the late-medieval and early-modern period mean that Scottish medicine was in fact European medicine? Did the increasingly British and, later, Imperial, context from the early nineteenth century mean that Scots were participating in British and Imperial medicine? Does the highly technological nature of twenty-first-century medicine, which has virtually no national barriers and is truly global, mean that historians must write about medicine in Scotland, and not Scottish medicine? There has been much debate among historians as to whether there was a distinctive Scottish Enlightenment in the eighteenth century, or whether there was merely Enlightenment in Scotland. The same dilemma is faced by historians of medicine.

All of these factors need to be taken into account, though it will be a major contention of this book that whereas the nature and precise manifestation of the Scottish factor changed over the course of the last two millennia, it is still possible to identify distinctive characteristics or aspects which, if not nowadays very different from British or Western medicine, have been influenced and characterised by Scots and by Scotland. At the beginning of the first millennium there were no Scots, but the various peoples who inhabited the territory which became Scotland lent their individual and group characteristics to the development of the nation and its people. Over the course of the next two thousand years the descendants of these people became Scots and inhabited a discrete territory, but also maintained contacts with England, Europe and ultimately the New World and the technological globe. The identity of the Scots is difficult to describe or assess. One view is that it was influenced considerably by two factors: the Christian religion and a continuous monarchy.[1] This may well be true of the medieval period, but different and more complex factors shaped modern Scots, so that by the end of the second millennium AD, the average Scot may not be either Christian or monarchist. Despite this, though, some factors do seem to remain, including the importance placed on educational opportunities. These changes are complex and the influence of the Scot within and furth of Scotland is less easy to identify, but it does seem that the complexities of the past have produced, whether by coincidence or intent, something which can be labelled Scottish, although the debate on what precisely this is will go on. In order to give some sort of interpretation it is necessary to contextualise both in the Scottish and the international sense. Chapters One, Three and Seven offer brief general historical surveys of the periods covered in each of the three main sections of the book. The 'Further Reading' and 'Select Bibliography' sections include reference to works on Scottish and British political, social and economic history, as well as to books and articles on medicine.

Chapter Two is a brief account of medicine as practised in the territories which would become Scotland and which would be peopled eventually by inhabitants called Scots. The modern Scot is a distant descendant of early ancestors who themselves had regional rather than national identities. A recently published book on Scottish identity highlights the difficulties of defining Scotland, particularly before the period when the territory became circumscribed and stabilised: 'Before the thirteenth century, Scotland meant different things to different people, and different areas to different people, and any idea of Scots as a distinct nation or people was not fully formed before the period of the wars of independence'.[2] However, even when the nation eventually became bio-geographically delineated, the identity, culture and ideologies of its inhabitants still depended to a great extent on their local identities, and not on an image or identity which has been constructed by historians and others at a distance of many centuries.

Chapter Three deals with medicine in medieval Scotland which was, as was most of the European continent, dominated by the overwhelming influence of the Roman Catholic church. The church dominated all aspects of society, and so the medical discourse was also largely the discourse of the church. Anatomists experienced difficulties in extrapolating from animal dissection to the human condition (human dissection being frowned upon), and the attitudes of fatalistic acceptance inculcated into the population affected the givers as well as the seekers of medical help. If a disease or injury were considered to be just desserts for sin, then individuals did not seek medical care from 'professionals', but rather treated themselves or used common cures, charms, spells and other superstition-based remedies, as well as the ministrations of the church, both sacred and secular. The medieval period in Scotland was, in the wider context, a time of consolidation of the nation under a more stable dynastic progression. The period was not without conflict; disputes among the nobility were settled by bloodfeud rather than litigation, and monarchs ruled by the sword as much as by the council or parliament. The medicine that was practised reflected this – Scottish surgeons were becoming highly skilled in the art of the quick – though certainly not painless – amputation; they gained repute not only in Scotland or in the courts of Scottish kings, but also in the armies and on the continent of Europe. Peter Lowe (c. 1550–1610), who wrote a student textbook on surgery[3] and was one of the founders of the Faculty of Physicians and Surgeons of Glasgow, had, before settling in Glasgow, served both the French army and the French royal house for a lengthy period. Connections of a more peaceful, trading, educational and cultural nature, were made with Europe, especially with France and the Low Countries, and these ties would continue and become very important for the progress of Scottish medicine in the early-modern period.

The medieval period was also significant in terms of the secularisation of medical training and practice. Although any grand idea of a sudden flowering of medical knowledge and progress is not appropriate, as secularisation did not bring about instant enlightenment, there were certainly wider opportunities for individuals to study medical philosophy outwith the confines of the religious houses. For several centuries medicine had been practised within the walls – spiritual and physical – of the church. Physicians and surgeons were also members of religious orders, and dispensed health care as part of the general hospitality offered by religious houses such as that at Soutra, situated on a strategically important overland route between Scotland and England, a medieval hospital site which has yielded much information on the structure and functions of such an institution during several years of detailed excavation and analysis.[4] The medieval enclosure of medicine perhaps characterised it not so much as Scottish, but as religious medicine practised by Scots, and one aspect to consider is the extent to which medicine, or indeed any aspect of culture, required to be secularised before it could acquire a national identity, traits or characteristics, or whether the Scottish version of the dominant religion was itself an influence in the development of a distinctively Scottish medicine. Scotland enjoyed special daughter status with Rome, there being no archbishop until 1372, and this may have allowed for the development of a peculiarly Scottish form of the universal church, which in turn shaped a distinctive Scottish medicine.

The early-modern period, covered in Chapter Five, was crucial to the formation and characterisation of the Scottish medical institutions, particularly the Incorporation of Surgeons of Edinburgh (1505), the Faculty of Physicians and Surgeons of Glasgow (1599) and the Royal College of Physicians of Edinburgh (1681). These bodies, together with the universities, would produce the Scottish medical practitioners of the eighteenth century, among whom were some of the greatest of the great Scottish doctors, notably William Cullen, Joseph Black, the Hunter brothers and at least the first two of the legendary dynasty of Monros. It may be argued that Scottish medicine could not be distinctively Scottish unless and until it was practised by Scots who had been trained in Scotland by Scots. This was not the case with physicians until 1726, with the foundation of the Medical School at Edinburgh University, though surgeons had always served local apprenticeships. Theories and concepts of professionalisation are complex and problematical for historians,[5] but it may be argued that the development of the early-modern period, despite heavy reliance on patronage and the continued need to pursue unqualified practitioners, saw the emergence of many of the characteristics and attributes now generally agreed as contributing towards the creation of a professional body. This is not a point of view which will find ready acceptance among those of a more postmodernist persuasion, but whereas it is very dangerous to look only for a process of cause and effect, it may be equally perilous to ignore at least the dialectic of changing circumstances. Indeed, one of the most significant features of the early-modern period was the process and effects of the Reformation. Although reform took several generations to penetrate the more remote corners of the land, and although the protestant ethic of work may have been an ideal rather than a reality, the more egalitarian, individual practice of religion had considerable effects on the Scots and their lives in general, as well as their academic or professional lives.

The seventeenth century was one of conflict, civil war and economic fluctuation. It also bridged the gap between the union of the crowns in 1603 and the union of parliaments in 1707. The process of urbanisation gathered pace (although by 1707 probably no more than ten per cent of the population of Scotland lived in towns of any size, Edinburgh being some four or five times larger than the next largest town). Edinburgh, Aberdeen, Perth and Dundee were the main urban centres, with Glasgow beginning to catch up by the end of the century, as the focus of Scotland's overseas trade shifted from east to west. Apart from Edinburgh, though, most of the other towns were still too small to sustain medical organisation or education to any significant or lasting extent. Much of the rest of Scotland was, as yet, relatively unaffected by professional medicine. Qualified physicians were scarce, even in the larger towns, and country residents who could afford – or who wanted – to consult them were confined to the nobility and gentry, and perhaps their households. A further complicating factor which has to be considered, then, is whether any Scottishness attributed to medicine can be, or should be, applied to the totality of medical care and practice, including the amateur, rather than to the important, but as yet restricted, formal medicine on offer. Did the wise woman in the highlands, or the rural parish minister, dispense remedies which were informed by their culture, or were home cures independent of regional or local influences? Certainly the popularity of healing wells owed much to pre-Christian as well as to imported Christian influences. Highland formal medicine was very different from lowland formal medicine, though highland physicians had access to Gaelic versions of medieval medical treatises, including those derived from Arabic as well as Graeco-Roman origins.[6]

Chapter Six looks at the Enlightenment period, which perhaps saw the peak of Scottish medicine in terms of its role as world leader and pioneer. This was the era of the great doctors, the moderate *literati* in the Scottish church, and the towering intellects of the Enlightenment, as well as the age of Scotland as North Britain, as part of Great Britain and as part of the embryonic British Empire. This was the time when

Scottish universities attracted medical students from all corners of a shrinking globe, and also when Scottish-trained practitioners took Scottish medicine back to all corners of that globe. Scots occupied many medical posts in London, while the influence of Scots in America is well documented. Scottish medicine was unique in many ways at this time, but what was that uniqueness? Much of the impetus for the Edinburgh Medical School had come from Europe. The early professors in the Medical School were Europe-trained, so, was the Scottishness European, or European clothed in Scottish national dress? All of this took place against a background of, in the early part of the eighteenth century, uncertainty regarding the dynastic succession to the British throne, as a result of the efforts of the Jacobites to restore the Stewarts as well as the unfortunate obstetric history of Queen Anne, whose seventeen pregnancies resulted in the survival of only one child, the Duke of Gloucester, who died at the age of ten, plunging the nation into a succession crisis. Politics was dominated by a few influential individuals. Henry Dundas, perhaps the most prominent political individual of the century, earning the epithet 'Harry the ninth', was consulted by the Edinburgh medical institutions on a number of occasions when legal advice was required, and as the nineteenth century approached, Scottish medical practitioners would become drawn increasingly into British national politics and British national medical politics. This period was also one in which attitudes to diseases of the mind were changing, and when caring for the mentally-afflicted became part of the broader sphere of medical treatment rather than a problem of containment within local communities or institutions.

The final two substantive chapters deal with the modern period. Chapter Eight considers medicine in the nineteenth century. Here there were two major new areas: firstly, the significant medical and surgical advances which were enabled by the introduction of anaesthetics and the use of antiseptics, which allowed patients to survive conditions that had been impossible to treat or cure hitherto; and secondly, the nineteenth century witnessed the evolution and increasing application of 'state medicine' in the form of public health enquiries, surveys and legislation. The confluence of various factors such as the charitable ethos, state action and medical and surgical progress produced some rapid advances, although state funding of medical care for the whole population would have to await the final century of the second millennium. The Victorian period had its share of great doctors, just as the eighteenth century had had its share. James Syme, for example, developed an operation for amputation of the foot, which continues to be performed. There were other giants of Scottish medicine comparable to their eighteenth-century counterparts, notably James Young Simpson. Eponymous operations and medical conditions routinely performed or treated in the late twentieth century found their eponyms in the nineteenth-century medical world, including Hodgkin's disease and Bright's disease. Roentgen discovered X-rays, and Marie Curie was a pioneer in radium treatment. There were many other such developments. The suffering caused to troops fighting in the Crimean war stimulated Florence Nightingale to set up the beginnings of the nursing profession, although she was by no means the only major stimulus. It is, perhaps, a little more difficult to identify a Scottish aspect by this time, although many prominent Scots contributed greatly to world medicine. In the British context, the Medical Act of 1858, which sought, after much bitter controversy, to standardise medical education and registration, did much to create 'British' medical practitioners, but were any particularly Scottish characteristics still identifiable? Was it, by this time, 'medicine as practised by Scots' or was it still 'Scottish medicine practised by Scots' and was it influencing the wider community both at home and abroad?

The twilight of the second millennium witnessed perhaps the most profound changes in medicine, particularly as the century drew to a close and technology removed many barriers and obstacles to a global medical practice. Consideration of these changes forms the core of Chapter Nine. The aftermath of two world wars affected medicine in a number of ways. Expertise in the treatment of wounds and other afflictions gained pace, among the notable features was the pioneering work in plastic surgery carried out by individuals such as Archibald McIndoe. Scottish medicine has for centuries been influenced and affected by the current state of war or peace and the stage reached in the technology of war. In earlier times surgeons faced new challenges when the bullet replaced the pike; at the end of the period the technology of war is still stimulating changes in the technology of medicine. Materials and techniques developed for other branches of science are being put to medical use. The scourges of poliomyelitis and tuberculosis replaced the cholera epidemics of the previous century, but their effects were no less troublesome. Alongside the progress in medical and surgical techniques was the new political situation after the Second World War. The definitive labour victory at the first post-war election set the scene for the advent of the National Health Service (NHS), the grand aim of which was to provide treatment 'free at the point of need'. This had enormous implications for the organisation and receipt of medical care. In the last few decades the NHS has been under considerable strain and has experienced a number of reorganisations, which have had varying degrees of success. Meanwhile, technological medicine has progressed beyond the wildest imaginings of past generations.

This brings in new challenges, particularly to the relationship between practitioner and patient, when machinery, minimal-access surgery and diagnosis by computer can be seen readily as alien and threatening. With the flourishing of new technology has come the proliferation of para-medical practitioners of many sorts, from ambulance technicians to radiographers and physiotherapists, many of whom are women who have thus strengthened the female professional side of medicine.

As the second millennium closed, Scotland once again had a parliament with powers over the provision of health care. It remains to be seen what effect this will have both on ideas of national identity and on the progress of health care. This book will, therefore, try to achieve the almost impossible: to account for major influences on two millennia of medical practice and treatment in Scotland; to account for changes in medicine itself, in terms of Scottish influences, and in terms of the current historiographical debate. This is not a book for the dedicated postmodernist. It looks unashamedly for causal factors, or at least the creative effects of combinations of factors according to period, as well as action and interaction between the nation and its medicine, but in a manner which will, it is to be hoped, pre-empt accusations of Whiggishness.

Roy Porter's recent monumental work on the history of medicine[7] does in some ways achieve the impossible, charting medical progress in the world from ancient times to the present. However, its index is very revealing. Entries under the heading 'Scotland' number only two, and relate to death rates for coronary heart disease and to a Roman hospital excavation. Edinburgh rates one entry on medical education, and one each on the Royal Infirmary and women in medicine. This ignores the fact that Scotland has long been a major influence on medicine in Britain and beyond.

Since this book is intended to provide an overview of Scotland and medicine over a very long time period, it is not possible to deal in any great depth with many of the issues, which themselves merit scholarly monographs and much more detailed assessment. The aim is to highlight major influences and trends, not close chronological detail. The reader will not find minute detail on every topic covered, as this is not the aim, nor is the book heavily footnoted. The Select Bibliography indicates major works on a number of topics, and the Further Reading section suggests avenues for further, more detailed reading. It is hoped that at least some of the ideas put forward here will be taken up and expanded on by others sharing an interest in the medical history of this small, but extremely complex and important nation. The title of the book is crucial – it aims only to highlight themes and possible interpretations and influences, not to offer a detailed chronicle of either the nation or its medical history. The aim is to offer a framework upon which detailed work on aspects or localities of Scottish medicine may be developed.

CONCEPTS AND THEORIES

Historians nowadays are confronted by many theories. Theories of history, theories of social structure and theories of the process of change mean that it is no longer possible – or at least it is deemed not to be possible by sociologists and the authors of book reviews, among others – to write history without reference to the abstract as well as the gathering, contextualisation and analysis of evidence.[8] There are theories about spheres, about structuration and theories about the impossibility of theorising or deducing longitudinally. These theoretical approaches do stimulate the historian to take a new view of history and are valuable so long as they are not allowed to dominate the history to the extent that the history is submerged. One theoretical framework which may be appropriate for at least parts of this study is that of the interaction of spheres of knowledge, influence and social status. This theory, enunciated by Jürgen Habermas, relates much of the social dynamic, particularly in the eighteenth century and onwards, to significant changes in the location and use of information. Habermas claims, for example, that scientific knowledge became much less restricted and available to a much wider range of the population, in a large area of middle ground located between the very private sphere of the royal court and the general public sphere.[9] This theory has implications for the study of the history of medicine and nation. In terms of the history of medicine, this relates to the relationships between lay and professional medical practitioners; between patient and both types of practitioner, and the evolution of exclusive medical institutions. Increasing access to previously restricted medical knowledge had the result of stimulating the institutions to re-emphasise and confirm their rights to be exclusive within this broad and widening public sphere of knowledge.

To take this to a more specific level, one area in which spheres evolved rather than coalesced comes from the evolution of hospitals as a significant part of medical care and treatment. Some aspects of medicine were no longer practised or influenced wholly in the home, but apart, in the often alien environment of a hospital, which altered significantly the balance and dynamic of the patient-practitioner relationship. Another important dynamic of interacting spheres was the changing role of women both in nation and medicine. Women in early Scotland were highly regarded medical 'practitioners', but this was a very different medicine and an equally different regard from that which is held of women physicians, surgeons and members of paramedical professions nowadays. Women acted as charmers, healers, witches and wise women, and were regarded as essential elements in the cosmology of care. The trials and tribulations of Sophia Jex-Blake and others in the nineteenth century point up the very different rates at which the individual spheres grew and interacted with each other and with the nation in general.

In terms of the nation and nationality, Scotland evolved from a collection of very separate but interacting regional spheres of influence to become a national sphere (but one which was certainly not a homogeneous entity). This national sphere became part of a larger British sphere, and in turn the British sphere became the core of an empire. Scots at the dawn of the third Christian millennium are, perhaps, just a little uncertain as to the precise location of their nation within the British and global spheres. Similarly, Scottish medicine is in something of a flux.

Another potentially useful approach might also be the social construction theory put forward by Jordanova. This involves the consideration of the complex combinations of factors which underlie developments in medicine, science and their practice and application.[10] It may be said that this is merely emphasising the need to contextualise, but context is of key importance in any account of any aspect of medicine and society in any period. It is clear that throughout the history of Scotland and Scottish medicine the changing and complicated backcloth was not just a static, empty canvas, but was at the same time an instigator of change, a feature of change and a result of change.

In addition to the consideration of spheres or social construction as possible theoretical foundations for the study, it is also possible to consider long-term factors and trends, such as the creation and defence of a medical orthodoxy, or claims for custody of medical and surgical knowledge. It seems that as time went on, exclusive ownership of knowledge and its application was a major factor which was fought for by various groups of practitioners (and is, of course, linked to the professionalisation process). In its turn, new knowledge helped to create a new orthodoxy, or orthodoxies, and claims to ownership and defence of these changing orthodoxies may also be a structural framework for the book. In terms of theories of emergent nations, it should be rewarding to consider this in terms of the consolidation of the territory, the subsequent defence of the territory, and the functions of that defended territory within the expanding context of Britain, the Empire and the late-modern world and, of course, devolution.

Theories, though, must never dominate to the extent that the real process of history (insofar as it can ever be known) is obscured merely in order to satisfy a perceived need to theorise in the abstract.

What is, essentially, the core of the book is an assessment of factors which influenced and shaped medicine and Scotland, principally Western medicine in a predominantly Christian territory. The major spheres of influence and concepts which would seem to be important include:

1. The Scottishness of the nation, of its medicine, its practitioners and its people.
2. The nation and its evolution in the context of region, nation, multiple kingdom, empire and, possibly, nation again.
3. The diseases of the people – what, when and how did diseases occur, progress and become treatable or were eliminated? What old ills went and what new ills came? Can these be accounted for in terms of the evolution and development of the nation and the complex interaction of spheres of influence?
4. The cures and the providers of these cures – medicine and surgery; medical and surgical training and practice; new medical knowledge and the fate of old medical knowledge; the institutionalisation of medicine; rural and urban medicine, lay medicine, industrial disease; epidemic and endemic disease.
5. The interaction of spheres throughout the centuries. The sphere of the nation was very different in 2000 AD from what it had been in 1000 AD or 1 AD; within that, the multitude of constantly changing factors, including war and peace, custody of knowledge; cosmology and beliefs; government and governed; healer and healed; town and country; male and female; religious and secular. The binary nature of many aspects of change and continuity offers a balance which changed markedly through the ages but which remains, none the less, a balance, however precarious.
6. The issues of professionalisation, professional exclusivity, public accountability, private practice and the caring ethos which was, or should have been, at the core of all of these things.
7. The technology of medicine through the ages and how it influenced medicine and medical treatments.
8. The changing nature of the consultation process throughout the period.

The book is certainly not an attempt to impose any sort of rigid sociological or philosophical construct on Scottish medicine or the Scottish nation. Models by definition are temporary, trial structures for the larger, more permanent whole, but if used circumspectly may have a positive influence on the analysis of the historical processes and their interactions.

NOTES

1. Webster, B., *Medieval Scotland. The Making of an Identity* (London, 1997), 3.

2. Broun, D., 'Defining Scotland and the Scots before the wars of independence', in *Image and Identity. The Making and Re-making of Scotland through the Ages*, (eds) Broun, D., Finlay, R. J. and Lynch, M., (Edinburgh, 1998), 11.

3. Lowe, P., *A Discourse of the Whole Art of Chirurgerie* (London, 1599).

4. See *Sharp Practice* series of reports published annually by the Soutra Hospital Archaeoethnopharmacological Research Project (SHARP, Edinburgh), from 1987.

5. Burnham, J. C., 'How the concept of profession evolved in the work of historians of medicine', *Bull. Hist. Med.* 70 (1) (1996), 1–24.

6. Bannerman, J., *The Beatons. A Medical Kindred in the Classical Gaelic Tradition* (Edinburgh, 1986).

7. Porter, *Greatest Benefit.*

8. General works on historical theory include Marwick, A., *The Nature of History* (Basingstoke, 1989); Tosh, R., *The Pursuit of History. Aims, Methods and New Directions in the Study of Modern History* (London, 2000).

9. Habermas, J., *The Structural Transformation of the Public Sphere. An Inquiry into a Category of Bourgeois Society*, trans. Burger, T. (Cambridge, 1989).

10. Jordanova, L., 'The social construction of medical knowledge', *Social History of Medicine* 8 (3) (1995), 361–83.

PART ONE

A NATION IN THE MAKING

Medicine in Scotland from Earliest Times to c. 1500

CHAPTER 1

SCOTLAND AND SCOTS IN THE MAKING

As the Bronze Age melted into the smelter of the Iron Age, the peoples of Scotland were no more united or settled than they had ever been. They were still largely nomadic within their tribal areas; their nationality in terms of allegiance to a territorial entity was essentially one of locality, and their loyalties were given according to the prevailing tribal hierarchy, customs and cosmology. It is likely that general levels of violence increased in this time as territorial disputes intensified and as weapons of war became easier to manufacture. Medicine and surgery would have changed little from the age of the more brightly coloured metal or the age before there was any metal, or at least any metal derived by human process. Wounds of all sorts, infections caused by wounds or by diseases, and the disabilities caused by inadequate nutrition formed the major part of primitive medicine. The age of a new metal did not mean a different country or different peoples, and the spheres of influence continued to be local, though perhaps a little less nomadic. There was, as yet, no Scotland in the modern sense of the term. There were people who would become known eventually as Picts, or Caledonians, or Albions, but no-one could claim to be Scottish. Medicine and surgery were just as localised, as most early people did not have access to the sort of sophistication which characterised early Greece, Rome or Egypt and their medical practitioners and teachers. The dawn of the Christian era would see the legacy of these sophisticated early cultures disseminated to some parts of Scotland in the baggage trains of the Roman armies, but pre-Christian Scotland was essentially a collection of localities, tribes and ancient traditions. Indeed, the early Christian period was characterised by the combination of elements of pagan and Christian within rituals and customs. So, pagan medicine did not disappear; rather the important places and practices of pagan medicine were adapted and reshaped, though the official Christianisation of the nation certainly did not mean that most, or even some of the people wholly abandoned earlier beliefs. It is a characteristic of Scotland that the origins and heritage of the people were hybrid; the beliefs were hybrid and the medicine was equally hybrid.

A major external influence on Scotland and its early peoples was the Roman invasion led by Emperor Claudius in 43 AD. This brought the indigenous people into contact with a highly sophisticated culture as well as efficient and comprehensive military domination, at least for a time. The Roman presence in the territory which would become the British Isles lasted until 407, when the Roman army withdrew finally. This was a confluence of very different spheres, and one which would have some influence on medicine and medical practice. Around 83 AD the Romans first appeared north of what is now the border between Scotland and England, led by the infamous Agricola, and early domination centred on the important, fertile and accessible area between the Forth and Clyde. The first three centuries of the first millennium saw much conflict between the indigenous peoples who were competing with each other over territory, and between them and the Roman invaders.

When discussing the history of Scotland from earliest times to the medieval period or, perhaps more accurately, the history of early Scotland, the Picts are never far from the centre. Ironically, though, there is no real consensus as to who the Picts really were.[1] There is some debate as to whether the religious leaders of the Picts were members of the historic confraternity of druids, who conducted rituals and organised pre-conflict sacrifices, but these individuals, referred to by Pliny as *genus vatum medicorumque*, were key individuals in the medical cosmology of the day, which was very much part of the general, complex cosmology of early-Christian Scotland. Among the beliefs they enunciated was the view – and possibly the hope – that the soul was not fixed to a single individual, but could pass after death to a new external shell and continue in this way indefinitely.

After the disappearance of the Roman invaders, Scotland was plunged into darkness, or so the label for the next few centuries of the so-called Dark Ages would suggest. The period is, in historical terms, dark, because of the lack of surviving evidence, particularly written evidence, but in terms of Christianity the period saw the gradual enlightenment of large tracts of Scotland, following the paths set by St Columba and his followers and successors. The advent of Christianity did not, though, unite the country, which was as fragmented and un-united as it ever had been. The localities still dominated, and there was as yet little sense of a wider identity or a central ruling structure. The title of Alfred Smyth's book *Warlords and Holy Men*[2] gives a good indication of what 'Scotland' was like. Holy men such as St Columba endeavoured to convert the inhabitants to the Christian religion, while at the same time the warlords sought to establish themselves and expand their territories. In terms of the sense of kingdom or nation, there was clearly very little, and this would be the case for some considerable time to come. The term Dark Ages has many implications, and in terms of both the progress of the territory and the health of its people, darkness was an apt term. The Romans may have had central heating, public toilets and dispensing chemists,[3] but their influence was too localised and temporary to have much of a lasting effect, particularly on parts of the land which their centurions and symbols had not reached or influenced. The particular legacy of Roman medicine to Scotland is equally difficult to determine, although it may be assumed that variations of trepanning and combinations of drugs used by Romans and native 'Scots' would be introduced. It is clear that Gaelic translations of Greek and Roman texts were available in Scotland by early medieval times, indicating the extent of the classical medical world. Whatever the case, it is claimed by some historians that by the end of the first millennium Scots had become much less outward-looking and more concerned with defence and enclosure of themselves and their property. Archaeological evidence from hill forts, crannogs and other structures confirms this perceived need for defence against intruders or assailants. The invader was by now Viking rather than Roman, and the Vikings would not be the last ethnic group to infiltrate the territory and contribute to the shaping of the early nation.

The year 832 was of some significance in Scottish history, as it marked the start of an established 'national' monarchy in the persons of Kenneth McAlpin and his successors, although no monarch could claim complete security of tenure for several centuries to come. From then, until the beginnings of relatively more settled rule from the time of Malcolm I who became king of Scots in 943, the people endured both the Dark Ages and the onslaught of the Vikings, who achieved an important victory over the Picts in 839. By the year 1000, though, the 'post-Roman peoples had amalgamated under the ascendant Scots of Dalriada into the Kingdom of Alba'.[4] This kingdom was certainly not stable, but was more of a single entity than at any time previously.

It was during the reigns of Queen (later Saint) Margaret and her son King David I (1124–53) that clearer progress was made towards shaping the nation and, particularly, its religion and social structure. The so-called Normanisation of Scotland was underway. Margaret was deeply religious and brought members of religious orders to Scotland to set up a number of religious houses, such as the Augustininans and Tironensians. These establishments not only fostered the spread of the Christian religion, but also helped in the dispensing of medicine as part of the hospitality of the religious houses. David's influences were many, but it was during his reign, and beginning with his initial gifts of charters, that the burgh network of Scotland began to take shape. The royal burghs would become a significant, and unique, urban phenomenon, and these burghs would house the first tentative medical and surgical institutions. Burgh populations were small in the early periods, but these growing concentrations of individuals who were not bound by feudal ties in the same sense as on the land, would prove crucial in the development of urban institutions of a religious, secular and medical nature.[5]

From this period until the era of the Stewart kings and the transition of Scotland from the medieval to the early-modern phase, the major focus for the people was not the repulsion of Vikings, Picts or Normans, but of the English. Successive English monarchs tried – and failed – to dominate and conquer Scotland. It is, however, not surprising. The emergence of the feudal system of landholding and property transfer allowed wealthy and high-ranking individuals in all parts of what would become the British Isles to hold substantial tracts of land by gift of kings or other nobles.[6] Thus, noble Scots held lands and titles in England, for which they were required to submit and pay homage to the king of England. Similarly, Scots held lands in France, particularly in Burgundy, and in other parts of Europe. So, it was certainly not yet the case that an individual of substance living in the Scots territory considered himself to be wholly loyal, either in a practical or a philosophical sense to that territory. His 'national' identity was the common identity of rank in a developing European feudal society.

From the modern perspective, some Scots tend to maintain the view that the recurrent conflicts between England and Scotland in the twelfth and thirteenth centuries were simply a direct confrontation between two opposing, but unequal, powers. This view is much too simple. What was really happening was that there was conflict between England and those Scots who opposed the policies of the English kings, and by no means all Scots were in the latter group.[7]

The medieval period was important to Scotland in several ways. There was ongoing conflict, particularly with England, but also conflict involving European countries. The nation was unsettled in terms of territory and in terms of monarchy. The kings of the Scots ruled over disparate peoples and over frequently changing territorial areas, and tried to construct a history in order to justify their position and actions. The origin-legends of the Scottish nation are many and varied, and often involve an allegedly unbroken chain of monarchy back to the daughter of an Egyptian pharaoh (it is a little ironic that in later times gypsies, or 'Egyptians', were looked on with scorn).[8] The wars of independence (or, more correctly, the wars to maintain the independence of Scotland from

England) were bitterly fought and the age of Wallace and Bruce was of considerable significance to the progress of the nation, though in the longer-term view perhaps not as significant as recent film-makers would claim. The much-romanticised Wallace and Bruce period did much to consolidate royal power and establish a relatively stable dynastic progression, and from the early fourteenth century it is much easier to claim Scotland as a more or less settled territory, ruled by more or less dynastically settled kings (and occasionally queens). The consolidation of the Bruces and then the Stewarts[9] meant that there was progressively less threat of full-scale civil war over the succession or over the territory. Succession was never easy, though, and few of the early Stewart kings managed to die in their beds. Relations between kings and nobles continued to be problematic and often dangerous and the highland and border areas would continue to be problematic for centuries.

By the turn of the fourteenth century most of the territory which formed Scotland had been delineated. The northern and western isles still belonged to Norway; however, most of the rest of the territory (apart from the vacillations of the town of Berwick) was by now under the jurisdiction of the monarchs of Scotland. The monarchs themselves were in the process of trying to establish and consolidate both their dynastic integrity and power over their territories and subjects. At this point it may be justifiable to claim that the identity of the Scot was a local identity within a confirmed national boundary and a single ruler (apart from the territory more closely controlled by the Lords of the Isles until the end of the fifteenth century, the lordship being finally forfeited in 1493). Horizons were still narrow for the majority of the population, although those individuals on higher levels of society no doubt had a better sense of the larger nation, its structure, governance and international contacts.

Perhaps by the end of the medieval period, though, it was time for the territory of Scotland and its inhabitants to share a name, if not a completely settled or homogeneous identity. Localities continued to be of crucial importance, whether highland or lowland, and the noble or the clan chief held sway over his people. Inter-family disputes were still worked out by bloodfeud, even mortal combat on occasion, and there was an increasingly complex network of loyalties and identities which shaped both the control of the territory and the character of the Scots. Webster claims that two of the most important factors which shaped the Scottish identity were the Christian religion and a stable dynastic progression.[10] The situation may have been more complex.

The highland problem was and would continue to be a problem for a number of reasons. Firstly, the territorial configuration was very different;

the land was sparsely populated and inhospitable. Secondly, the loyalties of the people were not necessarily to the monarch, they were much more likely to have been to the clan chief. Until well into the medieval period there was a rival 'monarchy' in the highlands, in the person of the Lord of the Isles – a title with romantic overtones but an institution which was a threat to the centralisation policies of several monarchs. Most of the lands which were dominated by the Lords of the Isles, who were the descendants of Somerled of Argyll, were held from successive monarchs (ironic, perhaps, that monarchs would grant such rights over territories). Most of the lands were on the western seaboard and the outer isles, and the lordship was consolidated from the mid-thirteenth century, following the Treaty of Perth, concluded in 1266. The tangible legacy is a series of stone castles built to symbolise the domination of the territories. The Lordship and its influence declined after 1475, but had been a powerful influence in the highlands, which prevented moves to integrate the distant territories more fully into the corporate nation.[11]

The highlands continued to be a significant problem even after the dissolution of the Lordship and full absorption of the whole territory of Scotland under the crown. From the accession of the Stewarts and particularly once the dynasty had been consolidated under the monarchs named successively James, the territories proved to be difficult to govern in the same manner as the rest of Scotland. This had implications on a number of fronts. Firstly, if national identity needs to be the same in all parts of the country, then this highland–lowland dichotomy prevented more rapid progress being made towards any sort of corporate identity – although it would be quite difficult for many centuries, if at all, to claim a single corporate logo for Scotland and the Scots. Secondly, as the Stewart dynasty tightened its grip on the throne (despite the fact that only one of the first five Jameses managed to die in his bed, and the only one not named James, but the mother of a James, also suffered a violent and endlessly romanticised end), central to their policies of government was to centralise – to bring control of most aspects of Scottish life to the centre. This centralisation resulted in ongoing conflict with the very different highland way of life. The clan system was very different from the pattern of kin networks in the lowland areas and, consequently, much more difficult for the monarchs to control or direct with any degree of continuity. Thirdly, and again related to the problem of national identity, the ongoing attack on Gaelic culture and language can be seen as part of this assimilation policy. Detrimental remarks had been made for centuries about the perceived barbarity of the highlanders, notably in Fordun's chronicles and other early printed works.

Whereas before the turn of the first millennium there had been in effect a clutch of peoples living on a piece of land, who gradually drew together and forged partnerships, loyalties and conflicts, the early centuries of the second millennium saw Scotland becoming characterised more and more by the characters and actions of successive monarchs and the well-established feudal structure of society and economy. By 1424, when the first of these kings bore the name James (James I, 1406–37), the Stewart dynasty was strong but by no means secure. What would become central to both the consolidation of the territory and the dynasty, though, would be the relationships which existed and developed between kings and nobles. Large parts of Scotland, particularly the highlands, remained aloof from much of what was happening in the central and eastern lowlands, but the political and dynastic focus was very much on the kings and nobles. The development of feudal society was both the result and the product of this type of ongoing relationship.

In terms of kingship and the governance of the people, by the end of the medieval period the Stewart dynasty was well established and there was a clear – though often conflicting – bond between king and nobles and between nobles and their peoples. Although few of the Stewart monarchs managed to die in their beds peacefully, there was no sustained threat to the survival of the dynasty. Medieval Scotland was both very stable and very unstable, but the nation itself was much more cohesive that it had been a thousand years before. Structurally, society evolved on feudal lines, which produced the relative stability of mutual dependence, despite bloodfeud and conflicts between and among noble houses and the seemingly congenital inability of kings to die naturally. By the end of the medieval period also, Scotland was coming to the peak of its 'Europeanness', in terms of trade, education, culture, noble and royal marriage, and the common territorial interests of kings and nobles. It is not at all surprising that once medicine escaped the stifling and claustro-phobic atmosphere of the monasteries and the church, Scots acquired their medical knowledge and training in Europe. So, the period ended with Scotland looking outwards, relatively confidently, as an important part of the European continent. Relations with Scotland's contiguous territories were another matter entirely.

In terms of the economy of the territory, by the end of the thirteenth century strong trading routes had been established with mainland Europe. Connections of a less welcoming sort had been made with the Viking onslaught in the opposite direction, not to mention the Roman invasion of many centuries before that. The potential of the Scots to boost their economy was not great. War, Black Death and other scourges affected most parts of the country at various times throughout the period. Most of the items traded were the primary products of the land, particularly wool, hides and fish. As time went on, and as the tentative process of urbanisation began to take place, so Edinburgh gradually assumed the lion's share of trade. This was partly geographical, given the location of Edinburgh and its port of Leith; and partly due to sheer size and increasing political importance.[12]

In summary, at the close of the medieval period there was a more or less discrete territory ruled by a more or less stable monarchy. There appeared to be a sense of national purpose if not a fully formed or articulated identity; there was a strong European focus and a developing burgh network. All of these factors combined to create the background circumstances, or the elements of social construction, which would underlie and shape early medicine and surgery.

The two main chapters in this section will consider, firstly, the fragmentary evidence of medicine in early times, and, secondly, the medieval period, in which the territory became fixed and the nation came under the twin forces of feudalism and the Roman church.

NOTES

1. Lynch, *Scotland*, 12–25.
2. Smyth, A., *Warlords and Holy Men. Scotland AD 80–1000* (London, 1984).
3. Maxwell, G. S., *The Romans in Scotland* (Edinburgh, 1989).
4. Armit, I., *Scotland's Hidden History* (Stroud,1999), 23.
5. For account of burgh development see Pryde, G. S., *The Burghs of Scotland: A Critical List* (Oxford, 1965).
6. Recent account in Barrell, A. D. M., *Medieval Scotland* (Cambridge, 2000).
7. See new appraisal in Watson, F. J., *Under the Hammer. Edward I and Scotland, 1296–1305* (East Linton, 1998).
8. Broun, 'Defining Scotland', 4–17.
9. Dynastic progression from 843 illustrated in Lynch, *Scotland*, 487.
10. Webster, *Medieval Scotland*.
11. Grant, A., *Independence and Nationhood. Scotland 1306–1469* (Edinburgh, 1984), 200–20.
12. Account of early economic development in Whyte, I. D., *Scotland Before the Industrial Revolution c. 1050–1750* (London, 1995).

CHAPTER 2

EARLY MEDICINE IN EARLY SCOTLAND

INTRODUCTION

It is, perhaps, overly trite to state that wherever there have been people, there has been medical practice, but since man evolved by whatever route, there have been diseases and injuries which have required some sort of intervention in order to restore the individual concerned's capacity to hunt, make tools, work a plough, fight in a war, care for household and family, drive a train, lead a nation or invent ever more complex computer systems. This book is concerned with the history of Scottish medicine, or of medicine in Scotland, which implies that the major focus is on the fixed bio-geographical entity as now exists. However, some brief consideration of medical matters in relation to the territory and peoples who eventually formed the Scottish nation is necessary in order to provide as comprehensive a view as possible of medical practice. What this book is mainly concerned with is the progress and development of Western medicine in a predominantly Christian nation, although of course as time went on, elements of other religions and alternative medical practices entered the national and medical spheres. Coverage of the very early period is of necessity constrained by the selective and sparse survival of mostly non-written sources. Archaeological evidence is important here, and the bulk of what is known about iron age or bronze age medicine or, indeed medicine in Roman or Dark Age Scotland comes from physical source materials and ephemera rather than from any written record.

The very early history of the territory which came to be known as Scotland is almost equally uncertain. Various peoples lived in ancient tribal groupings ruled by tribal or regional kings, or *Ri*. Very little can be known about these times, but it is fairly safe to assume that any medical treatment given would be based on folklore or rituals passed down through the generations, and would be very closely bound up with tribal or group rituals, relating perhaps to the seasons, or harvest, the celebration of reaching adulthood, or preparation for war with a neighbouring tribe.

The dynamics of daily life related to the seasons, not to fixed calendar dates, and so the thrust of medicine was also seasonal, to the extent that cures and prevention were applied according to season, astrology and legend. It is difficult to make much of the Scottishness of medicine at that time; its influence would, though, permeate down through many centuries, even, perhaps, to the nineteenth-century folklore of the north-east of Scotland.[1] In the early centuries AD, there cannot really be ascribed a distinctively Scottish aspect to medicine. Any medical treatment was, for the most part, given and received in a very restricted sphere, of tribe or people, of locality, of tradition, of folklore, of herbs and plants common to the area, in other words, medicine was local, traditional, oral and lay, and not separate from other belief systems, though in areas which had been touched by other worlds, such as those dominated by the Romans, a further influence was brought to bear. The social construction of medicine and nation was at the same time narrowly based but surprisingly complex.

One of the main facets of medical treatment for much of the early period, and indeed for the next two millennia, was the treatment of wounds of all sorts sustained in conflicts of all sorts. The Scottish nation would be forged by the sword as well as by the feudal system, and early medical practitioners were required to try – often in vain – to save the lives of those wounded in battle or bloodfeud. Before the days of litigation, many disputes were settled by bloodfeud or mortal combat. This chapter will attempt to assess the fragmentary surviving evidence about medicine and medical treatment in this period, before Scots were Scots, and before Scotland was Scotland.

EARLY EVIDENCE

Medical evidence from other parts of the globe tells us something of the diseases which afflicted early peoples. Osteo-arthritis was commonly found among Egyptian skeletons, for example. Recent widely publicised finds of frozen, mummified corpses at high altitude have told us much about the life, lifestyle and death of individuals over five thousand years ago. It is clear that environment, the type of food available and customs of war and peace had great influence on the cause of death of such individuals. It is necessary, therefore, when looking at medicine at any period of the emergence of the Scottish nation, to take the changing environmental factors into account.

The high levels of general violence and the instruments used to inflict wounds produced injuries which resulted in severe skeletal damage, evident in axe-holes in skulls and broken bones. Any conflicts relating to territorial matters must have produced ample work for those members of the communities whose role it was to treat injuries and attempt to cure diseases. An example of this sort of medicine, which is closely bound up with the progress of the nation and its peoples, comes from a bronze age find in Fife, which showed that the individual concerned had been gravely wounded by a major wound to the side of the skull and a second wound, probably from an axe, which had almost severed part of the cervical spine.[2]

Archaeological evidence shows that the primitive peoples of early Scotland were not as primitive as might be thought. They produced high quality flint tools and arrowheads, and demonstrated high levels of craftsmanship in working with the easily damaged flint. These tools were used for many purposes, not least of which was in conflict, but equally important were farming, construction of dwellings, domestic activities and, of course, the origins of surgery.

The most often-quoted surgical procedure from these times is the operation of trepanning, or making an aperture in the bony cranium in order to let out evil spirits or evil matter; another area where the flint tool was useful. The surviving evidence suggests that the skull was scraped and penetrated by just such implements. A particularly good example has survived in a bronze age skull unearthed near Rothesay. The skull shows evidence of an expertly carried out procedure, with evidence that the bony wound had healed (indicating that the patient had survived the operation for some time and had not died immediately as a result of shock or infection).[3] The complex and difficult nature of the procedure would tend to suggest some degree of specialisation by individuals who could gain enough experience and expertise in the procedure to allow a reasonable hope that the patient would survive. The procedure was carried out for many centuries thereafter and, indeed, is still performed today in operations to deal with intracranial problems. The difference nowadays is that the procedure is undertaken to deal with a physical problem and not with the purpose of releasing evil spirits.

A comparison may be made here with the later operation of lithotomy for the attempted cure of bladder stones, which were a major affliction at all ages and at all levels of society. Orthodox surgeons avoided attempting the procedure, presumably because of the slim chance of survival. The problem was so pressing, though, that some individuals were prepared to submit themselves *in extremis* to surgery carried out by 'amateurs', often itinerant lithotomists claiming expertise. These individuals often had no right to practise surgery but perhaps because of the regularity with which they tried the procedure, a patient may have had more chance of surviving than with a trained surgeon who had little or no previous experience. (Two millennia later this same dilemma faces the managers of orthodox medicine. One such example is the question of maintaining a medical or surgical specialty in a remote area, where the single consultant may not encounter a sufficient range of cases to enable him or her to maintain an adequate level of expertise. To have a local specialist is convenient for patients, but they may not always provide the best or safest service.)

It is likely that wounds of all sorts would have been treated by the application of cooling and restorative plants and herbs, varying according to locality, season and the prevalent cosmological and astrological cycles. Just as would be the case in Christian Scotland, pagan Scotland operated in terms of a complex cosmology, in which the earthly and the supernatural forces which affected the land and its people were not considered to be unnaturally related in any way.

Druidic, or Pictish, medicine was truly cosmological in its beliefs, as far as they can be ascertained, but the practical application of these beliefs depended on location, geography, season and the types and varieties of plant and animal life at the disposal of those who attempted to heal the sick or eliminate evil spirits (very much the same thing). Among the plants used for treatments were water pimpernel, club moss and, of course, mistletoe, a plant potent and sacred to druids. As well as its symbolic importance, the plant was reputed to cure infertility and also to provide an anti-poison agent. Many of the plant-based drugs in use over the centuries have provided derivatives, or can be reproduced artificially, and are still in use. What has been removed have been the cosmological overtones; plant-based remedies are used because their chemistry is better understood. Perhaps particularly Scottish usages of certain plant-based remedies can be said to be tribal-derivative or locality-derivative rather than nation-derivative, but whatever the case, many ancient treatments provided, literally, the roots of modern medicine.

MEDICINE IN ROMAN SCOTLAND

One of the striking contrasts to be found in assessing the Roman period is between the very much superstition-based beliefs and practices of the indigenous peoples and the clinical efficiency of the Roman occupiers (though Roman gods were no less integral to life in all its aspects, including medical practice). The Roman armies were extremely well cared for, with, apparently, a surgeon provided for every cohort of 600 men, and well-organised and equipped field hospitals. These hospitals were constructed according to standardised plans, and a good example of such a hospital has been excavated at Inchtuthill. Casualties were operated on using finely crafted surgical instruments which would not be unrecognisable to modern surgeons.[4] It is very likely, though, that within the geographical area of occupation, the local population would have had some access to this type of care, and, indeed, that some elements may have been adapted and modified in line with local customs and practices. Among the procedures claimed to have been carried out by the surgeons of the occupying Roman forces were repair of hernias and cataract surgery, while a plethora of substances was used to concoct Galenical drugs and applications. Research on the use of drugs in ancient times has shown that the Romans used a number of derivatives of the opium poppy, as poultices, pills or potions, and there is no reason to suppose that invading forces did not bring supplies of the commonly used remedies to Scotland.[5] Other medicinal compounds came from chalk, belladonna, eggs and other animal, vegetable and mineral derivatives, and although the influence of the Roman invaders did not reach the remoter corners of the territory, their wide range of medicines must have influenced the treatment practices of the indigenous populations in their 'catchment area'. Roman physicians also made use of what they found in their conquered territories. Those physicians who practised in Scotland began to use iris, juniper and mistletoe as well as substances with which they were more familiar.[6]

As the nation, or, at least, the peoples living in the territory continued to interact and defend their territories, so medical practice continued largely unchanged. There was little to be done other than to use the products of nature in combination with qualifying seasonal, religious or superstitious conditions to treat the various epidemic, endemic and violence-derived conditions. The clinical efficiency of Roman times faded away and medicine became a little more embedded into the 'Scottish' ways and traditions. With the Romans came the first hints of the written record of Scotland, and although the influence of the Roman invaders on the whole territory was perhaps negligible over the span of two thousand years, evidence of Roman medicine confirms that both the knowledge and practice of medicine by these invaders were the best that was known or available. It was not so much any advance in knowledge or surgical technique that marked out Roman surgeons or physicians; rather that their basic and limited knowledge was enhanced by the sheer efficiency, literacy and organisation of the apparatus of the Roman Empire, wherever it happened to be located.

THE DARK AGES

Dark Age Scotland was a curious mixture of the descendants of Pict, Scot, Roman, Celt and others. There was as yet no real concept of nationality, rather one of loyalty to locality and territorial chieftain and resistance to invasion, in this period principally from the Vikings. There could not, therefore, be a specifically national identity to medicine or medical practice, unless the very amalgam of origins is taken as a token of an identity. In terms of belief, though, the gradual and pervasive Chrstianising process in the footsteps of Columba and other early Christian evangelists meant that there was an increasing homogeneity of core belief, at least in the more easily accessible, lowland areas of the country. Certainly in this period the territorial disputes among the various regional leaders and between regions and invaders would become more bitter and provide large numbers of the casualties of territorial violence to be treated by the medical practitioners of the time. This was an age when major wounds were caused by hand-held weapons, or projectiles such as catapults. Hand-to-hand combat undertaken by eclectic groups of individuals not particularly expert in war or tactics meant that those who treated the casualties of these human-powered implements had, in general, two functions: the amputation of parts which could not be saved, and the treatment of wounds and the infections which they caused. Roman surgeons had well-equipped medicine chests; Pictish or Scottish practitioners did not. The cure of wounds depended almost as much on the astrological picture, or local superstition (or expertise) as on any standard medical knowledge or standard treatments for certain wounds or conditions. In those parts of the country which had been touched by the Christian message, the sick looked to God for deliverance. In other areas, the wounded looked to gods, or to the stars, or to some local religious icon or holy place. Whatever the perceived source of sustenance and help, the important point is that earthly power alone was not regarded as sufficient in itself. A dip in an ancient Pictish well, or in one newly de-paganised and renamed for a Christian saint, was important because of the belief that good was contained therein. It did not really matter to the sick or injured individual whether the good was pagan or Christian. The wearing of lucky charms or the carrying out of rituals were other aspects of this animistic, or holistic, view of disease and its causation and treatment. Objects to which preventative or healing powers were attributed included the bezoar stone (a concretion from the alimentary tract of some animals and thought to counteract poison), stones of particular shapes, or glass of a particular colour.[7]

There is, understandably, very little in the way of reliable evidence about medicine or medical practitioners in a largely rural country with little in the way of communication or contact with other inhabitants even a short distance away. This was inevitably the birth-place of the many legends, folk tales and outlandish cures which have survived surprisingly unscathed in some instances, almost to the present day. The people lived differently; there was much endemic violence and no knowledge of cleanliness or disease prevention. What is not disputed, however, is that the cosmological sphere of Dark Age Scotland was complex and closely connected to seasons and the phases of the moon. The standing stones on Lewis or Orkney may have been there for centuries before the dark descended; their significance and implications were possibly better understood in 200 AD rather than 2000 AD. Whatever the real purpose of man-made artifacts like this, it is very clear that the whole life cycle, of health as well as disease, was connected inextricably to supernatural, unearthly forces and influences. Just as man learned to sow and reap according to season, so certain forces became dominant at certain times of the year, and had their own particular effects. Crop failure or dearth were believed to be due to the action of supernatural forces and these would be attributed increasingly to supernatural Christian forces, once the tenets of Christianity had been superimposed upon older beliefs to form a hybrid entity. So, it did not really matter whether the early 'Scot' was converted to Christianity or not; he or she would seek out 'holy' places and carry out rituals with or without the introduction of Christian terminology.

In the health and disease sphere – it is perhaps more appropriate to refer to these than to 'medicine', which implies something specialised and applied – supernatural forces played no small part. Even with the advent of the printed word in some of the more advanced areas of Europe towards the end of the first millennium, one of the most popular medical illustrations was that of 'zodiac man' – a representation of a human being, together with the symbols of the zodiac placed on the part of the body which would be affected if the individual became ill during the span of a particular sign. For example, if someone became ill in April, under the sign of Taurus, it was considered most likely that the neck would be affected, or would be the seat and cause of the disease.

In addition to man-made holy places, natural places became 'holy' in the broadest sense of the term. In this connection, water was particularly significant. Holy wells and sacred streams were long part of ancient pagan rituals. It was very easy for the promoters of Christianity to subsume these within the ambit of Christian holiness, so that certain wells or springs took on the names and patronage of saints and the good that was perceived to be drawn from them could then be attributed to

Christian miracle or the intervention of the saints. Saints and places developed medical specialties. The ancient well of St Triduana, on the outskirts of Edinburgh, for example, acquired a reputation for the treatment and cure of eye afflictions.

Since nobody, and certainly not isolated Scots, had uncovered the inner working of the physical body, any individual who professed to have the gift of cure regarded it as precisely that – the gift to recognise and deal with imbalances in the spirits which affected the mechanics and functions of the body. If ailments and indeed the environment in which people lived were controlled and governed by supernatural forces, then it was natural to claim that healers were also possessed of gifts which were not available to the general population. The concept of the witch doctor survives in many corners of the globe in 2002. In 1000 AD the Scottish equivalent may not have been referred to in these terms, but in effect he or she was in all other respects a normal member of the community, with no special training, but the recipient of special gifts of prophecy and cure. This is perhaps one of the fundamental aspects of pre-medieval medicine in relatively uncivilised parts of the world – those who cured were not trained to cure in any modern sense; rather they were recognised as having been given *powers* to cure. In 2002 AD those who minister to medical needs have 'powers' which have been acquired after lengthy periods of specialised study; in 1000 AD individual healers became identified by other means.

So, while the healers themselves could not readily explain the origins and nature of their curative powers, the cures which they offered could only derive from reference to the natural and supernatural worlds in which they lived, and in which the mind and body were one. Cures were also of necessity regional and seasonal, using the plants and other substances which were available at any particular season. Afflictions were treated by a combination of incantation, ritual and the application or ingestion of herbal concoctions. The incantations and rituals were crucial, otherwise the internal medicines or external applications could not work. Over the centuries, and as the peoples of Scotland became more mixed and hybrid, so the cures and their attendant rituals became more and more complex and influenced by more and more varied beliefs, so it was perhaps not too surprising that when certain practices related to both healing and malevolence became known as witchcraft and treated as crimes, those accused of witchcraft were often precisely those individuals who had been assumed by local communities to have special powers of healing. Rituals which seem to the modern eye to be ridiculous in the extreme, none the less were carried out in good faith. It was believed, for example, that when gathering club moss for medicinal purposes, it should be gathered by the right hand passed through the left sleeve of the gatherer's tunic, and the tunic itself had to be white and the gatherer barefoot.[8] There seems to be no rationale for walking seven times round a well backwards, but auto-suggestion seems to have played more than a little part in treatments at this time (as indeed it may well do in the third millennium AD). Most early medical illustrations contain overt allusions to the supernatural, particularly in the Christian period, when patients are normally portrayed in prayer, whatever aspect of their treatment is being illustrated.

THE WESTERN MEDICAL TRADITION

Apart from the period of Roman influence in Scotland, it is difficult to make very definite distinctions between the eclecticism of medicine in early Scotland and the classical elements of the so-called Western medical tradition.[9] This is partly because there were really very few differences in the practice of medicine under the banner of ancient Celtic cosmology and that labelled classical Western. The origins of the Western medical tradition are traceable to a small Greek island, now more famous perhaps for lettuces than Hippocrates. The key elements of Western medicine are credited to Hippocrates (c. 460–c. 377 BC), whose name may still be uttered, at least symbolically, by medical students before embarking on their careers as doctors. Hippocratic medicine was essentially holistic and untrammelled by complex or noxious medicines. Hippocrates' way was to assess the patient and his or her affliction in global terms, taking into account not only specific or localised symptoms, but also the patient's lifestyle, eating habits, temperament, the seasons, the weather and the current astrological picture. His philosophy was one of holistic approach and holistic treatment, the latter composed primarily of advice regarding diet and lifestyle rather than any attempt to deal with a local-ised cause. His views on diagnosis included advice that the physician should:

> observe thus in acute diseases: first, the countenance of the patient, if it be like itself, for this is the best of all; whereas the most opposite to it is the worst, such as the following: a sharp nose, hollow eyes, collapsed temples; the ears cold, contracted and their lobes turned out; the skin about the forehead being rough, distended and parched, the colour of the whole face being green, black, livid, or lead-coloured ... It is a mortal symptom also, when the lips are relaxed, pendent, cold and blanched.[10]

Advice on treatment was handed down through the generations in the form of axioms, usually referred to as aphorisms, such as: 'whosoever having need of purging have pains above the midriff, it is a sign that he must be purged upwards, but the pains which are under the same, show a purging downwards to be needful, for which way the humor naturally desire to go, that way you must by the help of medicines send it'.[11]

Once the Greek dominance had ceded to Rome, so also Greece gave way to Rome in medicine. When Galen (129–c. 216 AD) succeeded Hippocrates as the centre of medicine and medical philosophy, drugs, or Galenicals, began to be introduced in addition to advice about environment and personal conduct. Most of the Galenicals, quite naturally, were quite natural. Herbs and plants made up the majority of such 'drugs' and were administered in the context of a continuing holistic philosophy. It would not be until the arrival on the scene much later (during the Renaissance) of an individual rejoicing in the name of Theophrastus Phillipus Aureolus Bombastus von Hohenheim (Paracelsus, c. 1493–1542) that chemical medicines would begin to enter the sphere of prescription more frequently. This would mark one of the first influences on the separation of amateur and official medicine, but was long in the future. Galen, meanwhile, tried to make progress in the elucidation of the structure and function of the human body, but his dissection of animals and false extrapolations led him to several errors, such as describing the human uterus in similar terms to that of the dog.

But while the dominant empire may have changed, medical practice had not. As Porter states, 'Personal in Greece, medicine remained personal in Rome'.[12] The nature of medical philosophy meant that it had to be individual; the equally individual and unregulated nature of medical 'training' provided opportunities for all sorts of people to practise many different forms of medicine. 'Official' doctors learned their craft from the most notable philosophers and teachers of the day, not in universities, which were a phenomenon several centuries in the future.

Since the Western medical tradition was based essentially on nature and natural progressions, the medicine practised in early Scotland shared many of its characteristics, not necessarily because Romans brought the message, but because this sort of treatment had been in use for centuries anyway. Early peoples were very much more in tune with nature and the earth than we are today, so it was quite natural that early Scottish medical practice should mirror many of the core elements of classical medicine. What was superimposed or super-added, though, were the regional overtones. These regional overtones were not necessarily particularly Scottish, because at the time there was no such thing as Scotland. What they were, rather, were applied beliefs and superstitions which had evolved over the centuries in particular localities.[13] These overtones may still be seen in regional variations of 'old wives'' tales or cures for diseases or afflictions like the common cold. Cosmological effects and their attendant beliefs and superstitions varied according to locality and local folklore.

Although it is the case that, as Comrie states, 'medicine in the southern part of Scotland has always remained more "orthodox" than elsewhere',[14] none the less, it would appear that at least the core 'orthodoxies' of the holistic approach can be detected in even the most apparently bizarre of treatments. In many cases, the more bizarre or esoteric elements related to the attendant rituals or incantations, rather than the administration or ingestion of bizarre or esoteric ingredients (although in fact many of the elements of Galenical drugs contained items which would be included in the bizarre category, such as earth-worm broth, crushed beetles or roasted moles).

THE GROWING DOMINANCE OF CHRISTIANITY

It may be claimed that religion (in its broadest sense) shapes a nation. It is also possible to assert that religion shapes medicine. Both of these claims would appear to have credence in relation to early Scotland. The process of Christianisation had profound effects on the beliefs and actions of the people and, therefore, on the collective attitudes and actions of the nation. The advent of the Christian era also brought many influences to bear on medicine and the application of belief as part of the medical package of the time. Not all of these influences would be for the good of either nation or medicine. As the Christianisation of Scotland progressed, in the wake of Columba and other missionary pioneers, and as the names and reputations of Columba and some of the other early saints became more widely known, so then their names were often added to places which had had a 'holy' reputation in the Celtic or pagan past. Their functions were historic by reputation, but they now acquired the more current trappings of the Christian faith to justify that reputation rather than the earlier pagan connotations. In the south-west of the country the influence from English saints, such as Cuthbert, was also strong. Once the monastic establishment at Iona had been founded, in 563 AD, and as the community became settled, the monks turned their attentions to the planting and cultivation of a variety of herbs and other plants, which could be used to compound medical treatments. The settlement also, apparently, had a small infirmary and a dispensary. So, the spheres of influence and knowledge derived from pagan times, Roman times and Christian times began to interact and exchange traditions and practices. The eclectic mix which would characterise the Scottish people in later centuries was already at least partly in place by the turn of the seventh century AD.

The long tradition of the cure by the touch of kings or saints was also becoming well established by this time. By the seventeenth century it was still common for the monarch to allow his garments to be touched in order to effect a cure for scrofula (tuberculosis). Stones or other objects blessed by saints were also thought to have acquired special powers. The broken femur of Maugina, 'a saintly virgin' was said to have been healed by the application of water in which had been immersed bread blessed by Columba.[15] There are many other examples of such cures by secondary intervention. So the sphere of influence of an early saint or monarch was not confined to acts carried out in his or her immediate presence.

In early times, and quite understandably given its central function in the maintenance of life and the provision of nourishment, water took on especial significance. Watery places thus also acquired legends, and pilgrimages were made to sites which were deemed to be particularly effective in the cure of many diseases and afflictions, both mental and physical, and of animals as well as humans. In pagan times, water spirits were believed to have had both benevolent and malevolent functions. Once the watering holes were adopted by Christians, the spirit was that of God, working through the elements.[16] In addition to the importance of wells and natural elements in the healing process, the veneration of objects which were thought to have acquired special powers was another important facet of the complex sphere of early medicine in early Scotland. This was particularly the case with saintly relics, which were important not just in medical matters but also to those who wished to claim saintly justification for the cohesion of the nation. Whereas, for example, relics of St Columba were carried in an ornate, but portable carrier, the *Brecbennach*, the large stone shrine at St Andrews Cathedral, perhaps destined to contain the bones of the national saint, could not be carried around the country, but may, as has been claimed, mean that the significance was to the imagery of central power rather than of missionary zeal.[17] Saintly relics could, thus, be used to justify the policies of kings, nobles and priests as well as physicians, surgeons and lay healers of all sorts.

Whatever the problem to be dealt with, medical, surgical, or psychological, any treatment given and received in this era involved a natural combination of the natural and unnatural or supernatural. No self-respecting medical practitioner would fail to consult the astrological charts or invoke some sort of healing power, whether by physical ritual, spoken charm or intoned incantation. Herbal remedies were prepared superstitiously, that is, with careful attention to what was appropriate for the month, season or state of the moon. In pre-Christian times various gods would be credited with the potential to cure specific diseases or conditions. In the Christian era, especially in the early centuries, there was a combination of pagan and Christian influences, the former often being adapted quite unself-consciously to the scope and compass of the latter. Once the Christian church began to dominate Scottish society, though, the effects on Scottish medicine would be those of stagnation and hindrance. Medicine in medieval Scotland reflected this, as the tentacles of the church penetrated and influenced all aspects of life.

PLANTS AND HERBAL MEDICINES IN EARLY SCOTLAND

As has long been assumed, the core of medical treatment was natural, and mostly plant- and animal-based in its composition. The condition-specific usage of certain plants evolved from a combination of legend, folklore and empirical factors. There may not have been double-blind controlled trials of digitalis and other plants; what there was, though, was a gradual build-up in the communal experience of the effects of the ingestion or external application of an immense variety of substances, either singly or in combinations. In this sense, there was probably very little difference between the usage of plant-based remedies in ancient, medieval and, indeed, in early-modern Scotland. Excavation of an ancient grave in Perthshire found a bronze age male with a chest wound which had been filled with sphagnum moss, preparations of which were apparently used for their antibiotic potential until after the First World War.[18]

A welcome new addition to the literature on this topic explores the flora of ancient Scotland and the use made of plants for all aspects of life, not just for medicinal purposes.[19] From this, much useful information can be derived about medicine in ancient times. The late Bronze Age has yielded evidence of the medicinal use of skullcap (anti-inflammatory), dead-nettle (burns), juniper (diuretic, treatment of rheumatism), while in later periods, during the Viking and Pictish periods, juniper was still in use, as was henbane and celandine, and garden angelica acted as an antibacterial agent as well as an expectorant. It is clear that the inhabitants of Skara Brae on Orkney made use of the iris plant to treat a variety of conditions. From later investigations, it seems that the plant had a variety of uses, as an astringent, a purgative, a clotting agent and a cold cure, and that iris was still being used for these purposes in the highlands and islands in the nineteenth century. Similarly, the Orcadians apparently made use of puffballs to staunch the flow of blood, while surgeons in the nineteenth century were using puffball powder for exactly the same purpose. So, from neolithic to Victorian times, there can be claimed to be a real 'healing thread' of herbalism. The difference over the centuries has centred on the gradual dilution or elimination of the non-physical aspects to these treatments. The balance of importance between the treatment and the cosmological elements has altered greatly, but who is to say categorically that medicine taken with ritual or incantation was not more effective, given the acknowledged importance of auto-suggestion (controlled trials involving the use of placebos demonstrate this well)?

CONCLUSION

There is little doubt that the inhabitants of ancient Scotland handed down to their Pictish and medieval Scottish descendants a formidable array of medicinal remedies, many of which remained in use until very recently or, indeed, may be still in use, and not just in the remotest parts of the country. In terms of interacting spheres, medicine in early Scotland may be said to have operated within a single, general social sphere. A feature of Scottish medicine and, indeed, of Scotland as the book and time periods evolve, is that more and more complex spheres, with more and more complex interactions serve to characterise the nation, its peoples, its external relations and its medicine. Medicine in pre-medieval Scotland was simple – it would continue to be so for several centuries. It was tuned in to nature rather than politics or professions; it gained its knowledge from the traditions of Greece and Rome, altered to suit the people and their belief systems. The country itself may have been primitive, unformed and inhospitable; the cosmological entity within which the country existed certainly was not. Physical cures and medicines had to be derived from the substances which were available; their application was directed not so much by a single physician, rather by a kind of universal physician, to be found within the essence of the earth and its people. By the end of the pre-medieval period the tentacles of the Christian church were penetrating deep into the territory which was not yet Scotland; in time this church would dominate the newly consolidated country, its people, its rules and its medicine. The main conclusion on early medicine, though, must be that it was perhaps more in tune with the people and their beliefs than would be the case in the future.

The main thematic elements, then, were the common use of natural substances in combination with ritual elements, but with regional variation. The influence of the more formal tradition of Roman medicine was important, but localised, while the effects of the process of Christianisation were to begin to clothe disease and affliction in the black garments of divine retribution. In all cases, though, physical medicine was not sufficient. The attendant rituals and incantations were essential. By the end of the Dark Ages the overtones were Christian, and this would have the effects of stifling progress in medical knowledge, but also of bringing a more common element to the beliefs, practices and lifestyles of the peoples living in the territory which was almost, but not quite yet, Scotland. The social construction of medicine in early Scotland derived from the confluence of a multiplicity of local, regional and foreign influences, which also helped to shape the social construction of the people as a whole.

NOTES

1. Buchan, D., *Folk Tradition and Folk Medicine in Scotland. The Writings of David Rorie* (Edinburgh, 1994).
2. Comrie, *History*, i, 28.
3. Ibid., 27; Hamilton, *Healers*, 1–2. Eighteenth-century account in Mynors, R., *A History of the Practice of Trepanning the Skull; and the After-treatment: With Observations upon a New Method of Cure* (Birmingham, 1785).
4. Comrie, *History*, i, 33–5, illustrates Roman surgical instruments. See also Hamilton, *Healers*, 2–3; Porter, *Greatest Benefit*, 69–82; Simpson, J. Y., *Archaeological Essays* (Edinburgh, 1872) contains a section on Roman medicine.
5. Scarborough, J., 'The opium poppy in Hellenistic and Roman medicine', in Porter, R. and Teich, M. (eds), *Drugs and Narcotics in History* (Cambridge, 1995), 4–23.
6. Darwin, T., *The Scots Herbal. The Plant Lore of Scotland* (Edinburgh, 1996), 12.
7. Boyd, D. H. A., *Amulets to Isotopes. A History of Medicine in Caithness* (Edinburgh, 1998), 5.
8. Comrie, *History*, i, 30.
9. Conrad, L. L. et al., *The Western Medical Tradition 800 BC–1800 AD* (Cambridge, 1995); Porter, *Greatest Benefit*, 6–8.
10. Clendening, L., *Source Book of Medical History* (New York, 1960), 2–1.
11. Sprengell, C. (ed.), *The Aphorisms of Hippocrates and the Sentences of Celsus, with Explanations and References to the Most Considerable Writers in Physick and Philosophy, both Ancient and Modern* (London, 1708).
12. Porter, *Greatest Benefit*, 77.
13. Good account for the modern period in Beith, M., *Healing Threads. Traditional Medicine of the Highlands and Islands* (Edinburgh, 1995).
14. Comrie, *History*, i, 38.
15. Ibid., 43. See also Macquarrie, A., *The Saints of Scotland: Essays in Scottish Church History* (Edinburgh, 1997).
16. Detailed list of holy wells in Scotland in Anderson, J., *Scotland in Early Christian Times* (Edinburgh, 1881), 193. See also Morris, R., *Scottish Healing Wells: Healing, Holy, Wishing and Fairy Wells of the Mainland of Scotland* (Sandy, 1982).
17. Lynch, *Scotland*, 36–7.
18. Darwin, *Scots Herbal*, 11.
19. Dickson, C. and Dickson, J., *Plants and People in Ancient Scotland* (Stroud, 2000). This book is a very rich and rewarding source of detail and information about many medicinal and other plants in all areas of Scotland.

CHAPTER 3

MEDICINE IN MEDIEVAL SCOTLAND

INTRODUCTION

In terms of the evolution of medicine in Scotland, the medieval period would, increasingly, prove to be one of stagnation, as the Roman Catholic church gradually and efficiently exercised close control over all aspects of religious and secular life. Attitudes towards illness and disease, and to their treatment, became imbued with the heady but stifling mix of religious belief, religious practice and the actions of those in religious orders. 'Professional' medicine and surgery became the province of the monastery. Religious houses offered hospitality in its broadest sense, and included in this hospitality was the offer of medical treatment. However, given that diseases were thought in many instances to be the consequence of sin or the will of God, the sort of medicine that was given was very much along the lines of palliation and symptomatic treatment. Knowledge of the structure and function of the body did not improve to any great extent, and indeed humoral medicine as derived from the Greek and Roman tradition fitted very well into this increasingly dominant religious background. Humoral medicine had long been centred on symptomatic treatments, following expulsion – by whatever means and in whatever direction – of evil matter or humor. Medieval Scotland was, in medical terms at least, more than a little closed in on itself. The church dominated society socially, politically and also economically (the monasteries were also among the major sheep-farmers of their day), and the population relied on churchmen and those in religious orders to provide the range of services which would by the seventeenth century be the province of lay professionals. Meanwhile, though, as well as catering for the religious well-being of the Scots, the church in its many forms provided legal, medical and educational services as well as social control and the punishment of offenders against the social norms as defined or articulated at the time.

An essential factor in the construction of a secular and professionalised medicine and surgery was the evolution of secular and professionalised institutions. Towards the end of the fifteenth century, as towns, particularly Edinburgh, began to grow in population and occupational groups became sufficiently large, a number of craft incorporations and merchant guilds began to appear.[1] The main purpose of these organisations was to create and maintain occupational privileges; to act as social protectors of members and their dependants, and to – in some instances – maintain an altar dedicated to a suitable saint. The small community of barbers and surgeons of Edinburgh was no different, and in 1505 petitioned the Town Council of Edinburgh for permission to set up an incorporation. Permission was duly forthcoming and the group received its charter, or Seal of Cause, ratified the following year by James IV, a monarch who expressed great interest in medical and scientific matters.[2] If a long-term view is taken, it is not implausible to see the seeds of the future highly organised, learned and technological modern surgical profession here, although of course the changing and evolving social, political and economic background would also create new situations and new stimuli to progress. By the turn of the seventeenth century, Glasgow also had its uniquely combined medical and surgical organisation. This was, however, well in the future, and by the time that Robert the Bruce had helped to ensure some sort of continuity of monarchy in Scotland by the turn of the fourteenth century, medicine was in the process of secularisation, but not yet under the corporate *aegis* of any recognisable institution. Development was relatively limited in terms of elucidation of body structures, functions or diseases, but progress and change did come with the beginnings of the process of secularisation and institutionalisation of medicine and surgery.

During this period, dominated by the Roman church, Scotland was consolidating as a territorial entity, though riven with destructive conflicts and a continuing opposition to English attempts to encroach and impose domination. These conflicts, naturally, produced many casualties and much experience for the medical attendants of the time. As medicine and medical training became more and more secularised and practised outwith the walls of the monasteries, thus it was possible for the beginnings of a return to Hippocratic classicism to take place, and also for the two emerging branches of medicine and surgery to begin to go their separate ways. This chapter will, then, examine the giving and receiving of medical treatment in a period of consolidation for the nation and of divisions in medicine between official and unofficial.

MONASTIC MEDICINE AND SURGERY

The monasteries may have been closed, inward-looking institutions, but monastic medicine was important for the future of medicine in Scotland as well as for medicine in medieval times. In terms of the excavation of evidence from this period, the historian must be prepared to consider much more of an interdisciplinary approach, utilising the expertise of environmental historians, archaeologists and others. A major case-study, and one which has offered much evidence on what actually happened in a religious institution is centred on the archaeological investigations of the monastic hospital at Soutra.[3] This was situated in a remote area, but on one of the major overland routes south. The terrain was inhospitable and the isolation meant that those who were treated there were mostly travellers. Much useful information on medical practice has been gleaned, which cannot be obtained from other sources. This was a monastic foundation, which had books, but the books have not survived. What have survived, though, are the bones of infants or fetuses, grains of grain, utensils and other debris and detritus. What this evidence provides is an insight – limited but none the less useful – into the experiences of the sick and the traveller; the common diseases, the herbal remedies, and the sheer variety of the latter. This was, clearly, an important site, set strategically on an important overland route across what would become, eventually, the border between Scotland and England. The evidence confirms that medicine was practised, and in considerable quantities.[4] The medieval Scottish medical practitioner or surgeon, though not qualified formally in medicine or surgery, did offer a service which was separate from, if not greatly different from, lay practice in the period.

There is evidence, for example, of traces of blood in a number of locations at Soutra, although it is difficult to relate this directly to blood-letting practices. Small amounts of flax and hemp fibres were also found, and confirmation of the use of these plants in British medieval religious houses comes from the records of Whalley Abbey in Lancashire and Battle Abbey in Sussex.[5] It is likely that practices were relatively similar in monastic hospitals, with variation depending on available plants or medical tracts. There is some evidence of a similar, but smaller-scale 'spital', dedicated to St Magnus, on the east Caithness coast.[6]

However valuable Soutra might be, some of the evidence needs to be taken with a degree of caution. It has, for example, been claimed that the discovery of a number of tiny skeletons confirms that an 'abortion clinic' was in operation, despite the dominance of the Catholic church. This is a difficult conclusion to defend. Given the many factors of isolation, weather conditions, problems of travel, mortality rate and size of full-term medieval infants and the precarious medical and general condition of their mothers, it would be impossible to prove whether these were the skeletons of newborn or stillborn infants or near-term fetuses which succumbed to circumstances rather than to any element of maternal desire, coercion or obstetric accident. Just as medieval sheep were much smaller than modern ones, so it is to be assumed that medieval babies were not, on the whole, strapping ten-pounders as many are today. This type of evidence is, though, in many instances, the only available source of information, and such investigations are of great value to the historian, provided that the conclusions are derived with a good measure of caution and attention to the circumstances of the period and the location. What it does confirm, however tenuously, is that the sphere of the church almost wholly contained the sphere of medical practice as delivered outside the domestic sphere by other than family members or local worthies.

Within the global sphere of the church then, was a microcosm of medicine and surgery. Those in religious orders provided religious instruction, Christian hospitality and medical care to those individuals who came into contact with the fairly numerous, but scattered, Scottish monastic institutions.[7] It is little wonder, then, that new ideas or treatments, or indeed new belief systems, had virtually no chance of being even discussed, let alone tried out or adopted. This is not, though, to deride what was done for the sick in the medieval period. Treatments were given on the basis of fairly insubstantial logic for the most part (though deemed at the time to be entirely logical), and it may indeed be the case that many patients died for iatrogenic reasons rather than from the original disease, but the care was given with the best intentions. However, if both medicine and nation were to strengthen in the second millennium, the influence of the church in both areas had to be moderated, although it remained crucial in secular political terms for several centuries thereafter. For the moment, the social construction of medicine was the religious construction of medicine.

In terms of power and influence in the general sphere, the Scottish church was dominant. As mentioned, some of the monastic foundations were crucial to the economy, being among the most successful sheep farmers in the country. Church and state were one, and thus those in religious orders had important secular influences. In medical terms, the church was dominant.[8] It may be said that 'orthodox' medicine in this period was 'church medicine'. Churchmen were not trained specifically in medicine, but they did have access to the available medical literature, and as part of their holistic responsibilities, treated the sick who were within range of their foundations. The sick were treated because it was part of the Christian ethos to offer sustenance and support to the weaker members of society. Monasteries had herb gardens which supplied produce for food but also for the preparation of medical potions. It is likely that any surgery that was performed was of the most primitive and basic nature – as it would be, indeed, for a long period after the secularisation of medicine. A recent analysis of material excavated from cemeteries adjoining Carmelite priories in Aberdeen, Perth and Linlithgow has concluded that in percentage terms the number of fractures was relatively similar to the pattern today, but that rural life produced a higher rate of such injuries. It also seemed to be the case that fractures of the long bones had been treated well enough for them to have healed in relatively good alignment, indicating a fair degree of skill among surgeons or lay individuals who treated the patients. The excavations also produced evidence of the practice of trepanning.[9]

The importance of monasteries to Scottish medicine may be dated as far back as the reign of Queen (later, Saint) Margaret, who was instrumental in the 'importation' of monks from France, thus providing strong French influence on Scotland's religious and medical life.[10] Conspicuous piety was a feature of the time. As the monastic institutions evolved, infirmaries became part of the residential and farming complexes, and a number had an elemosiner, or almoner to oversee hospitality, charity and care of the sick.[11]

For those who did not have access to monastic medicine, there was no alternative but to try the wide variety of folk and superstitious medical 'practice' which formed an important part of the cosmology of the time. It is important to remember that belief in a Christian god did not negate or dilute more general beliefs in the supernatural and in unexplainable forces which brought disaster – or good – to the population. It was perfectly acceptable and natural to combine Christian belief with long-held belief in the powers of individuals in society who had been given some sort of higher power. Witchcraft, charming and superstitious cures were applied, not merely because no other source of more rational treatment was available, but because they were a fully accepted and rational part of the ethos of the time.[12] In later periods there would be concerted political campaigns against witchcraft, but there is good evidence to confirm that belief in, and treatment in terms of, the supernatural, were widespread and would continue to be so long after the end of the medieval period.

SECULARISATION – NEW SPHERES?

One of the major, long-term factors in the emergence of orthodox Scottish medicine as a separate sphere of predominantly professional practice and influence was the separation of the learning and practice of medicine from a number of spheres to which they had been linked intimately for many centuries. From the end of the first millennium the process of separating medical and surgical practitioners from their earlier ties to the church began. In common with lawyers and teachers, medical men were also religious men and religious men carried out a multiplicity of functions, by virtue of their literacy and education. The gradual secularisation of literacy would be a crucial step in the secularisation of any of the major, modern, secular professions. In terms of the custody of knowledge and claimed rights to sole custody of knowledge by professionals, the twin processes of secularisation and literacy would prove to be of singular importance in the redefinition of medicine and the ongoing struggles by medical men to lay claim to sole custody of the increasing body of available knowledge. Similarly, the less definable but necessary process of secularisation of the body, its functions and diseases, was a pre-requisite of the discovery of its workings and possible treatments. By the latter decades of the eleventh century there was the beginning of the view in religious circles, or at least at the epicentre of religion, the papacy, that surgery at least was not an occupation which should be carried out by clerics at any level. Finally, or, more correctly, initially, the impetus towards secularisation came from the papal bull *ecclesiae abhorret a sanguine* issued in 1163. This edict declared that clerics should no longer let the blood of others in the cause of medical treatment. This date and this decree may be cited as one of the most important signposts at the crossroads of medieval society, religion and medicine. The problem for the secular medical and surgical practitioners was that there were two signposts at the crossroads, the high road leading to academically trained physicians and the (perceived by physicians at least) low road of practical apprenticeship towards qualification as a master surgeon. The view that it was no longer part of the responsibilities of religious orders to give invasive medical treatment was, in the long term, to allow for the liberation of medicine. It is perhaps not too outrageous or overly Whiggish to claim that enlightenment in medical terms started in 1163, rather than in the second half of the eighteenth century with the usually capitalised version of the term. What did happen, though, was that medical students began to attend secular universities in order to learn about the philosophy of medicine. What they learned may not have been at all liberating or stimulating to the intellect, but the important point is that they were, despite many universities being founded by religious orders, able to consider and study classical Graeco-Roman medicine, and also to be aware of the Arabic strand which had been developing in parallel.[13] It would take until the eighteenth century at least for the body to be understood in any of the complex manners in which it is today. It would take even longer for this knowledge to be translated into new methods of treatment. The crucial factor is that, in a country where religion was deeply important and permeated all aspects of society, medicine was no longer constrained by religious dogma. If the medieval period lightened the darkness of the Dark Ages, so the secularisation of medicine would prove to be even more illuminating.

Some caution needs to be expressed, though, in order to demonstrate that university medical philosophy was little different from lay beliefs, traditions and practices. The University of Salerno was ahead of its time in some ways, particularly because it admitted female students and also apparently had females on the teaching staff, but in other ways it was barely distinguishable from the rest of the global sphere of medicine.[14] A long and detailed poem on health issued from the Salerno School in the fourteenth century contains the following stanza:

> Three speciall months (September, April, May)
> There are, in which 'tis good to ope a veine';
> In these three months the Moone beares greatest sway,
> Then old or yong that store of bloud containe,
> May bleed now, though some elder wizards say
> 'Some dayse are ill in these, I hold it vaine:'
> September, April, May, have dayse a peece,
> That bleeding do forbid, and eating Geese,
> And those are they forsooth of May the first,
> Of other two, the last of each are worst.[15]

These sentiments, coming from a leading continental university reflect the essence of belief and practice at the time. In early seventeenth-century Scotland, remarkably similar advice was still being offered, this time not in an erudite medical tract, but in a Poor Man's Guide:

> For letting of blude there be three perrellous dayes in the yeir. Thair be thrie days in the yeir in the quhilk no man sold lat him blude nayther for infirmyties nor yet none other evills, nor these dayis to take no drynks though they be medycynabill. These be the dayis following. The last day of Apryll, the first Monday of August and the last Monday of December. These three dayis be forbidden for they be all the wayes full of bode of every man, and therefore if a women or man be letten blude on these dayis they sal dye within xv days.[16]

Needless to say, in the case of Scotland, the Reformation was a process of no little significance in altering the whole ethos of the nation and its people. John Knox clearly did not provide new medical knowledge; it took several generations before the Reformation could be said to have been fully established in the furthest corners of the land. However, physicians and surgeons were able to discuss the body and its functions in much more detail without the threat of religious condemnation. The so-called 'Protestant work ethic' may be something of a myth, just as the 'lad o' pairts' may have been a hope rather than a reality on the part of some Scots. That is not to condemn either factor as of no significance; they probably were. Certainly, the high regard in which education has long been held is both part of the complex make-up of the nation and a reason why Scottish medical practitioners were highly regarded and can be said without a trace of xenophobia to have led the world by the end of the eighteenth century.

However, secularisation or liberation in itself was not enough to produce a body of qualified, professional practitioners. From the thirteenth century the continental universities, such as Salerno and Padua, followed by Paris and, later, Reims and Leiden, would provide the necessary institutional and academic context for physicians to learn their medicine and, eventually, for new science to be developed. In Scotland from the late fifteenth century, as the burghs became more numerous and, in a few cases, larger, groups of craftsmen of various sorts began to organise themselves into craft incorporations. Their motives were simple: they wished to create a demarcation barrier around themselves and their trade, in something of the same manner in which merchants dominated overseas and internal trading. This was a fortuitous development for surgery, particularly in Edinburgh and, later, Glasgow, and to a lesser extent in Aberdeen and Dundee, as it enabled the barbers and surgeons in these places to form similar groups and thus set up the institutional basis for the training of professional surgeons. So, then, the process of urbanisation in Scotland created yet another sphere of influence, which itself created sub-spheres of occupation-specific institutions. This process would seem to be a good example of the Jordanova social construction theory.

Burghs or no burghs, though, the secularisation process in terms of the availability to the population of anything other than traditional, lay medicine was slow, patchy and not complete until well after the medieval period had melted through the early modern period into the so-called modern, enlightened age. One papal edict could not, at a stroke, secularise or professionalise medicine. The surgical incorporations could not evolve until burgh settlements had themselves evolved sufficiently to allow more than one or two practitioners to make a living within their walls. So, the importance of the secularisation of medical training in the medieval period was not so much for its impact on the people of medieval Scotland, but rather in setting in train the process which would lead to the professionalisation of medicine, surgery and their practitioners over succeeding centuries. Although medicine would gradually emerge from the sphere of religion, it did not do so immediately.

MEDICAL PRACTICE BEFORE PROFESSIONALISATION

In Scotland before 1505 there was no real organisation of medical practitioners of any sort. The only 'official' medical men were also religious men, and the surgery was performed by individuals from many walks of life, including those who officiated as barbers or tonsurers to the monasteries, priests or monks themselves before they were debarred from letting blood after 1163, and various itinerant operators who claimed special powers or abilities. Perhaps the major manifestation or defining feature of medicine in this period was precisely that it could not be defined or compartmentalised according to any notion of all medicine being practised or controlled by individuals who did not do anything else, and had been trained in the arts of medicine and surgery. The treatment of injuries and ailments was very much part of the 'normal' cycle of life with all its attendant dangers, beliefs and superstitions. Illness and disease were not distinguished as being outside the sphere of life. Quite the contrary, illness and disease were very much part of the all-embracing system of beliefs and traditions, based on many things, from the cycle of the moon to the seasons and the effects of divine retribution or favour.

Despite the fact that the Roman church was all-pervasive in its influence over Scots and their lives, it was not within its powers to eradicate other beliefs and traditions, which had evolved over long centuries of 'darkness'. Scots found no conflict in combining Christianity with pagan ritual, healing ceremonials and witchcraft (though the latter would not become significant politically until the early-modern period, when monarchs and nobility sought to increase their controls over the people). Witchcraft itself was a complex phenomenon – before the political era of witches and their powers and threats, charming and healing rituals and spells were an integral part of the cosmological sphere within which the Scottish nation was contained. Such beliefs were held particularly strongly in the more rural areas and before the burgh network began to consolidate, and indeed before roads alleviated communication problems. As news of any sort took come considerable time to pass over relatively short distances, then the stories, naturally, became embellished and lengthened, so that some minor item grew into magic. The supernatural world was just as much a part of medieval Scottish medicine as the more worldly Christian church.

Scots in the early medieval period coped with their illnesses and injuries in ways which are not entirely clear, precisely because the legacy of the Dark Ages is so dark and obscure. There is little doubt, though, that within the fragmented and disparate communities scattered over the territory which would become Scotland, there was no attempt to separate the unexplainable elements of cure from the explainable. No-one understood how the body worked; it was, therefore, not surprising that no-one attempted to explain the cure of diseases on the relatively rare occasions on which a serious affliction might have been alleviated by a combination of herbs, incantations and physical ritual such as walking backwards round a holy well.

The nature of applied cures – concoctions of herbs mostly – depended on a number of factors. Different parts of Scotland produced different herbs and plants. Different herbs and plants appeared in different seasons. Different seasons were supposed to cause different diseases and afflictions. So, any disease was treated according to the season, the cosmology of the season, and the fruits of the land produced in that season. It is quite possible, therefore, that the cure for a fever in the remote Scottish islands in the winter was very different from the treatment given to a fever in Edinburgh in summer, or in the remote south-west in the autumn. This dependence on the natural cycle of the earth produced a folklore and 'calendar' of medical treatments. It became commonplace to take preventative steps according to the season too. Once it became known that scurvy could be helped by scurvy grass, people took it to try to prevent the onset of an extremely debilitating disease. Various tonics were thought to be helpful at various times for various diseases. Thus grew a complex, interlocking framework of cures, at the same time flexible and pragmatic, but also seeing the beginnings of action rather than reaction. It needs a significant leap of the imagination to make a connection between spring bloodletting or the taking of scurvy grass to the current campaigns to vaccinate the entire young population of Britain against meningitis. Postmodernist historians would throw up their hands in horror at any such suggestion. The discourse of each age is, of course, of its age and should not be forced into the role of causal determinism. None the less, connections can, and indeed must, be made if the narrative is to have cohesion. Cause and effect can be overplayed indeed, especially if the effect is claimed more than a thousand years later. The point is, though, that medicine *evolved*. It was of course influenced by many factors of locality and of general knowledge and the evolving state of the country.

This evolution apart, what kind of cures and treatment were used? The evidence is, of course, limited, and the legends are separated with great difficulty, if at all, from what really took place. Medieval medical practice was humoral, holistic and varied in general only in terms of geographical location and local versions of superstitious belief or availability of plants. The main aim in most cases was to rid the body of evil matter and restore the equilibrium by means of Galenical remedies or locality-specific cures. Prophylactic venepuncture, purges and doses of scurvy grass were common. A proliferation of cures for toothache have survived, perhaps indicating the scale and severity of the problems. The following cure was recommended. For 'stynking teeth': 'Take two handfull of comyn and stampe it small, and seith it in wyne and geif them to drynke xv dayes and it sall make thame hole'; 'For the toothache and thy gummes [that] do swell: Tak the joyce of the reid nettyll and they quhit of ane egge and quhyt meill and make ane plaister and lay it to the sore quhairever it bay, and it sall swage and heill'.[17]

Some of the cures involved considerable animal cruelty, as witnessed by the following treatment for convulsions:

> Take a quick mole and putt it into a hot iron pott neare to be red. Close the pott closs till it be full dead then take a girdle and putt it on a soft cleare fire with the back of it down and dry the mole a while on it till the most part of the wetness of it be gone, then take it and cutt it in small pieces and dry it on the girdle again till it be so dry as to be beat in powder, then beat it in powder and divide it in nyn shares and take three of the shares and mix them with three drames of the powder of amber.[18]

This sort of cure may not have been prepared in the more rarified atmosphere of the monastic foundations, but the principles behind the cures in all areas were similar.

SURGERY

Once the process of secularisation of medieval medicine was underway, surgery became more and more the manual, non-intellectual aspect of medicine. Perhaps because of the impossibility of achieving much without the benefit of anaesthetics or antiseptics, and also because the training was essentially and necessarily practical, surgeons were regarded as inferior to physicians in all aspects, social as well as occupational. Although the beginnings of corporate organisation of surgeons and barbers date from the very early years of the sixteenth century, much of the surgery carried out in most parts of Scotland was performed by amateurs of all sorts, from monarchs right down to gardeners and labourers. Treatments were given in rural communities by anyone with some sort of cognate skill, however tenuous the connection. Simpler things like the pulling of teeth could be done by anyone brave enough to try; wounds could be treated by anyone with rudimentary knowledge of herbal remedies; arrows were pulled out of victims on the field of battle by fellow soldiers, and all of this was done under the shelter of a multi-coloured canopy of super-stition, ritual and legend and, of course, the all-seeing eye of God.

THE MEDICINE AND SURGERY OF WAR

In the development of any nation, violent struggle is the norm rather than the exception. In the case of Scotland, matters were no different. From the conflicts with Vikings, Saxons or indigenous Picts or Scots, to the famous and infamous battles such as Bannockburn (1314) or, later, Flodden (1513), the progress of national delineation and dynastic supremacy resulted in many casualties and much work for medical men who served the armed forces of all sides. In the medieval period under consideration here, the weapons which produced injury were propelled either by hand or by machine (the effects of boiling oil can only be imagined with a great deal of effort). Most of the injuries dealt with by medieval military surgeons were the result of stab wounds, sword injuries, depressed fractures of the skull caused by clubs, penetrating wounds inflicted by lances, and other consequences of close fought, hand-to-hand battle and of the devastating effects of cannon and other war machines, though the latter would more likely result in instant death rather than survivable injury. There is also some evidence of punitive amputations, according to a case documented in English sources about three men directed by Edward II to be cared for; 'the Scotch rebels having inhumanly cut off his hand while engaged in the King's service' (at the battle of Bannockburn).[19]

In many cases the surgeons could do little. The vivid descriptions of the wounds and sufferings of battle casualties by the eminent French surgeon Ambroise Paré leave little to the imagination. The strong Scottish connection here is that Peter Lowe, who would be one of the co-founders of the Faculty of Physicians and Surgeons of Glasgow, spent many years working as a surgeon in France and was influenced strongly by Paré's work – to the extent of plagiarising some of his illustrations in his own publications.[20] One of the major contributions made by Paré to military surgery was his introduction of the use of bland dressings to cover amputation stumps, instead of the application of hot pitch or tar, which had been the practice hitherto.

Once firearms entered the field of battle, they entered the field of battle surgery too, and the following case describe by Paré must have been typical of those encountered by Scottish surgeons at home or abroad:

> He was wounded ... by a pistol shot at the joint of the left arm, fracturing the bone, which was as badly comminuted as if it had been broken on an anvil, because the shot was made at close range. By the violence and force of the blow, several complications developed: violent pain, inflammation, fever, swelling, crepitation of the entire arm ... and the great danger of gangrene.[21]

Treatment was by compresses, drains and incisions to drain ulcers, and the removal of sixty bone fragments. The patient recovered.

It has been claimed by one author that the continued use of Latin as the means of communication among the educated of Europe meant that Scots surgeons would find employment easily in the service of the armies of European heads of state.[22] This may well have been the case, but the passage was eased by strong trading connections and also the complex and highly important European marriage market, which had ensured that educated Scots were well used to travelling to Europe, living in Europe and being drawn into the employment and service of European masters. The heyday of the Scots surgeon abroad would be later, in the early-modern period, but the initial connections were indeed there. Also, if Latin were the means by which Scottish surgical practitioners could gain access to Europe, this is confirmation that it was possible for individuals not of the highest social rank to gain sufficient education. When the Incorporation of Surgeons of Edinburgh was founded in 1505, one of the stipulations noted in the charter, or Seal of Cause, was that entrant apprentices must be literate in Latin.

As with other aspects of medicine, though, no matter how highly educated and Latin-literate any surgeon was, the horrors of battle were the same in any language, and the treatments that could be offered to casualties were limited. Surgeons became expert in amputation, often the only option available. They could not carry out complex reconstructions or do abdominal surgery to any extent. All they could do was deal with wounds to the best of their limited ability and try to bring about some degree of pain relief. Evidence from Lowe, however, indicates awareness of the need to try to lessen pain as far as possible. In a detailed account of the technique for carrying out above-knee amputation, Lowe stresses the need for application of a tight tourniquet for amputations, as 'first, it holdeth the member hard and fast, so that the instrument or incising knife may cut more surely. Secondly, that the feeling of the whole parts may be stupified and rendred insensible'.[23]

Lowe's work also confirms that surgeons were debating methods, however limited the options might be, indicating that some 'counsaileth to cut in the joynt, alledging it to be more easie to be done ... others think best to cut four inches from the joynt, either above or under, according to the circumscription of the putrefaction, which is both more easie and surer than in the joynt'.[24] Clearly some thought went into choosing the most appropriate technique, and early examination records from the Edinburgh surgeons show that amputation was a frequent topic.

As with most aspects of medicine, the circumstances and possibilities of the time helped to shape both the experiences of the patients and the aims, objectives and methods of their medical attendants.

SCOTLAND AND EUROPE

One of the factors which provides a particularly close link between medicine and nation is the strong and fruitful links which existed for centuries between Scotland and mainland Europe. In many ways Scotland was much more of a European country than a 'British' country (although of course the concept of Great Britain was yet to come). Trade with Europe formed the backbone of the Scottish economy; the European marriage market was crucial to the formation of the pan-European nobility, a group which had its own common identity despite the individual nationality of any couple or family; military service by Scots in European forces was a long-held tradition; and young Scotsmen travelled to the continent to further their education, either in mercantile or academic pursuits. The Auld Alliance forged in 1295 was a factor in the continuity of relationships rather than starting them from scratch. However, it is also perhaps true that in the minds of those living on the mainland of medieval Europe, the Scot was indistinguishable from others from the pan-Celtic groups such as the Irish, Welsh or Cornish.

These connections would be crucial in shaping the nature and direction of Scottish medicine until well into the Enlightenment period. This is an overarching factor in Scotland in general and medicine in particular. In some ways, it may be claimed, this is one explanation for the less than comfortable relationship between Scotland and its contiguous southern territory. Historians of medicine have recognised this close relationship with Europe, but what has perhaps not been emphasised fully enough is the distinctive nature of the relationship between Scotland and Europe. In the formative centuries of Scotland as a fixed territorial entity, this connection was at its strongest, and the legacy to medicine in Scotland was of considerable importance and cannot easily be underestimated. This is also connected very closely to the religious traffic between the two land masses, both before the Reformation, when the religion was shared, and during the Reformation period, when Scottish protestantism was influenced by Calvin and Luther. The influence was focused through the Scottish filter of John Knox and his adherents, but was none the less very European in nature.

From the twelfth century on, a number of Scots had travelled to Europe to study at the *studia generalia*, or early universities, and among those was perhaps the most prominent and notable, who was known as Michael Scot (Michael from Scotland), in the same manner of appellation as, for example, John Duns Scotus. Michael Scot comes down through the centuries as both reality and legend. The legend concerns Michael Scot of Balwearie in Fife, who was alleged to have been able to do such awesome things as divide the Eildon hills in three, or fly unaided. The reality of Scot's European sojourn is more typical and conventional for the time. He was apparently employed as a linguist in Toledo before entering royal service.[25] His publications, including *Liber Physionomie*, benefited from developments in printing, to allow several editions to be made available. Scot died around 1236, and his subsequent reputation was constructed as a famous physician, though like most such individuals he was probably more of a polymath or jack of all trades and master of all professions too. There is also considerable doubt as to whether or not he really did practise as a physician.

The European connection brought a common thread to medical training, however limited it may have been. Whatever the nationality of the students, the language of study was Latin. This was a considerable advantage in terms of communication, but the amount of material communicated was severely limited and consisted mainly in the absorption of the contents of the few medical works available at the time. It is likely that these took the form of an amalgamation of Hippocratic, Galenic and Avicennic traditions. Students of Scots origin therefore experienced what most other students experienced. However, there is little in the way of evidence that any of them was able to make a significant or seminal contribution to medical knowledge. The number of Scottish medical students who went to Europe was small; many of them chose to remain abroad to travel and undertake further study. So, in terms of the influence on the development of Scottish medicine within Scotland, it must be admitted that this was limited in this period. There were instances, though, of European medical practitioners being summoned to treat high-level patients in Scotland,[26] indicating that those with power and influence felt it necessary to do this, and that the regard for Scottish practitioners was relatively low, wherever they had obtained their medical knowledge.

A further factor which linked Scotland and Europe, and the effects of which cannot be overstated, is the advent of the printing press and its eventual introduction to Scotland by Walter Chepman in 1507. Print would be the medium of progress henceforth. The printed word would be the key to knowledge, enlightenment, records, transactions, trade, industry and, of course, medicine.

GAELIC MEDICINE – THE HIGHLAND CONDITION

As with many aspects of Scotland from earliest times until the present, what happened in the highlands was often very different from events in the lowland areas. The highlands had been a continual and irritating problem to successive monarchs once the territory of Scotland had become finally delineated. However, in many ways Gaelic culture was much more sophisticated than anything to be found in the lowlands, at least in the time before the Renaissance and before courtly culture became the artistic centre of excellence. The Gaelic language was ancient, Gaelic poetry complex and often sophisticated, and importantly in this context, Gaelic medicine was advanced and often ahead of anything available in the rural lowlands. Everything highland was different from everything lowland, and this was no less the case with respect to the training and practice of medicine in the area.

Gaelic medicine was a family thing. Most aspects of highland life were family things – often involving the wider family of the clan, but still local and constrained within specific spheres of influence. Gaelic physicians were almost exclusively the sons of Gaelic physicians. Knowledge was passed down through the generations, and the highland physicians led a peripatetic life, dispensing medicine in the localities through which they passed. Their knowledge was, though, in some ways not quite so different from the knowledge possessed by physicians trained in different ways in different places. A number of Gaelic medical texts survive, which are translations of Arabic and Greek manuscripts. The whole foundation of Western medicine, at least what would become orthodox, professional or legitimate Western medicine, lay in the warmth and sophistication of classical Greece. Hippocrates and Galen wielded influence that permeated the entire known world for over a millennium. Arabic medicine had connections, but rather more tenuously. Gaelic medicine clearly combined strands of each, and it is impressive that individuals in such a remote, inhospitable and apparently intellectually barren region of a poor country could acquire and use this sort of knowledge. Acquire it and use it they did, though. The physician was highly regarded in this culture, and customarily occupied the seat next to the bard at the chieftain's table – an honoured position, particularly so in an age where symbolism was visual and of crucial importance.

One of the best-documented medical families in the highlands were the Beatons. They were a powerful family, and practised and taught medicine for several generations. According to the very detailed genealogical investigation carried out by Bannerman, the Beatons were of considerable importance in this area.[27] The influence of orthodox highland medicine diminished as communication with the lowland areas improved. However, highland folk medicine was quite another thing, and survived with its own set of idiosyncracies and peculiarities for centuries, indeed in some instances to the present day. For example, snails are still used to cure warts, and the juice of roasted snails is reputed to cure lung diseases.[28]

It could be said, then, that the demise of a separate and distinctive highland medical tradition ended a separate sphere and brought the highlands into the national medical sphere. However, the provision of qualified physicians in medieval and early-modern Scotland was really an urban provision. Physicians were itinerant in circumscribed spheres, delineated more by travel constraints and their own social rank rather than by other criteria. In medical terms, the assault on Gaelic culture had the detrimental effect of snuffing out a tradition of excellence. One of the major effects of this process was to allow free rein to folk and traditional medicine. The influence of the seer or other apparently charmed individual would supersede the classical knowledge of the Beatons. In effect, then, the dark ages of medicine in medieval Scotland owed much in the lowlands to the stifling effects of the Roman church; in the highlands, matters were a little different. Highland medicine was stifled by attitudes and by the policies of monarchs to a much greater extent than by the grip of the church on the lives of the people.

In the early-modern period the highlands would be even more of a battle ground than in the medieval period, perhaps not in terms of pitched battles, but in other attempts to blur the distinctions between highland and lowland ways of life. The attempted plantation of the Isle of Lewis, the Statues of Iona of 1609 and other measures meant that it was increasingly difficult for clan chiefs, clan physicians or clan poets to maintain any sort of separate sphere of identity. On the other hand, this can be seen as part of the process of the creation of Scottish medicine, as opposed to highland and lowland medicine, although as time went on, Scottish medicine was mainly available in the lowlands, and the highlands were left largely to their own traditional and unorthodox devices.

SOCIETY, ECONOMY AND THE BLACK DEATH

Continuing the themes of Europe, Scotland and religion, in more practical terms the economies of the various areas of Europe depended very much on the general state of war or peace within and between countries, and also the state of the environment in terms of dearth, harvest failures and episodes of plague and other epidemic and endemic diseases. Scotland's main trading was with northern Europe and the Baltic states, and consisted of primary products derived from animals and fish.[29] Communication was difficult and trade was interrupted by pirates just as much as by war or natural disaster. Coastal and overland trade with England were also important and also influenced, and to a great extent controlled, by cross-border relations. In this period the general trend by the early fourteenth century was towards economic decline, inflation and, most particularly, the devastation caused by the Black Death, which swept Europe in the middle of the fourteenth century.

The plague eventually reached Scotland in 1349, allegedly the result of contact between a Scottish army and its infected English counterpart in the border area. Whatever the cause, the affliction spread rapidly and caused significant mortality. The rampant nature of the disease was such that victims, according to the chronicler John of Fordun, 'dragged out their earthly life for barely two days'.[30] There is no doubt that the poor and most malnourished in society were affected to a greater extent than the better off, and that poor weather and bad harvests served to compound the problems. The plague was considered by most to have been some sort of divine retribution, and this attitude was slow to disappear. However, by the time of some of the later visitations, in the first half of the sixteenth century, and stimulated also by the growth of burghs and, therefore, larger concentrations of population, measures were taken to try to control the outbreaks. Once the contagious nature of the disease was beginning to be understood, towns simply shut down during out-breaks. Interpersonal contact in burghs and elsewhere was reduced to the absolute minimum and draconian punishments were meted out to those who were thought to have spread the disease either deliberately or accidentally. Overseas trade was severely affected by quarantine regulations, and gibbets were set up in burghs to demonstrate the application of the law to the people.

Some burghs took measures akin to the more recent procedure of appointing Medical Officers of Health. Robert Henryson was perhaps the original Medical Officer of Health.[31] He was appointed, at a salary, by Edinburgh Town Council in 1578 to advise the magistrates on what best to do to deal with these recurrent and debilitating outbreaks.

Not only were burgh governments trying to do something about containment of the plague, the medical men were also putting their minds to the problem. By the early sixteenth century it was becoming easier to produce the printed word. The first printing press in Scotland had been set up in Edinburgh in 1507, but there were also greater opportunities available in Europe, in Paris, Antwerp or Amsterdam. A defining feature of the continuing progress of 'orthodox' medicine would be the increasing practice of publication. This was certainly so in the case of Gilbert Skene. Mediciner to the University of Aberdeen, Skene published what is thought to be the first medical treatise in the Scots language, *Ane Breve Descriptioun of the Pest*, in 1568.[32] In this work, Skene describes the causes, manifestations and a variety of treatments for the condition. Despite being a medical man and a university mediciner, learned in physic, Skene states quite unequivocally that 'the first and principal cause may be callit, and is ane scurge and punischment of the maist iust God'.[33] Listed as 'inferiour causis' are 'standand water, sic as stank, pule or loche moste currupte; erd, dung, stinkand cloisettis, deid cariounis vnbureit'. Skene was clearly aware of the environmental hazards, though not apparently of the means of transmission of the disease. Environmental portents of an imminent outbreak are said to be 'contineuall weit in the last part of the spring or begyning of Sommer without vindis, great contineuall heit or Meridonal Vindis, with turbide mistie Air'. Skene backs up his views by reference to Hippocrates and other ancient outbreaks. Eclipses, comets or shooting stars are also indicators.

Diagnostic signs of the disease are outlined in considerable detail, and include coldness of the exterior of the body but internal heat, 'grangring of mowthe, detestable brathe, greit dolour of heid, dolour of stomak, inlak of appetite, vehement doloure of heart, intolerable thrist, frequent vomiting of divers colours'. Other signs might be a black tongue, turbid urine, and 'last of all and maiste certane, gif with constant feuer, by the earis, vnder the oxstaris or by the secrete membres maist frequently apperis apostums callit bubones'.[34]

This was clearly a disease of epic proportions to the individual, and it is worth covering Skene's work in some detail in order to illustrate how devastating the disease was, and the major problems it posed, perhaps not for the medical profession but for local authorities. Although acknowledging the impotence of man against the omnipotent will of God, Skene gives detailed advice on appropriate prophylactic measures, again stating that 'the principal preservative cure of the pest is to returne to God'. More worldly measures included, in classical humoral fashion, the elimination of 'superfluite or corruptioun of humoris' by the usual means; bloodletting using the 'Vaine callit Mediana of the richt arme';

and of course a plethora of herbal concoctions including rose water, calamint, juniper, myrrh, origanum, mint, vinegar and a host of other ingredients.

This case study of the plague is particularly useful, not just because plague was socially and economically devastating. It illustrates very well many of the classical features of medicine in Scotland and the workings of burgh society in the later medieval period.[35]

THE CONSTRUCTION OF AN ORTHODOXY

In terms of the evolution of an orthodoxy in Scottish medicine, the medieval period, or at least the later part of it, saw the beginnings of a period of transition from the enclosed orthodoxy of medicine as practised by members of religious orders, to the early seeds of a secular orthodoxy which would gradually supersede the multiple cosmological orthodoxies of religious and lay medical belief and practice. If the interacting spheres of Scottish medicine were to bring about custody battles over ownership of the orthodoxy, then before this could happen, the orthodoxy itself would have to be defined, refined, and confined to its custodians. In other, more simple, terms, the trained practitioner who acquired knowledge based on empirical study of the body and its functions, as well as knowledge of developing philosophical standpoints (such as the iatro-mechanical and iatrochemical theories of body function current at the end of the seventeenth century), would become recognised by increasing proportions of the population as the possessors of the 'true' or legitimate body of medical and surgical knowledge. Until this came about, it would be difficult to sustain the claim that trained medicine was orthodox medicine. Indeed, there is almost a case for claiming that in some ways what became the orthodox had long been, for practical purposes, the unorthodox aspects of medicine and medical and surgical practice, particularly in the remoter parts of Scotland and other countries.

It may be claimed, then, that until the secularisation of medical knowledge and practice, the major sphere of practical influence lay outwith the walls and gates of the religious foundations. That is not to say, of course, that these institutions did not provide a much needed service; what is clear, though, is that that service was of necessity restricted to the immediate vicinity of the foundation, and to travellers who were fortunate enough to gain hospitality and medical treatment there. Hospitals like Soutra were few in number, but often located on strategic overland routes. So, in some ways, the medical Scottish traveller had greater access to the orthodox than the town dweller or resident of some remote, rural community.[36]

CONCLUSION

The medieval period was important for Scotland in many ways, and not just for medicine and its practice. The country went through a period of great change, despite the all-consuming influence of the Roman church. The wars of independence had maintained Scots in their country, ruled by Scottish kings; the nobles were busy strengthening their ties with Europe, particularly in terms of the useful and very important marriage market. These connections, together with important and longstanding trading links, would set out the path towards the Reformation, the Renaissance and the flowering of Renaissance culture and ideas in many forms and in many areas. Scottish arts and architecture would be influenced increasingly by what was happening in France, Italy and the Netherlands; in turn Scottish medicine and surgery would benefit from these relationships. Surgery would be taught and written about by men such as Peter Lowe, who based his work on that of the famous French surgeon Paré. Similarly, the study of anatomy would be revolutionised by the publications of Andreas Vesalius and other anatomists of the Renaissance period. So the medieval period was not just a time of relocation and redefinition of the medical orthodoxy, and, perhaps revision of long-held beliefs about the structure and functions of the body, it was a time of closer ties with Europe and also internal developments at home.

One of the reasons why lay, religious and secular institutional medicine bore such marked similarities to each other was the very close relationships deemed to exist between the workings of the human body and the functions of that body in relation to the earth and to the wider universe. As Roy Porter puts it with his usual aptness, 'while often aloof and dismissive, professional medicine has borrowed extensively from the folk tradition'.[37] It is true that once medicine began to be secularised and 'trained', every effort was made to discredit folk medicine, particularly that indulged in by women, but until the new orthodoxy was based on a fully understood and reasoned science, it could not be wholly eclipsed or shown to be false. If the social construction theory is applied here, the construction of medicine in medieval Scotland was predominantly religious and European in terms of shaping what would be claimed as the orthodoxy, while in other spheres an equally complex combination of locality, belief systems and seasons helped to construct what was still the orthodoxy for most of the people.

NOTES

1. Colston, J., *The Incorporated Trades of Edinburgh* (Edinburgh, 1891).
2. Full account of origins and progress of Edinburgh surgeons in Dingwall, H. M., *Physicians, Surgeons and Apothecaries. Medical Practice in Seventeenth-Century Edinburgh* (East Linton, 1995), 34–99.
3. Moffat, B., 'SHARP practice. The search for medieval medical treatments', *Archaeology Today* 8 (4) (1987), 22–8.
4. An ongoing series of reports from the excavations, carried out by the Scottish Archaeoethnopharmacological group, is published annually under the title *Sharp Practice*.
5. Moffat, B. et al., *SHARP Practice 3. The Third Report on Researches into the Medieval Hospital at Soutra* (Edinburgh, 1989), 10, 19, 23–30.
6. Boyd, *Amulets and Isotopes*, 7–8.
7. For a dated but still useful antiquarian account see Walcott, M. E. C., *Scoti-monasticon: The Ancient Church of Scotland: A History of the Cathedrals, Conventual Foundations, Collegiate Churches, and Hospitals of Scotland* (London, 1874).
8. Barrell, *Medieval Scotland*, 42–66.
9. Maclennan, W. J., 'Fractures in medieval Scotland', *Scottish Medical Journal* 46 (2000), 58–60.
10. Dilworth, M., *Scottish Monasteries in the Late Middle Ages* (Edinburgh, 1995), 5.
11. Almoners have been noted at Dunfermline, St Andrews, Paisley and Arbroath. Dilworth, *Scottish Monasteries*, 69. See also Cowan, I. B. and Easson, D. E., *Medieval Religious Houses in Scotland*, 2nd edn (London, 1976).
12. There is an expanding body of knowledge on witchcraft in Scotland. The standard work until now has been Larner, C., *Enemies of God* (Edinburgh, 1983), but more recent studies are adding considerably to the topic. Miller, J. H. M., 'Cantrips and Carlins. Magic, Medicine and Society in the Presbyteries of Haddington and Stirling, 1603–88' (unpublished Ph.D. thesis, University of Stirling, 1999), is an important study of the general cosmology of healing in the early-modern period). See also Levack, B., *The Witch Hunt in Early Modern Europe* (London, 1987); Maxwell-Stuart, P. G., *Satan's Conspiracy. Magic and Witchcraft in Sixteenth-century Scotland* (East Linton, 2001); Sharpe, C. K., *Historical Account of the Belief in Witchcraft in Scotland* (London, 1884).
13. Porter, *Greatest Benefit*, 92–105.
14. Powicke, F. M., Emden, A. B. and Hastings, R. (eds), *Universities of Europe in the Middle Ages* (Oxford, 1987).
15. Clendening, *Source Book*, 69.
16. EUL, Dc.8.130, *Ane Gude Boke of Medicines*.
17. EUL, MS Dc8.130, *Ane Gude Boke of Medicines*, f.xxv.
18. EUL, MA LaIII, f3.
19. *Calendar of the Close Rolls Preserved in the Public Record Office under the Superintendence of the Deputy Keeper of the Records. Edward II AD 1313–1318* (London, 1893), dated a few weeks after the battle.
20. Lowe, P., *Discourse of the Whole Art of Chirurgerie*, first published in 1597, contains several illustrations identical to those in the works of the French surgeon Ambroise Paré.
21. Hamby, W. B. (ed), *The Case Reports and Autopsy Records of Ambroise Paré* (Springfield, 1960), 63.
22. Blair, J. S. G., 'The Scots and military medicine', in Dow, D. (ed.), *The Influence of Scottish Medicine* (London, 1986), 20.

23. Lowe, *Discourse*, 90.
24. Ibid., 89–90.
25. More detailed account of Scot and his activities in Galbraith, J. D., 'The mediaeval traffic with Europe', in Dow (ed.), *Influence of Scottish Medicine*, 3–15.
26. For example, the Archbishop of St Andrews was treated by Italian and Spanish physicians in the mid-sixteenth century. Comrie, *History*, i, 178–9.
27. Bannerman, *The Beatons*.
28. Beath, *Healing Threads*, 184.
29. Whyte, *Scotland before the Industrial Revolution*, 47–54.
30. Skene, W. F. (ed.), *John of Fordun's Chronicle of the Scottish Nation* (Edinburgh, 1871), ii, 359.
31. Dingwall, *Physicians, Surgeons and Apothecaries*, 22.
32. Skene, G., *Ane Breve Description of the Pest* (Edinburgh, 1568).
33. Ibid., 3.
34. Ibid., 12.
35. For account of situation in Europe see Porter, *Greatest Benefit*, 122–6.
36. See Cowan, *Medieval Religious Houses*, for more detailed account of such establishments.
37. Porter, *Greatest Benefit*, 39.

PART TWO

A NATION ASCENDANT?

Medicine in Scotland from c. 1500 to c. 1800

CHAPTER 4

SCOTS AND SCOTLAND IN BRITAIN

The title of the New History of Scotland volume which covers much of this period is *Lordship to Patronage.*[1] This title implies that it was during this period that Scotland experienced some sort of transition from a medieval nation to something different. This is an important implication. Certainly the much romanticised period of the wars of independence and Wallace and Bruce has stirred up great sentiment among modern Scots. Whether the contemporaries of Wallace and Bruce thought the same thoughts about their territory is quite another matter. The construction of a national identity is more problematic perhaps than the physical delineation of that nation. Historians must rely on discourse about nationhood to make judgements about the state of development of that nation, but caution must be exercised in imposing modern interpretations on the discourse of earlier periods. Ideas of national identity continued to be shaped by a number of factors, including, certainly by this period, the Christian religion and the consolidation of the royal dynasty.[2]

This period saw arguably the most crucial phases in the development and evolution of the Scottish nation. The reigns of the various good, bad and indifferent Stewart monarchs, and those of the first few Hanoverian incumbents of the British and imperial thrones produced difficult, steady but by no means inexorable progress. At several points the monarchy was under real threat, and the looming presence of the southern neighbour was problematic for much of the time. This period includes two of the most infamous battles in Scottish history – Flodden in 1513 and Culloden in 1745 – both of which were devastating defeats for the Scots. However, closer and more co-operative contact was enforced by, firstly, the union of the crowns of 1603, followed a century later by the more controversial and still bitterly debated union of the parliaments in 1707 (which survived by only four votes in the House of Lords in 1713). Thereafter, the fate of Scotland was tied to that of the United Kingdom, united physically but perhaps not emotionally nor intellectually. By the turn of the nineteenth century, Scotland would be not only part of a multiple kingdom but also an important player in the pursuit of Great British empire-building, which would occupy the energies of the country for some considerable time. The embryonic empire would offer many opportunities to career-minded upwardly mobile Scots in many occupations, not least in medicine.

The question of national identity throughout this long period is controversial and not at all simple. The end of the wars of independence, or, more accurately, the wars to maintain independence from England, achieved for Scotland what had been desired – continued independence from England. The various Stewarts, mostly named James, held on to their thrones and territories with considerable difficulty until, in 1603, Scotland was united with England under the rule of a single monarch. This was something of a problem for England too – most countries united under one crown did so under the crown of the larger nation. In this case, the world was topsy-turvy and not a good omen for future co-operation. For most of the seventeenth and eighteenth centuries, Scotland and England were in some sort of political or religious conflict, marked especially, of course, by the Bishops Wars and subsequent Civil War; the execution of the legitimate monarch (in which the Scots were uneasy participants precisely because Charles I was indeed the legitimate monarch); the short but bitter period of 'republic' under Cromwell in the 1650s; the restoration of a damaged but still powerful monarchy in 1660; the less than smooth accession of William and Mary to the Scottish throne in 1689; the hard-won presbyterian religious settlement of 1690; the acrimonious debate over the question of parliamentary union, which eventually took place, in 1707;[3] the Jacobite phenomenon and the long period of political management which characterised the eighteenth century.

RELIGION AND THE SCOTS – CONFLICT AND CHANGE

It may be claimed that the progress of any nation is affected deeply by the religious persuasion of its inhabitants, particularly those in positions of power and influence over the lives and fates of the general population. Scotland is, perhaps, the ultimate example. The first millennium saw the ancient Celtic churches gradually overtaken by the Roman church, though Celtic influences were by no means lost completely. Scotland was a special daughter of Rome, and the Roman church in Scotland was peculiar to Scotland.[4] The influence of Rome was well nigh all-consuming, with the politics of religion and the religion of politics almost indistinguishable. Scottish kings used the church for their own ends; and the Scottish church was not slow to manipulate kings and to participate in politics. A notable example is the support given to Robert the Bruce by the church hierarchy, despite his having committed murder, not just in a church, but in the sanctuary. In this, and in most ages, the spheres of politics and religion were closely related and the social construction of both was complex.

In the case of Scotland, if religion is a key aspect of national identity, then the events of the mid-sixteenth century must have played a crucial part. The Reformation did not change Scotland overnight (it did in St Andrews, but took much longer elsewhere, indeed several generations in places such as the highlands)[5] but it undoubtedly in the long term helped to mould the Scottish nation and character. Presbyterianism and its ramifications were at the centre of politics and the political nation throughout the period of transition from indeterminate territory peopled by Scots to determinate territory leading the intellectual world and participating in the building of the British Empire. It is debatable, however, whether this key role derived from the deep beliefs held by Scots about themselves and their relationship with God and the monarch, or from the shelter of the presbyterian doctrine as an umbrella of convenience which protected a number of groups who were at various times disillusioned with part or all of their experience as Scots or Britons.

The Reformation came to Scotland late compared with other parts of Europe. The Roman church was in the process of a period of self-examination, and various proclamations by its Reforming Councils were trying to curb the perceived excesses of the clergy and to reform the church. However, the main problem, that of finance, was not tackled, and the scenario was the typical 'too little, too late'. The events of 1559–60, though, were not concerned wholly with religion, but with noble ambitions. It is fairly safe to claim that throughout most of Scottish history the major events which had some sort of permanent result could not have occurred without the participation of the nobility, or a substantial number of them.[6] The effects of the changes took at least a generation to filter through society, and in some remote areas, much longer. It was all very well to declare that protestantism was to be the nation's religion, but transforming the beliefs of the people was quite another matter. The complex array of beliefs held by Scots included, but was not altogether dominated by, religion. Witchcraft, superstition, folklore and the remnants of pagan beliefs and rituals were all part of the complicated, but well understood, context in which the Scots lived, worked, fought and experienced cures and treatments. By the middle of the eighteenth century the Scottish church was fully established but had already begun to fray at the edges. The close links between religion and politics were beginning to pull the church apart, so that individuals who were more moderate in their outlook and were willing to accept a more Erastian polity came into conflict with those of a strictly evangelical bent. The first split from the established church took place in 1733 and from that point it is debatable whether indeed the long fought-for state church could be said to encompass the state in its widest sense. The presbyterian settlement reached with William and Mary in 1690 ran contrary to William's preferred solution of moderate Anglicanism through-out all of his kingdoms, but it did ensure that the kirk of and in Scotland would be presbyterian. A small number of Episcopalians remained, and they still remain as part of Scotland's increasingly complex profile of religious adherence. So, Scotland in 1700 was perhaps becoming a little more 'British' in outlook, but was it becoming any more Scottish? Small groups of Roman Catholics and Episcopalians remained outside the state church, and the latter group received a fair measure of toleration under the terms of the Toleration Act of 1712. Bitter disputes between the moderate and evangelical wings of the Kirk resulted in dissenting groups leaving the state church to form their own organisations. So, if corporate religious adherence is claimed to be a pre-requisite of a national identity, then prospects towards the end of this period looked bleak indeed.[7] By 1800 the pessimism was justified, as the state church had fragmented almost irretrievably.

In terms of religion and its effects on medicine in this period, the links are rather more tenuous. The secularisation of medical practice and, in some senses, the secularisation of the body, had long taken place. By the end of this period diseases were thought less often to have been the result of God's anger, although days of national prayer and fasting were still taking place well into the third quarter of the eighteenth century. The Scottish church itself was in the process of fragmenting, and from this time the main influence of the sphere of the church on the sphere of health would lie not in sermons on sin (although the demon drink was another matter altogether) so much as in exhortations to philanthropy and attempts to relieve poor social conditions, which were the cause of so much illness and suffering. Unlike England, the kirk in Scotland retained responsibility for poor relief until the 1840s.

UNIONS AND CONFLICTS

In terms of assessing Scottishness and the role of Scotland in the broader sense, one of the crucial events of this whole long period was without doubt the union of the crowns in 1603. This, contrary to the usual scenario, resulted in the monarch of a small nation succeeding to the throne of its larger neighbour. James VI and I was the prime legitimate claimant, and acquired his non-Scottish thrones without bloodshed, but the situation thus created affected Scotland both directly and indirectly. James VI and I was still the king of Scotland and the Scots; however, he was now also king of England, Wales and Ireland. While he wished to portray himself as a key figure on the European kingly stage, he had also to continue as far as possible as a Scottish king of Scotland, a country now linked to England by a shared monarch, but separate in almost every other way. If it can be assumed that characteristics of national identity are formed or influenced by national institutions, then the fact that Scotland retained a separate parliament for a further century, and continues to retain distinctive religious, legal and educational systems, must maintain Scotland as a discrete national entity, whether or not the identity can be kept distinctive and real. In other words, and in terms of the complexity of interacting spheres of influence upon which this work is postulated, the sphere of Scotland was concentric with that of England, but with sufficient 'native' characteristics to ensure that concentricity would not lead to full absorption.[8]

The century following the union of the crowns saw much conflict, but ended with confirmation of the distinctive nature of some aspects of Scotland's national life and organisation. Scotland witnessed many conflicts and problems, although combined with this were several crucial steps in the development of the institutions of intellect and professions, particularly in Edinburgh. The religious problems continued and were focused on the bitter struggles faced by the Covenanters in their mostly fruitless attempts to preserve the purest form of the Calvinist doctrine possible. The National Covenant (1638) (just as the Declaration of Arbroath centuries earlier) was seen as a document of national intent, although again care must be taken in over-interpreting these key documents in the context of more modern concepts or ideas of the core of corporate identity. The bitter wars between 1638 and 1651 were about Scottishness on several levels. The Scots were reluctant colluders in regicide, in line with their historic regard for the indefeasible status of the rightful monarch, and welcomed Charles II warmly on his restoration in 1660. Matters came to a head, though, with the overt Roman Catholicism espoused by James VII, and his determined attempts to fill high offices with adherents to his faith, which led ultimately to his being forced from the throne and into exile in France.

After a long century of conflict, Scotland and England were linked even more closely with the much debated and by no means certain (until almost the last minute) union of parliaments, which took place in 1707. The historiographical debate over this is still heated,[9] and in the infancy of the newly restored Scottish parliament, continues to be so. Sufficient here to say that this new union had many effects on Scotland, Scots and, of course, their medicine, although most effects (like those of the Reformation) were very slow to penetrate the furthest circumferential points on the Scottish sphere. The union of parliaments brought the sphere of politics into the British context for the first time, in the sense that Scotland was now to be governed (at least ostensibly) from Westminster. A meagre total of forty-five MPs would now look after the interests of the Scots in the House of Commons, and sixteen 'representative' peers would cater for the landed and noble interests.

What really happened, though, was that the political fortunes of the Scots lay within the twin constraints of the corrupt and inappropriate electoral and constituency system, and the efficient 'management' of Scotland on behalf of the government by a succession of political managers, notably the second and third Dukes of Argyll, and then Henry Dundas, whose nickname 'Harry the ninth' says a great deal about his perceived influence.[10] Against a background of change and adjustment to the union, not to mention the threatening cloud of Jacobitism, the first medical school in Scotland was set up in 1726, and for a short while Scotland led the world in medicine, if not in other ways. There was, though, a considerable time lag between the setting up of institutions and professional structures and the translation of this into new or more effective treatments. What was happening was that the framework for the creation, possession and defence of the orthodoxy of medicine was being established.

As the first century of parliamentary union progressed, the stability of the monarchy in a period where successive incumbents of the throne bore the name George rather than James was threatened periodically by the recurring, but unsuccessful Jacobite campaigns. These campaigns had considerable potential to destabilise not only Great Britain but also Scotland itself.[11] The composition of the Jacobite forces and supporters was just as complex as any other aspect of Scotland and its history. By 1750 the threat had largely subsided but had been very real (and had implications for medicine – the new Royal Infirmary of Edinburgh, opened in 1741, was commandeered as a casualty hospital in 1745). Once the threat had effectively evaporated, the monarchy was largely unchallenged and the assimilation of Scotland into Britain and subsequently the Empire was underway.

Economically Scotland did benefit in a number of ways from this fuller union. The economy had been precarious right through the period covered here. Inflation in the fifteenth and sixteenth centuries, followed by limited recovery in the seventeenth century (punctuated by episodes of plague, harvest failure and the notorious 'ill years' of the 1690s), together with the politics of trade barriers and the limitations of war and piracy gave way gradually to a more stable situation. Access to foreign colonies meant that by the middle of the eighteenth century Glasgow and the west of Scotland were the location of the economic boom. There had been a gradual but definite relocation or re-orientation of the direction of Scottish trade. The very strong economic ties with Europe did remain but in a rather weaker state, while the pull of the Americas helped to ensure the very rapid expansion of Glasgow and its satellite towns. The burgh network had always been important and distinctive; by the 1750s Glasgow dominated economically while Edinburgh was the professional and service centre of the country.[12] The effects of agricultural improvement underpinned much of this economic change.

ENLIGHTENMENT

The Enlightenment as a European phenomenon is generally dated in origin to the third quarter of the eighteenth century.[13] However, there is a view that in Scotland the process had much deeper roots in the past, roots which were nourished by aspects of Scottish society which facilitated openness of mind and the dissemination of knowledge and its application to the lowest levels of society. Certainly, the establishment of the medical school in Edinburgh, followed soon after by the first Infirmary, was tangible evidence of progress. There had also been the beginnings of economic improvement in terms of new agricultural techniques and practices, though this would flourish later in the eighteenth century. The high regard for education and the promotion of education for all, which was a core feature of religion in Scotland, was an important factor in characterising the Scottish Enlightenment.[14] Indeed, Robert Sibbald, perhaps the most famous Scottish doctor of the seventeenth century, had tried to set up a philosophical society which would have included individuals with an array of talents, not just in the field of medicine. Sibbald was himself a polymath and served, among other things, as the Geographer Royal. The age of the polymath and the scientific progress of the later part of the seventeenth century were also crucial building blocks for the more concentrated period of intellectual flowering towards the end of the eighteenth century.

However, before the shining light of the late eighteenth-century Enlightenment, Scotland underwent what may be seen as a period of transition in intellectual terms. Changes within the universities started from the 1690s, so that the old-fashioned regenting system was replaced with a specialist professorial system, allowing subjects, including medicine, to be taught at greater depth and encouraging empirical studies. Allied to this, and very important in its time, were the effects of royal patronage of Scottish intellect. The key figure here was the Duke of York, the future James VII and II, who spent a great deal of time in Scotland in the early 1680s following the Exclusion Crisis. His support for the intellectuals of Scotland had a purpose; he was canvassing support for himself. None the less, his influence facilitated developments in a number of crucial areas.[15]

By 1800, much had changed. The later medieval period saw the identity of Scotland largely in terms of the identity of the Roman church, which had a stifling and stagnating effect on many aspects of society, not least in medicine and medical practice. The identity of Scotland in the seventeenth century was related closely to concepts of presbyterianism and the idea of the covenanted nation. These ideas brought Scotland into a bitter civil war and the eventual religious settlement did not take place until 1690. Once the union became somewhat closer and, in the view of some, much less balanced, the first half of the eighteenth century saw perhaps just as much uncertainty about who or what Scotland and the Scots were. In terms of the fostering of Scottish national identity there were other, major factors to be taken into consideration. The identity of Scotland was now inextricably tied up with that of Great Britain.[16] The construction of North Britain, mostly an elite concept articulated by Scots who could participate in this wider nation, added a further dimension to the character of the Scots, but may not have proved to be a unifying factor in the longer term. The second half of the eighteenth century saw the repressive aftermath of the Jacobite campaigns, when measures were taken to tame the highlands. Ironically, though, the banning of the tartan may have served to reinforced the idea of the highlander as the essence of the Scot. This was a nineteenth-century construct, and one which, it may be argued, did little to elucidate the true identity of the modern Scot.

In summary, the very long period from James IV to George III contributed a great deal, not only to the consolidation and defence of the Scottish territory, but also to the foundations of intellectual freedom and, ironically, of the constrictions of medical institutions and creation of the new orthodoxy. Much did not change at all, particularly in the remotest parts of the nation, and it is important to recognise that geographically a region evolves at a rate in inverse proportion to distance from the centres of power, progress and change. The rate of change in the Scottish highlands was slower and very different from that in the lowlands.

The two main chapters in this section of the book will consider, firstly, the processes which characterised early-modern Scotland, and, secondly, the different factors which helped to shape, construct and define medical training and practice in the period which has come to be known as the Enlightenment.

NOTES

1. Mitchison, R., *Lordship to Patronage. Scotland 1625–1746* (Edinburgh, 1983).
2. Webster, *Medieval Scotland*, 3.
3. Concise account of the regal union in Brown, K. M., *Kingdom or Province? Scotland and the Regal Union, 1603–1707* (London, 1992).
4. Despite many attempts, Scotland had been unable to achieve an archbishop, being accorded instead the status of 'special daughter' of Rome. Finally, though, in 1472 the first archbishop was installed in Scotland.
5. Lynch, *Scotland*, 198.
6. For a full account of the Reformation process as it affected Edinburgh, the centre of religion, politics and medicine, see Lynch, M., *Edinburgh and the Reformation* (Edinburgh, 1981).
7. Brown, C., *Religion and Society in Scotland since 1707* (Edinburgh, 1999), is a scholarly survey of the progress of religion in Scotland.
8. Many works have been written about James VI and I, his role, aims and effects on Scotland. See, for example, Lockyer, *James VI* (London, 1998).
9. For a useful and concise survey of the historiographical debate, see Whatley, C. A., *Bought and Sold for English Gold* (East Linton, 2000); Ferguson, W., *Scotland's Relations with England. A Survey to 1707* (Edinburgh, 1977) and Smout, T. C., *Scotland's Trade on the Eve of Union 1660–1707* (Edinburgh, 1963) provide the more mainstream political and economic perspectives.
10. A revisionist and largely positive view of Dundas and his activities is contained in Fry, M., *The Dundas Despotism* (Edinburgh, 1992). For a more traditional view of the politics of the period, see Ferguson, W., *Scotland 1689 to the Present* (Edinburgh, 1968).
11. Many works have been written about the Jacobite phenomenon. Recent, concise account in Pittock, M., *Jacobitism* (Basingstoke, 1998).
12. See Devine, T. M. and Jackson, G. (eds), *Glasgow, Volume I: Beginnings to 1830* (Manchester, 1995); Whyte, *Scotland before the Industrial Revolution*.
13. See 'Further Reading' section for detailed reference to literature on the Enlightenment.
14. See Phillipson, N. T. and Mitchison, R. (eds), *Scotland in the Age of Improvement* (Edinburgh, 1970) for coverage of some of these aspects.
15. Ouston, H., 'York in Edinburgh: James VII and the patronage of learning in Scotland 1673–1688', in Dwyer, J., Mason, R. A. and Murdoch, A. (eds), *New Perspectives on the Politics and Culture of Early Modern Scotland* (Edinburgh, 1982), 133–55.
16. Colley, L., *Britons. Forging the Nation, 1707–1837* (Yale, 1992) is a challenging view, based on the need for the nation to unite to defend itself from foreign threat.

CHAPTER 5

MEDICINE IN
EARLY-MODERN SCOTLAND

INTRODUCTION

Early-modern Scotland may be characterised more by developments within the nation as it had been consolidated by that point, rather than by the need to defend or expand the territory, although the country would of course experience a variety of conflicts, wars and revolts during this period. The Stewarts were well established on the throne, and would soon, ironically, acquire the throne of the contiguous nation to the south, against all previous historical trends. What was happening within the country had considerable bearing on the future of Scotland as a nation with an identity and also in terms of medicine and medical practice. The Reformation of 1559–60 would change the face of the nation permanently, and not just within the narrow confines of presbyterian religious belief and practice. Equally, the Renaissance touched most aspects of Scottish life, and the beginnings of the scientific revolution would also be crucial.

Once medicine had emerged from the closeted cloisters of medieval religious houses, the first steps could be taken towards the development of the secular profession, particularly in the urban setting. Rural and highland medicine were still very different and would continue to be so. However, the increasing secularisation of medical training and practice did not, yet, create Scottish medical training (surgery was rather different). Scots who wanted to become physicians experienced a combination of general education in Scotland followed by specialised medical education in Europe. There was, technically, some medical education available in Scottish universities, but in reality the only reputable (in terms of its own time and state) medical education available was on the continent. This trek to Europe to find good medical teaching followed many of the same, well-trodden routes which had been carved out over the centuries by Scottish merchants, nobles and soldiers. At this time, despite the union of the crowns in 1603, Scotland was culturally and economically still very European in orientation; at least, lowland Scotland was. The highlands were very different, and medical training there was also very different.[1]

General patterns of change in Scotland affected medicine. The gradual process of urbanisation altered the balance of the population both in terms of urban/rural distribution and in terms of north/south population. In the early-modern period the population of Scotland was more evenly distributed than it would be in the later eighteenth century and beyond, and by 1700 around half of the people still lived north of the highland line. This made highland medicine in some ways just as important as lowland medicine. Access to qualified, professional medicine was generally in inverse proportion to distance from an urban centre. So a major socio-economic trend in this period was the consolidation of the urban network and a gradual increase in the percentage of the population living in towns. The other major change was, of course, the union of the crowns of 1603 and its impact on the development of Scotland as a nation, followed by the perhaps more significant union of parliaments in 1707.

The Edinburgh physicians made at least three attempts to achieve an organisation, and finally succeeded in 1681, helped greatly by the patronage of the Duke of York, who would reign briefly as James VII and II. Once founded, the College set out to do many of the things that had been done by the surgeons almost two centuries previously.

With the establishment of the College of Physicians, and the continued development of the Glasgow Faculty and the Incorporation of Surgeons, there was the beginning of an important trend in medicine, and a trend that would last for at least two centuries: the trend towards the sharpening of the differences between rural and urban medicine. In effect, what was happening was that urbanisation helped to alter the balance of the population as a whole, and it also helped to facilitate the emergence of medical institutions and, consequently, to alter the pattern of medical care in rural and urban areas. Hitherto, the treatments that had been made available to Scottish patients were very similar, wherever the individuals happened to live. The basic treatments did not change markedly, and would not do so until well into the eighteenth century and beyond; what did change in the urban setting was the numbers of qualified practitioners, their education and supervision. It is likely that in the urban setting better-off patients chose, if they could, to consult a qualified practitioner either as the only opinion sought, or in combination with one or more alternative sources of treatment.

In terms of patronage and its importance, early-modern medicine was closely dependent, at least at its academic and organisational centres, on the support and patronage of the monarch, whereas in later periods the patronage was just as important, but it was often more the patronage of senior political figures which was more crucial. Certainly by the mid-nineteenth century, which saw moves towards national standardisation of medical training and registration, the lead-up to the crucial 1858 Medical Act would see physicians and surgeons spending a great deal of time and money in acquiring the patronage of senior government ministers and other politicians and prominent lawyers.

The medicine that was practised and experienced by the early-modern practitioner and patient was still essentially humoral in philosophy and in application, with the addition of perhaps a wider variety of herbal and animal substances in use, and also the gradual introduction of chemical compounds in the Paracelsian mode. By the mid-eighteenth century some progress would be made towards the reclassification of disease and the more accurate elucidation of body structures and functions, but even then the experiences of the patients were still very much the experiences produced by humoral medicine. The late seventeenth century would see the emergence of rival chemical and mechanical theories of body structure and function, against a background of Newtonian and Cartesian ideas, but until the mechanics of the body and its variously integrated systems and parts could be described accurately, there was little the doctor could do apart from treat according to humoral advice. As with most theoretical developments which have to be applied in practice, there was a considerable time lag between elucidation of new theories and the translation of these theories into different or more effective treatments.

Therefore, the sphere of medical practice still included virtually the entire population. Within that sphere, though, groups were beginning to emerge and develop along lines which would, eventually, be termed professional. The particular juxtaposition of early-modern circumstances, which involved often complex relations among king, nobles, people and occupational groups, meant that developing medical exclusivity had to emerge and consolidate within a climate of the need for patronage in order to become exclusive, but also the need to somehow show that the trained practitioner could offer something different from that which had been offered by a variety of healers for many centuries.

This chapter will, therefore, consider the major themes of demarcation and continuity; war and its effects; urbanisation and its influence on society and medical practice; the establishment and consequences of formal medical training in Scotland; European influences; the Renaissance and Reformation; new science and images of the body; and also continuities with previous periods.

DEMARCATIONS AND THE FIRST SIGNS OF STRUCTURED POWER

In terms of changing power structures within the sphere of medicine, the first major development in Scotland, consequent upon the ongoing process of urbanisation, was the foundation of the first exclusive surgical organisation, the Incorporation of Surgeons and Barbers of Edinburgh. This foundation was a significant development in terms of surgery, but in itself was only one of a number of craft organisations which were established from the second half of the fifteenth century. As burghs grew in size and number, groups of individuals undertaking the same sorts of work began to combine in organisations which had the dual purposes of acting as friendly societies for their members, and as policing institutions to impose and enforce occupational and territorial demarcations. It was, therefore, not surprising that by the end of the fifteenth century the growing numbers of barbers and surgeons in Edinburgh sought to acquire similar privileges. It was fundamental to burgh structure and function that groups of merchants and craftsmen had sole rights of distribution or manufacture within the walls of the burgh, and the surgeons quite naturally wished to have the same rights and privileges. They were the first surgical group in Scotland to take such steps and again this is not surprising, given that Edinburgh was by far the largest and most complex urban settlement, and there were enough practitioners to warrant and enable an organisation to be set up and maintained. So, what may be seen as the first tentative steps towards the separation of medicine from lay practice, if not professionalisation, came about perhaps more because of what was happening in other spheres of society as much as any real surgical or medical rationale for the separation. In other words, the discourse, attitudes and practices of society in general brought about change in many occupations, not just surgery. The stage which had been reached by the growth of the burgh network was the main catalyst here. Surgeons and others merely wished to have the same rights as any other group. Even the lowly bonnet-makers had the same desire. Very soon after their incorporation, though, the Edinburgh surgeons began to pursue much more defined and exclusive aims.

The early centuries of the existence of the Incorporation of Surgeons of Edinburgh have been covered in detail elsewhere.[2] By 1505 the surgeons and barbers had sufficient numbers to be able to petition the Town Council for a charter of incorporation. This was granted in July 1505 and ratified by James IV the following year – an early instance of two major influences on the progress and fortunes of the surgical organisation. Support from the Town Council would be crucial for several centuries, while patronage and endorsement by royalty were of major significance in the establishment of intellectual and professional bodies and their maintenance and survival in a period where the favour of the monarch helped to overcome many serious difficulties. The Edinburgh surgeons would benefit greatly from this close relationship with the Town Council, though by the middle of the nineteenth century they considered themselves too intellectually superior to have the label and low-status implications of a craft organisation. That, though, was in the future. At this time the surgeons were only too glad to have support from the Town Council and, from 1583, to occupy one of the craft seats on the Council. This was the relatively inauspicious start of a process of attempted separation of medical professionals from lay practitioners and healers, a process which would evolve over the next few centuries and bring Scottish surgeons and physicians to world dominance.

From the start, the Edinburgh Incorporation of Surgeons and Barbers acted like most other craft bodies. It attempted – not always successfully – to prevent unauthorised practice. This was, of course, not easy in a period when the orthodoxy and its official custody had not been defined or, more importantly, agreed, by those who would henceforth be excluded from that particular sphere of 'general practice'. The organisation had the usual clutch of officials, headed by the deacon, who normally held office for two consecutive years in the first instance. Other office-bearers included the boxmaster or treasurer, and the 'keeper of the kist', the wooden chest in which important documents, charters, bonds and the incorporation's mortcloth and banners were stored. In addition, the Incorporation's charter, or Seal of Cause, contained strict guidelines about training of apprentices and testing their competence to practise surgery in the name of the Incorporation. It was made clear that a master surgeon must 'knaw the nature and substance of everything that he werkes, or ellis he is negligent'. In addition, apprentices were to be taught anatomy, particularly of the veins, and also the astrological signs (a perfectly natural part of medicine and general belief at the time, and certainly not an indication of ignorance). After the period of apprentice-ship was completed, before an apprentice could complete the rite of passage from apprentice to master, he was to be 'diligently and avisitly examinit and provit', in order to demonstrate his competence to the assembly of master surgeons.

Over time, the examination system was refined and the content expanded or made more specific. At the same time, the Incorporation tried very hard to make the transition from being a 'mere' craft body to being, in its own words 'a learned society'. The aim was there right from the start, and is reflected in a number of ways. The surgeons very quickly detached the barbers from any political influence within the Incorporation. The barbers were also prevented from operating in the innermost parts of Edinburgh, being banished to work in the suburbs, particularly Canongate (until there was an outcry from aggrieved Edinburghers who had to walk to the suburbs to partake of the services of the barbers). The final, official separation from the barbers would not take place until 1722, but it was made very clear from the start that the surgeons and barbers were not equals (though the surgeons were more than happy to keep control of the validation of barbers and collect their membership fees). It was of considerable advantage to the surgeons that their Incorporation was founded and supported by the Town Council for almost eighty years before the Town's College, or University was established. In Glasgow the medical institution came much later than the University, which was thus able to oppose the Faculty by dint of history and tradition for some time.

With academic aims in mind the Edinburgh and later Glasgow institutions took pains to acquire the physical attributes of the learned society. These attributes included the establishment of libraries and museum collections, and the eventual construction of suitably ornate buildings which served as an outward sign of the gravitas and intellectual status of these groups. The Edinburgh Incorporation set up its library in 1699, and the listing of the original collection demonstrates that master surgeons had access to most of the current standard medical and surgical works, mostly from the continent, but including Peter Lowe's important surgical text in the vernacular. One product of the Renaissance was the rapid progress made in anatomical illustration, and many books were produced in this period, ornately and classically illustrated, if still less than anatomically accurate. The anatomical revolution was enhanced by the work of anatomists such as Andreas Vesalius, whose *De Humani Corporis Fabrica* was a key element in anatomical progress.[3] Thus the general literary stimulus offered by the Renaissance and the culture of print had very real and positive effects on European medicine and, thus, on Scottish medicine.

In addition to their efforts to produce well-qualified surgeons and to elevate the status of their Incorporation, the surgeons were faced with repeated efforts by the physicians of Edinburgh to encroach on their territory and jurisdiction. This was where close links with the Town Council would be especially beneficial. At various points during the first half of the seventeenth century, the physicians of Edinburgh made determined efforts to achieve a collegiate organisation of their own (see below). Petitions were submitted to James VI, Charles I and to Oliver Cromwell, before the final bid was successful in 1681, helped considerably by support and patronage offered to the physicians by James, Duke of York, who had his own reasons for wishing to gain support in Scotland. As matters came to a head, battle lines were drawn: on the one side were ranged the Incorporation of Surgeons and the Town Council, on the other the physicians and the Court of Session, to which some of the disputes were taken eventually. The debate was not only over whether the physicians should have a college, nor even what, if any, rights they should acquire over the surgeons or the apothecaries of Edinburgh, but rather as to whether a decree of the Court of Session should take precedence over an act of the Town Council, or vice versa. The problem seems odd at a distance of several centuries, but it must be remembered that at this point Scots law, and its jurisdiction, was by no means clear or standardised.

The Edinburgh surgeons thus led the way towards corporate practice, and it would be almost another century before a medical organisation appeared in the west of Scotland. Glasgow at this point was still a small, underdeveloped burgh, which would not flourish in the economic sense until the end of the seventeenth century when the general focus of Scottish trade shifted from Europe to America. By the end of the sixteenth century, though, there were just enough medical and surgical practitioners to enable an organisation to be set up. Whereas in Edinburgh the main stimulus had been the sufficiency of numbers and the background of emerging incorporations, the catalyst in Glasgow was to a great extent the influence and efforts of two individuals, whose main stated aim was to improve the standards of practice in the west of Scotland, and to deal with fraudulent and incompetent individuals.

Although Glasgow was a small burgh, the Town Council, as elsewhere, was faced with the problems of dealing with epidemic and endemic disease and the casualties of conflict, and there is evidence that it employed individuals on an ad hoc basis to deal with particular situations (as indeed was the case in Edinburgh, particularly during episodes of plague). Among these was Allaster McCaslan, who was paid for 'curing of sindry puir anes' in 1596.[4] By the late 1590s there was growing concern on the part of the kirk and the Council about the standards of medical care available, and it was proposed to institute an enquiry to determine exactly what the situation was, and in the way of these things to the present day, the logical move was to appoint a committee. No sooner had this committee got to work than two key players, Peter Lowe and Robert Hamilton, petitioned the King, James VI, who granted them the authority to supervise and control medical and surgical practice in the area. They were given the designation of visitor, with powers to do just that – visit and validate.

Peter Lowe, rather than his lesser-known colleague Robert Hamilton, is generally the focus of historical assessment of these events. Several key factors influenced his actions and the formation of the unique medical and surgical organisation in Glasgow. His precise origins in Scotland are vague and impossible to establish accurately, but the important aspect of his career was that he had studied and worked in France for a number of years before returning to the Glasgow area, although again the details are a little blurred – he may well have treated casualties of the infamous Bartholomew's Day Massacre in August 1572. He also published a number of works, including his justly famous *Discourse of the Whole Art of Chyrurgerie*, the first edition of which appeared in 1597. This was a surgical textbook in the vernacular, one of the first such works to appear, which contains details of surgical procedures which would not be unrecognisable or alien to modern surgeons.[5] Importantly also, he was familiar with the academic nature of French surgical training, which incorporated a higher-level university element as well as the more familiar apprentice training. Academically qualified surgeons, known as surgeons of the long gown, were members of the College of St Côme in Paris.[6] It was not surprising, therefore, that he advocated a joint institution containing both physicians and surgeons.

Lowe therefore brought a number of key elements to the construction of 'official' medicine in the west of Scotland – his European contacts, his academic training in France, his royal patronage on both sides of the channel, and his academic contribution to surgical training. These key elements gave him the ideal set of attributes to enable him to successfully petition the Glasgow Town Council with Robert Hamilton for a charter to set up a medical and surgical organisation in the town, despite the fact that there were probably no more than six or seven practitioners resident in the area at the time. The charter gave Lowe and his colleagues sweeping powers of supervision and control of medical and surgical practice, eventually in a large area of the west of Scotland, not just in the burgh of Glasgow itself. As with the earlier Edinburgh Incorporation, the Faculty of Physicians and Surgeons (FPSG) set about establishing rules and regulations for the training of apprentices, the admission of physicians and surgeons and the maintenance of discipline and control. This organisation was unique in that it contained both physicians and surgeons, but as time went on, this produced a great deal of internal friction. In Edinburgh the conflicts would be between rival organisations; in Glasgow much of the difficulty arose precisely because of the united organisation which contained practitioners who pursued both academic medical careers and more practical, apprentice-based surgical training.[7]

Another contrast with the Edinburgh surgeons was that in Glasgow restricted licences were granted to individuals who had acquired some surgical skill but who were not fully competent in all areas.[8] In Edinburgh a surgeon was either a fully licensed master or he was not. Eventually the internal difficulties between the two wings of the Glasgow organisation and the need for closer support from the Town Council resulted in a charter being granted in 1656 by the Glasgow Town Council setting up an Incorporation of Surgeons, which was at the same time part of, but separate from, the Faculty. This charter gained parliamentary approval in 1672. There is no space here to give fuller coverage to either of these two pioneering institutions. They have been dealt with in full compass elsewhere, but for the present the major influences and creative forces which shaped and directed these bodies must be emphasised – the corporate nature of events in Edinburgh, and the role of individuals in Glasgow, but in both cases the need for royal and burgh patronage for the organisations to be set up in the first place, and to continue.

Although there were surgeons in other Scottish burghs, and although there is some evidence of the brief existence of an incorporation in Aberdeen, and some vague corporate activity in Dundee,[9] it was only in Edinburgh and Glasgow that lasting and relatively powerful institutions came into being. In all cases, though, the fate of the organisations depended just as much on what was happening in the burgh and wider community as it did on internal processes. If it happened to be in the interests of a Town Council or other authority to support a medical or any other organisation or group, then the support would be forthcoming. However, the reverse was also the case. Shortly after its formation, the Incorporation of Surgeons and Barbers of Edinburgh took steps to demote the barbers and confine them to the margins of the Incorporation, but the Town Council did not see fit to reprimand the surgeons or provide any backing for the barbers.

While the foundation of these incorporations was undertaken very much in line with the general process and sphere of urbanisation[10] and also with the wish to gain dominance over the pursuit of certain occupations, developments in Scotland were of necessity on a smaller scale than those in other European countries. The medical world in France was effectively controlled and directed by the Medical Faculty at the University of Paris, and depended just as much on the cultivation of patronage as in Scotland. As early as 1311 a group of Paris surgeons had gained a monopoly of practice, but by 1372 the Paris barbers were permitted to undertake surgical procedures, and thus two separate surgical groups were legitimated until the middle of the seventeenth century. As in Scotland, the medical community relied on contacts with and patronage from royalty, and the French royal surgeon held considerable influence over the control and practice of surgery throughout the country. Physicians had the benefit of readily available academic training in several locations, particularly Paris and Montpellier, and their sheer size and intellectual advancement served to make France a world leader in the early-modern period. In Paris there were two levels of surgeon – the surgeons of the long gown, who had experienced university training, and the surgeons of the short gown, who gained their expertise by apprenticeship. In Scotland, of course, there were not as yet the university facilities to make this possible, but what was happening in the early-modern period does seem to fit with Brockliss's and Jones's view that in France the 'corporative medical community' was evolving, which 'comprised a complex tripartite ensemble of physicians, surgeons, and apothecaries grouped into various legally recognised collectivities'.[11]

Although the university at Salerno had provided an institution well ahead of its time, by the early-modern period Italy had been to a great extent overshadowed by the Netherlands and France, in terms of medical and surgical training. A recent study of medical and surgical provision in the kingdom of Naples has confirmed that in that part of Italy at least, there was a plurality of medical provision similar to that available to the population of Scotland. Physicians, surgeons and apothecaries shared the medical market place with ecclesiastics, folk healers, quacks, midwives and saints. In a similar manner to the power enjoyed by the French royal surgeon, who had effective control over surgery in much of France, the Royal Protomedicato in Naples was a 'committee' which enjoyed considerable power and authority. Headed by the royal physician, this body was concerned, naturally, with matters relating to income and the collection of visitation fees from the many physicians under its control, with the exception of qualified practitioners, at least in this period. Although the royal physician had great prestige, he could not wield very much influence or control over public health in general.

By the early seventeenth century there were no fewer than fourteen medical Colleges in Italy, in the major cities, together with numerous guilds and organisations of apothecaries and other practitioners. The Protomedicato was influential in some of these cities, but it is apparent that the Colleges were not able to gain a complete monopoly in any location, but were forced to come to some sort of compromise between, for example, noble and non-noble physicians.[12]

In all of these countries, the close connections between physicians, surgeons and kings is evident. In France and Italy, these connections allowed the royal practitioners to wield considerable influence over medical and surgical practice in their countries. In Scotland, and in England, royal physicians and surgeons had equally close contacts with the monarchy, but their main influence was in the sphere of patronage rather than that of direct influence over the medical or surgical organisations. In this period the key to reshaping the medical and other social spheres was patronage, and the favour of monarch and court was crucial to the promotion of the Scottish medical and surgical bodies, but not so directly to how these bodies functioned.[13] In terms of causation, the relations between those in power in society in general, and those in power in medicine in particular, were of considerable importance in accelerating or, at times, preventing change.

The Netherlands, which has become a significant focus for historians of Scottish medicine in the early-modern period, was clearly of at least some importance. It was not just Hermann Boerhaave (1668–1738) who drew Scots in large numbers to Leiden. Scots had other connections, not least in trade and the elite marriage market. By the end of the seventeenth century the Scots – and the English and Irish – had a king, a Stewart, who was also king of the Dutch. Many Scots fought in his armies in his determined pursuit of war against the French. However, this period in the history of medicine in Scotland cannot be covered adequately without some new assessment of the function played by Boerhaave himself in developing medical teaching in the Netherlands and in Scotland. It has been claimed that what Boerhaave brought was reason and a quality of refinement to the philosophy of medicine. Medical students who attended his classes testified to the way in which Boerhaave had apparently been able to 'digest a heap of indigestible stuff' into something much more rational and understandable. Adam Murray wrote home:

> I came an ignorant into it, and if I know anything now in physick I owe it to a Dutch professor. I had always an inclination to sit with a book in my hand but was never taught how to use it. In a word, I never read fewer books in a year than I have done this past year, yet have learned more these ten months bygone than for twenty years before, the cream of which I have put in writing, and makes six volumes in quarto of annotations upon Mr Boerhaave's two books, his Institutions and his Aphorisms.[14]

This account certainly suggests a rationale and orderliness about Boerhaave's teaching. It says less, though, about the essence of his philosophy. Some historians have accepted the reason and eirenicism which seem to have been the major characteristics of Boerhaave's philosophy. It is also the case, though, that he was not an original scholar and made no significant contribution to medical knowledge. It has also been claimed recently that his philosophy was not based on reason at all, but rather on sensory experience, thus rather shaking the foundations of the Boerhaavian legend.[15] If this was the case, has he been given undeserved acclamation? Whether or not he was an original thinker, and whether or not he was a keen advocate of clinical medicine, enough Scottish medical students and practitioners seem to have had sufficient contact with Leiden and its system and general ambience to translate at least some of its characteristics to the melting pot of early-modern Scotland. Perhaps Boerhaave was simply in the right place at the right time. Whatever the case, the previous links between Scotland and Europe had set the scene for the adoption of practices which the Scots themselves must have considered to be worthwhile.

Given the unavoidable links of geography, it might be assumed that Scottish and English medical and surgical organisation, training and practice would be very similar. However, this is only true to a very limited extent. The Royal College of Physicians of London was founded by circumstances which would be mirrored in Glasgow at the end of the sixteenth century. One difference in London was that in 1512 an act of parliament was passed which prevented physicians or surgeons from practising in London unless they had been certified by the bishop of London or the dean of St Paul's, who were to appoint appropriate medical or surgical examiners. Although Oxford and Cambridge universities were to retain their licensing rights, these would no longer be exclusive. This brings in a rather different religious element to the situation, although it had been the case since the foundation of the surgeons' and barbers' incorporation that licences had to be granted by the bishop. Some six years later, Henry VIII granted a charter establishing the Royal College of Physicians. It is claimed by a historian of the College that one of the main reasons why Henry granted the charter was that there was considerable evidence that medical matters were organised and controlled much more efficiently elsewhere, particularly in Italy and France. In addition, the petition was presented by a number of his close medical acquaintances, including Thomas Linacre and two other royal physicians.[16] The second reason is perhaps more plausible, given the pre-eminence of patronage in this period.

From its foundation, the London College of Physicians built an organisational and administrative structure very similar to that in operation in most such institutions, and a further act in 1523 gave the London College rights of supervision and licence over the whole of England. Examinations were introduced and refined, and during the seventeenth century the College acquired licensing rights over the publication of medical books. Major contacts and conflicts between the Scottish and English institutions would come in the late eighteenth and early nineteenth centuries, when the battle for territorial domination over the whole island came to a head.

The London Barber-Surgeons evolved along very much the same lines as their Edinburgh counterparts, and indeed had a longer pedigree, although their key charter was granted by Henry VIII in 1540. Some evidence of a corporate organisation exists from as early as 1309, and there had apparently been two groups before the formal charter, one group of surgeons and the other of barbers. In 1540 the two groups came together as the Company of Barber-Surgeons, and organised themselves on the same lines as the Edinburgh surgeons. Curiously though, their educational aims seem to have become a little diluted when a few years after their foundation, they decided that knowledge of Latin was not necessary. Indeed, modified examinations were provided for the 'unlearned that cannot wryte nor reade'.[17] Although on a larger scale than in Edinburgh, the London surgeons shared similar organisation, practice and problems. Eventually, in 1745, prompted by the increase in numbers of surgeons and the focus on anatomy as the core of surgery and surgical knowledge, the surgeons broke away to form a separate Company of Surgeons, and in 1800 were granted a royal charter. It is clear, therefore, that although there were differences among the various European surgical and medical organisations, there were core practices and shared difficulties, and, importantly, the need for both initial and continued patronage.

SCOTLAND AND EUROPE

As in many other aspects of the development of Scotland as a nation in this period, the European influences were strong, defining and crucial in many instances. Culturally, the Renaissance had brought much to Scotland in terms of art, architecture, humanist philosophy and continuing trade.[18] As well as adopting the artistic motifs of the best of French, Dutch and Italian architecture, the expertise was also imported in the persons of craftsmen enticed to Scotland to demonstrate their skills, teach the local craftsmen and help monarchs and nobility to emulate and develop what they considered to be the very best of Europe. Towards the end of the seventeenth century the flow of skills into the British Isles was stimulated by the effects of the Revocation of the Edict of Nantes in 1685, which saw large numbers of Huguenot refugees leaving France and taking their skills with them. All of this was, of course, parallel to, and in many instances influenced by, the two ongoing strands of trade and the very important European royal and noble marriage market, which helped to strengthen all sorts of linguistic, artistic, political, economic and cultural influences. Scots merchants had long sailed from east Scotland to many parts of Europe, settling in considerable numbers in the Low Countries, importing bulk wood and iron from Scandinavia and – perhaps more importantly for some – large quantities of wine from France and, to a lesser extent, Spain. The substantial numbers of wealthy Edinburgh merchants were at ease in Europe and saw no barriers to these historic, useful and practical connections (intermittent wars aside). Common factors were also the protestant tradition in the Netherlands and Scotland, and the municipal nature of the universities of Leiden and Edinburgh, not to mention progressively-minded university principals in both locations.

The same was no less true of Scottish physicians. Despite the historic and ongoing desire to improve the education of Scots at all levels and of all capabilities, and despite the presence of a mediciner at King's College, Aberdeen from its inception in 1494, and fragments of medical teaching elsewhere, it was not possible for a Scot to study medicine and graduate as a physician in Scotland, at least by any means which would be accepted nowadays as legitimate. This would, of course, change, with the foundation, on a small scale, of the medical school at Edinburgh in 1726. For the moment, this lack helped to continue and develop the European face of Scotland and of Scottish medicine. During the early-modern period and particularly from the early years of the seventeenth century, the *cursus academicus* for the aspiring Scots physician comprised a general degree taken at home, followed by a period of travel and study in Europe, culminating in examination at a continental university to acquire the degree of Doctor of Medicine. The sphere of early-modern Scottish medicine was, therefore, truly European, both in terms of the continuation of Hippocratic and Galenic humoral medicine (though with some acknowledgement of Arabic medical history too) and of the source of training and experience of medical practice. Scots went to many European universities, such as Padua, Paris, Orange, Amiens, Harderwick and others. Increasingly, though, and very clearly by the beginning of the seventeenth century and lasting until training was available in Scotland, two universities began to attract the majority of Scottish medical students. These were the universities of Leiden and Reims. The Leiden influence would be – in the view of many historians of medicine – influential to a greater or lesser degree in the small-scale and tentative beginnings of the Edinburgh University medical school.

It is important to remember, though, that at this point the sphere of medical training, at whatever centre, was not confined or configured by the name or location of any particular university. It can be claimed, quite reasonably, that medical training was European in nature, not particular to any university. This was because university study was as 'open' as it is possible to be. The present-day Open University, one of the major

developments in British education in the twentieth century, comes
perhaps closest to the situation which obtained in the early-modern
period. Any student, at any place, could study where he chose, in several
locations if he wished, and then present himself to take the final medical
examinations at a university at which he may well not have spent any
part of his medical training. An MD degree at this time was a test of
knowledge. The means by which this knowledge was acquired were of
lesser concern. All that was required was that the medical student
demonstrate that he had sufficient knowledge to be able to practise
medicine thereafter. There was no formal curriculum or residence requirement at most universities, and little in the way of supervision, control or
confirmation of study periods. Medical students in effect created
individual 'medical schools' for themselves, and their choices were to an
extent economically driven. Because of the high cost of study abroad,
those students who were able to do so tended to come from relatively
wealthy backgrounds, though by no means exclusively so. European travel
had long been part of the youthful experiences of the gentleman, and
medical students were able to do this and study at the same time. A
student may have been examined and graduated at Reims (where the
examinations were reputedly cheaper and also easier than at other centres),[19]
but during his period of study abroad have spent time dissecting at the
Hôtel Dieu in Paris, and attended lectures there, or at Orange or Leiden
(or London). Rough and ready though it appears now, this system may
well have had its advantages, in that the students went to locations where
what they wanted was available. There were no large hospitals in Scotland
in the early seventeenth century – indeed there were no exclusively
medical hospitals at all – so it made good sense to go to where there was
a large hospital where, despite the potential religious objections, frequent
dissections were carried out and clinical contacts could be made.

What emerged at the other end of study, then, was a European rather
than a Scottish doctor, an individual of some private means, who had
travelled extensively and had – or so he hoped – encountered the best
medical teaching and practice possible, thus returning to Scotland in the
optimum condition to advance the cause of medicine in a nation where it
was not possible to find suitable medical education. The disadvantages of
this system were primarily in the enforced selection of medical students.
As in most ages, money was a prime consideration, and, had the 'lad o'
pairts' really existed in this period, it would have been very difficult for
him to experience 'pairts' other than those of mainland Scotland and
local education.

However advantageous, though exclusive, was the strong Scottish
medical connection to mainland Europe, by the beginning of the eighteenth

century strong moves were afoot to take some steps towards bringing a 'proper' sphere of medical education to Scotland. The means by which this came about were, as was often the case, a fortuitous combination of facts and circumstances which coincided at an opportune moment rather than by means of any carefully planned or logical progression. This is perhaps one instance where the arbitrariness of the postmodernist interpretation might have some currency in the interpretations of events and processes. Whatever the case, by the early years of the eighteenth century, a number of predisposing factors had engendered at least the disposition to act.

Scots who studied medicine in Europe, particularly in Leiden, and particularly towards the end of the early-modern period, studied the classics. The Renaissance in general produced the renaissance in particular of the classical medicine of Hippocrates and Galen, supplemented by the chemical elements of Paracelsus and the beginnings of clinical training. There was also the less definable, but important, factor of travel and exposure to other countries, other languages and other traditions, but at all times sharing the common language of intellectual communication, Latin. This was one area where Scottish education was of great assistance to those who could afford to travel abroad. It would be equally useful to Scots who could not afford the luxury of study abroad once medical training became available in Scotland in the early eighteenth century. Evidence of the considerable difficulties faced by aspiring doctors comes from a series of letters written home by a medical student in Leiden in the 1720s. Much of the content of this correspondence is not about medical matters but about the problems of subsistence. Adam Murray wrote in October 1725 that: 'I happen to be here in a very unlucky year when every thing in living is extravagant, the money low and colleges [courses of instruction] much dearer than usual'.[20] The effects of enforced travel were, therefore, that the potential to be a doctor was restricted. Once training became available in Scotland, this would not automatically open the gates of the universities to all, but it was a significant step, and would go some way towards preventing a brain drain of doctors who went to Europe to train and did not return to Scotland at all – a trend which had existed since the days of Duns Scotus and before.

THE EDINBURGH PHYSICIANS FINALLY MAKE IT

With continued apologies to adherents of postmodernism or poststructuralism, it does seem possible to identify in this period some of the longer-term antecedents of the modern profession, if it is deemed necessary for a profession to have an institution with powers of control, supervision and education. It may be claimed that it is possible to go back as far as 1505, when the surgeons and barbers of Edinburgh were awarded their initial charter, which encouraged the pursuit of knowledge and the restriction of surgical practice to those who had been tested and found sufficient in that knowledge. This may be too much for some, but it was certainly a fact, if not a causal factor. At various points during the turbulent seventeenth century the physicians resident and practising in Scotland made attempts to form themselves into an official organisation. The first attempt came in 1617, during the reign of James VI, but this came to nothing. A further attempt came in the early 1630s, when Charles I was approached by a group of physicians who wished to set up an organisation containing a selected number of physicians, who would enjoy sweeping powers in Scotland, not only over fellow physicians, but also over the surgeons, who were, predictably rather less than enchanted by the prospect.[21] Again this attempt failed. Not to be daunted, the next, and potentially the most successful, effort came during the period of the occupation of Scotland by the Cromwellian regime in the 1650s, but this effort again came to nothing, partly because of the early end to the republican experiment.

Final success did not come until 1681. Because of the nervousness created by the Exclusion Crisis in England, the Duke of York had been dispatched Scotland, where he canvassed political support and patronised various aspects of the arts and culture of the nation. His patronage was important in the setting up of the Advocates' Library, which collection would form the basis of what is now the National Library of Scotland. So, the important element of royal ambition coincided with the attempts to form an exclusive group of physicians who wished to control the training and practice of medicine and form a body which would further the cause of medical organisation and practice in the most important social and political area of Scotland.[22]

1681 was indeed something of a golden year for intellectual Scotland. In addition to the foundation of the Advocates' Library, Sir George Mackenzie of Stair published his famous *Institutes of the Laws of Scotland* (before being forced, with other notables such as Gilbert Burnett, into exile in the Netherlands because of his opposition to the incumbent monarch). This publication was the first real attempt to write down Scots law and was of considerable importance, both in the history of Scotland and in the creation and maintenance of distinctive Scots law and, of necessity, Scottish identity – if indeed it is accepted that the institutions of a nation are major determinants of its identity or, at least, distinctiveness from other nations.

It seems appropriate that the other major intellectual achievement in 1681 was the foundation of the Royal College of Physicians of Edinburgh. Starting on a relatively small scale, with a roll of some twenty physicians, the College progressed quickly to take its place among the major medical institutions. One of the more curious aspects of this development was that as part of the 'deal' to bring the College into being, the negotiators undertook that the College would not organise the teaching of medicine. This seems hardly credible from the long perspective of hindsight, but this was the seventeenth century. In order for progress to be made in most spheres, some sort of bargaining had to take place and concessions made in order for the crucial first steps to be taken. Despite their restrictions in the field of medical education, the College quickly established itself along the lines of most such institutions, initiating entrance examinations, supervising members, establishing a physic garden, holding seminars at which learned papers were given, and offering treatment gratis to the certified poor of Edinburgh.[23]

In terms of evidence of steady progress towards the establishment of formal medical training in Scotland, then, this did not seem to be at all promising. Indeed, for much of the subsequent decade the College was more concerned with matters of litigation and appeals to the Court of Session against the surgeons, on the thorny problem of which body should be granted oversight of the relatively small group of Edinburgh apothecaries (an amorphous group which would never acquire any sort of power, let alone the political might of the London apothecaries company, despite a brief association with the surgeons).[24] So far, then, the surgeons were busy training surgeons, the physicians had at last achieved an organisation, but nobody was teaching medicine effectively.

THE NEXT KEY STAGE – MEDICAL SCHOOLS?

Enter once again the Edinburgh Town Council, a formidable body of wealthy merchants and almost equally wealthy craftsmen, including a representative of the Incorporation of Surgeons, together with two other significant individuals, George Drummond (1687–1766) and John Monro, father of the first of the long line of Alexanders. Edinburgh, like Leiden, was a municipal town in every respect. The Town Council licensed the surgeon's incorporation and was also in control of the Toun's College, founded in 1583 and for the most part free of religious barriers. Ever mindful of the quest to 'improve' Edinburgh in all respects, the Town Council decided in 1685 to appoint three Fellows of the infant College of Physicians to serve as professors of medicine (to the Council, not the university). These Fellows were Robert Sibbald, James Halket and

Archibald Pitcairne. These appointments appear to have been sinecures rather than real posts, symbolic rather than practical or academic. The 'Town Council Three' were given neither teaching accommodation nor remuneration by the Council, and there is not a shred of evidence to suggest that they undertook any corporate teaching at all. Their main significance at that stage was that they demonstrated that the Town Council was showing some interest in the promotion of good medical training and practice.

At the end of the seventeenth century a number of forces had converged, the effects of which would be to bring about one of the most significant facets of the history of medicine in Scotland. Scotland at that point was in something of a turmoil. The presbyterian religious settlement of 1690 was the final act in the process of Scotland's acceptance of William and Mary as the next incumbents of the throne, although the first rumblings of Jacobite activity were not far from the surface. Indeed, Archibald Pitcairne, one of the most prominent Edinburgh physicians, left the College of Physicians to join the Incorporation of Surgeons (in itself some indication of the relatively high social regard in which the surgeons must have been held), and this was alleged to be due, at least in part, to his Jacobite sympathies. It is something of an irony that this was the case, given that the College in great measure owed its very existence to the help of the recently deposed Stewart king.

As with most historical processes, it took a combination of factors to bring about specific change and, indeed, to maintain continuity. By the turn of the eighteenth century Scotland was in something of a state of flux. The monarch had migrated south a century ago, taking with it most of the influence of the royal court; by 1700 there was the possibility, though by no means the certainty, of further, fuller union between the two countries, and the nation had experienced another enforced change of monarchy, though at last a religious settlement had been reached. It appeared that Edinburgh was about to lose at least part of its very special status within Scotland. So, what was in place by the early 1720s was a country which was both stable and unstable, certain and uncertain. What was stable was the country as a whole (though there had been a period of economic downturn in the 1690s), the monarchy, the church, the universities and the medical institutions (though none of these was without problems). What was unstable was the relationship between Scotland and Westminster, the Jacobite question, and the self-image of Edinburgh. There is a view among some historians of medicine that this image problem was a major reason why Edinburgh was able to establish a medical school at the time that it did, and also why it was formed in the way that it was.[25] The parallels between Edinburgh and Leiden have been cited many times, and cannot be ignored. However, this alone cannot account for exactly when the final, crucial moves were taken. The catalyst was probably not simply the fact that Edinburgh felt lost, unfocused or less important after the union of 1707. This is to assume that every resident of Edinburgh had been opposed to the union and that there was agreement that it was detrimental to the image of the Scottish capital. This position is not easy to defend. Although the desired elements for a medical school were in place, and although the Town Council had a vital role in most of them, it is easy enough to defend the view that the Medical School would have been founded whether the union had taken place or not. It could not have been established without the support and consent of the Town Council. It could not have been established without sufficient qualified physicians to teach. It could not have been founded without the ongoing changes taking place in teaching methods in the university. It could well have come into being even if parliament and court had still been in Edinburgh and dominating the social climate. Intellectual life depended to a great extent on individual patronage, but perhaps not so much on the corporate presence of the great and good of the land.

In the event, it would take the efforts of individuals to bring about change at that particular point. Just as individuals had been key to the foundation of the Glasgow Faculty, so in Edinburgh the impetus came from the formidable duo of George Drummond and John Monro. These two men managed to bring together the political and medical communities and enable progress to be made. Drummond was a long-serving and ambitious local political leader. He was provost on a number of occasions, and had grand ideas for the physical development of Edinburgh into a town of classical European significance. Monro was a surgeon who had experienced the Leiden system and, importantly, had a son for whom he was just as ambitious as Drummond was about Edinburgh. Monro Senior groomed his son Alexander for a career in anatomy, sending him abroad and also securing him an apprenticeship with an Edinburgh surgeon. Alexander Monro qualified as a master surgeon in 1719, and in 1720 as a result of some less than savoury political manoeuvring, succeeded as the Professor of Anatomy appointed by the Town Council. He occupied this post outwith the walls of the university until 1725, when a grave-robbing scandal broke, and Monro clearly felt threatened as it was alleged that bodies were being procured for the benefit of the anatomists. He petitioned the Town Council for accommodation within the walls; this was granted, and proved to be a key step in the establishment of the medical school itself. The following year, four professors were appointed to teach theory and institutes of medicine; all of whom had studied at Leiden. Doctors Plummer, Innes, Sinclair and Rutherford, together with Monro and, from 1729 a professor of midwifery, formed the teaching and, importantly, examining cohort of the new medical school. This latter point is crucial. Medical degrees had been available at Edinburgh since 1705, but the candidates had often studied elsewhere, and were examined externally by Fellows of the Royal College of Physicians, who, ironically, had not been allowed to teach them. If it is the case that a school must be able to examine as well as teach, then 1726 can be seen as an important milestone in the long road to the professionalisation of medicine as well as to the ultimate dominance of the university degree as the main port of initial qualification in medicine.[26]

The final piece in the Edinburgh Medical School jigsaw came just three years later when, in 1729, the first infirmary was opened with the first patient coming from Caithness. This hospital was modest in the extreme, containing only six beds with, therefore, very limited potential to do much, either in the sphere of teaching or of medical treatment or nursing care. However, it was a beginning, and, importantly, had been advocated by Drummond and Monro for a number of years. It was built on public subscription, an inportant factor in hospital development for some considerable time in the future. A central part of the Leiden system was clinical teaching, though as in Edinburgh the St Caecilia Hospital was not a large institution and there is controversy as to the extent to which Boerhaave himself had made use of its facilities. Clinical teaching would be instituted in the second infirmary building, which opened its doors in 1741, but was forced to close them temporarily when the hospital was devoted to the care of the casualties of the Jacobite conflict in 1745.[27] From that point, hospitals were set up in most of the major towns of Scotland, and this was the start of another important trend in the sphere of medicine – the creation of a separate, in many ways artificial, sphere, in which the sick were taken out of their home environment, with a concomitant alteration in the balance of power among patients, relatives and practitioners. The dynamics of the practitioner-patient relationship were also altered. The hospital phenomenon will be considered further in subsequent chapters.

This, then, was the situation in Edinburgh. The 'Cunningham argument' is now no longer wholly, or even partly, favoured by many historians, and it would seem that individual ambition and priority were just as important as any grand civic or national plan. The teaching system that was instituted was certainly similar to that in Leiden, but it does seem that it was more of a coincidence that the legacy of Boerhaave was one of refining and standardising and perhaps, therefore, eirenic or calming.

There is little evidence that the individuals who formed the initial core of teaching staff taught as they did because they felt that the nation as a whole needed to be calmed down in the wake of the union; they taught what they did because they believed it to be correct in approach and content.

The Glasgow Medical School was the only other medical school in Scotland to begin to develop significantly in this period, and did so for rather different reasons and against a different background. Some support for the 'post-union' argument as related to Edinburgh might be drawn from the fact that Glasgow was not at the centre of Scottish politics or elite culture, although was rapidly becoming the dominant commercial face of Scotland. It may be that Glasgow's civic pride emerged a little later than that of Edinburgh, or it may be because of the less than harmonious relations which existed between the Town Council, University and FPSG, or it may be that there was not the same potent combination of an ambitious local politician and a pushy parent. Whatever the case, the medical faculty at Glasgow University did not begin to consolidate in any real sense until well into the 1740s.[28] The progress of medical education in the major Scottish centres is considered in greater detail in the next chapter.

EVERYDAY MEDICAL PRACTICE

What was now happening in the general sphere of the giving and receiving of medical and surgical treatment? The qualified practitioners were only part of the equation; the vast majority of the population were the receivers of care and it is necessary to pay attention to practice as opposed to preaching of medicine. In this area what was practised depended to some extent on the state of the nation, in terms of political stability, state of war or peace, and condition of the economy and food supply, and the geographical location of the patients. All of these factors helped to shape both the diseases and injuries which required to be treated, and the extent to which patients could influence their treatment, consult qualified practitioners or resort to self-treatment and folk medicine.

One factor which had important effects on surgery in particular was the significant changes taking place in the theatres of warfare. Guns superseded weapons powered by human or bow-and-arrow projection and this brought in great change, both to the nature of the wounds caused by these new weapons and the treatments necessitated by bullet and gunpowder. Guns changed the nature of warfare radically; they also forced surgeons to confront new and very difficult problems. Early surgical textbooks contain detailed illustrations of the various types of arrowhead, axe and club with which horrendous wounds could be inflicted; the early-modern period saw equally devastating, but different, problems caused by lead shot and other missiles propelled at high speed. Surgeons had to adapt both their teaching and practice to take account of new technology. This was not the technology of medicine as would be the case some two centuries hence, rather it was the enforced medical and surgical reaction to the aggression and conflict between and among Scotland and her neighbours. A modern parallel here is that surgeons in Northern Ireland have become world leaders in the development of techniques to treat bomb casualties.

A graphic description of the consequences of gunshot wounds comes from the casebooks of Ambroise Paré, whose work was known to Scottish surgeons (and indeed to some extent plagiarised by Peter Lowe in his own textbook of surgery). There is no doubt that the circumstances described here would be seen on many occasions on the battlefields of Scotland, after Flodden, Dunbar, Prestonpans and, ultimately, Culloden. He describes a case from a conflict in 1538:

> A poor soldier was shot with an harquebus in the left arm near the wrist and the joint of the hand. The ball lacerated and broke several bones, tendons and other nervous parts. Gangrene developed, then mortification spread nearly to the elbow. Gangrene extended to the shoulder and great inflammation extended to part of the thorax ... I was encouraged to remove his arm at the elbow. I did this as rapidly as I could, removing the arm without a saw since the mortification was just beyond the elbow.[29]

The horrific experience of this patient would be very similar to those of the wounded in battles in which Scots soldiers were involved. The medicine and surgery of war were, therefore, driven largely by the technology of war. Scottish surgeons gained high reputation in their skills of amputation and the care of wounds, and were frequently invited to serve at court.

Day-to-day medical practice in effect changed very little, despite the phase of demarcation and institutionalisation which characterised the early-modern period. What did seem to become increasingly evident, though, were the effects of literacy and the advent of print, with the result that there was some stratification of the consulting aspects, both on the part of practitioner and patient.[30] The treatment given for most conditions was similar, but also stratified or characterised by social status and geographical location. Individuals at the highest levels of society had the closest contacts with the demarcated and institutional aspects of medicine. They were often literate and could communicate with practitioners by letter and also read medical books for themselves. This is not to say that they did not still share all or many of the superstitions current in society as a whole. The medicines prescribed by qualified doctors may have appeared to be different from those contained in folk recipes, but the ingredients were very similar. In urban centres those at upper and middle social ranks had better opportunities for face-to-face consultation; those in the rural areas with means could finance a visit by a qualified physician, while the armed forces and royal courts had a permanent supply of medical attendants to cater for their needs.

The consultation experience therefore did not depend solely on wealth, but on a number of other factors, and there was an inverse relationship between social status and location, and the ability to consult individuals who by this time claimed custodial rights over what they had determined to be the medical orthodoxy. While on the surface the process of institutionalisation would suggest that members of the institutions would offer a different medical practice, in reality this was most definitely not the case. There was certainly discussion about new science, about Newtonian physics, Cartesian philosophy, mechanical structures of the body, and the nature of fevers, but practice and treatment were not new, and would not be for a long time to come.[31] So, if an assessment is made of 'medicine from below', then there is little that can be claimed as real progress or as the direct, practical effects of Renaissance or Reformation. The following examples of medicine in practice serve to illustrate these arguments, and also to provide some flavour of life and treatment in early-modern Scotland.

The evidence which survives is of necessity selective and skewed towards higher social strata, although there is some evidence of practice in the areas of folk medicine, charming, healing and witchcraft. With qualified practitioners it seems to have been the usual practice to invite a medical attendant to review the case, and if he agreed to treat the patient, arrangements were made for consultation by letter or in person. Surgical fees tended to be agreed in advance, and often included a sum for board and lodging in the home of the surgeon. There did not appear to be any fixed charges for individual procedures. Other factors, such as the length of time necessary to effect a cure, or whether the patient was boarded in the surgeon's house had to be taken into account, although cases which were more difficult to treat tended to be more expensive. The testament of James Rig, a surgeon who seems to have operated mainly in rural south-east Scotland in the early part of the seventeenth century, gives some indication of the sort of costs involved. William Guild of Duns was charged £100 Scots for 'curing him of ane great wound in his hand', while Alexander Wishart had to pay double that sum for 'curing and mending of ane wound of his thorax being struchane nyne inches therin', and evidence of payment in kind is seen in the 'firlot of beir' which another patient paid for treatment to a fractured rib.[32] Physicians apparently took some pride in not stating a specific fee, but relying on the patient to give them adequate remuneration, although there is also some evidence of fixed charges being made. Following consultation, any prescription or recipe was either made up at home from ingredients purchased from an apothecary or gathered from the countryside or herb garden, or compounded by the apothecary himself, at least in the urban setting. For example, a lengthy account submitted to the Dundas household by apothecary John Hamilton in 1617 contained 'almond milk according to the doctor's advice', 'materials for fomentation to his breist' and 'puder for staying his host' (cough).[33]

The darker side of early seventeenth-century life is demonstrated clearly in a detailed account of the condition of Lady Balfour, signed by two physicians who stated forcefully at the start of their report that they were fully qualified and university trained, and had not acquired their degrees *per saltum* or *per dispensationem*. They concluded that Lady Balfour was afflicted by 'an inordinate and unsatiable desyre of venerous actions such as in old tymes was attributed to satyrs', and that the major reason for this problem was the 'violent, unmanlie, unmannerlie, preposterus and untymely beseiging of that claustrum before maturitie of aige'.[34] Sexual abuse is nothing new, apparently. No treatment was noted, but the physical explanation for the symptoms was 'a sharp burning or salt humor which to these pairites floweth incessantlie either through unkyndlie heat of her bak and veynes, or by disorder of dyet'. So, even in cases like this, the perspective was still one of humoral imbalance.

One aspect of the consultation ethos was that there was, at least at upper social levels, a much more equal balance of power between patient and practitioner. Patients offered their own diagnosis on occasion, or indicated that they had treated themselves before consultation, and there was no real sense of deference, understandably in early-modern society in a situation where the patient may have been of higher social rank than the physician. A good example comes from the illness of Sir John Clerk of Penicuik in the 1690s. Clerk corresponded at length with prominent Edinburgh physician Dr John Burnett, when he seems to have been suffering from kidney disease as well as gonorrhea. Clerk wrote that he 'found a little pain in my making water and a tendence to ane gonorrhoea simplex'. The symptoms had appeared 'six horas post concubitum', and he also described 'testiculi sinistri tumor abortus est cum dolore', changing with ease from the vernacular to Latin for the most sensitive parts of the description.[35] The medical opinion seems rather bizarre nowadays, but would not appear so then. It was the opinion of Dr Burnett that 'Sir John's riding much of late in cold weather and under night has occasioned all the disorders of his bodie and that his coching also late at night has occasioned a separation of sharp serous humours which has fallen on the testicle and seminal vessels where is the tumor testis sinistri and the beginning of a gonorrhoea'. Sir John had treated himself, and a second opinion given by Dr Gilbert Rule hints at the attitudes taken by physicians towards their role in relation to high status patients who seemed to have a fair degree of medical knowledge themselves. Rule and Burnett wrote that they really had little further to offer as Clerk's health was improving, but 'to show how ready we are to be serviceable to you in our Art, we have thought upon the following advice'.[36] There followed some prescriptions for herbal remedies, but the main impression here is that the physicians clearly felt they had to do something. This is very much akin to the current view held by many patients that if they do not come out of the doctor's surgery clutching a prescription, then they have not been treated adequately.

It was also customary for individuals to circulate proven cures amongst their relatives and friends, so that a recipe prescribed initially by a physician may well have been tried by people with whom he had no connection and for whom it may not have been at all appropriate. One of these recipes was 'The Earl of Marchmont's Elixir', which consisted of 'an ounce of rhubarb cut in slices, an ounce of aloes beat small, a large handfull of carduus stryd and cut small. Infuse all in a large chopin of Brandy, let it stand a week shaking the bottle three times a day then strain off the brandy'. A further measure of brandy was to be added to the residue and left again for some days, and the two quantities of liquid amalgamated. It was said to be good as a prophylactic against ague and could be made up easily.[37]

Good illustration of the role of other professionals in local medical care comes from the journal kept by Robert Landess, minister at Robroyston in the middle of the seventeenth century. His diaries contain interesting detail about individuals facing prosecution for holding conventicles, and also note that three of his four children had died at a very young age. At the end of the journal is a collection of recipes, including one 'to ease a pain of the head', which contained 'violet oyll and womans milk' mixed with the yolk of an egg, to be applied externally in the form of a poultice.[38] It is very likely that he gave general advice to his flock on medical matters, as well as using the recipes to treat members of his family.

Another means of circulation by the written word was the commonplace book. These were books in which their owners noted down matters of interest, significant local events, copied out parts of printed books and collected recipes for cooking as well as for medical treatment. These early ad hoc collections were added to and formalised later by the more 'official' printed household medical book, such as Buchan's famous *Domestic Medicine*, published by a physician in 1769.[39] The trend, thus, was from medical recipes noted as general interest, to medical recipes collected and printed, giving them an air of authenticity as the culture of print gradually permeated down through Scottish society. One of the earlier 'amateur' (unattributed) books contained 'Mistress Hubbards rare water for weak and distempered children', the major ingredients of which were snails, oats, pimpernell, water, agrimony, raisins, liquorice and aniseed.[40]

The following cures for insomnia appeared in an early 'Poor Man's Guide': 'take the beris of lorell tree and breke thame in a morter and lay thame in an cloute all about his heid, and he sall sleipe'. Close links with religion appear in a cure for migraine:

> Take foure penny wecht of the root of pellitory of Spayne, and half penny wecht of spygnard and grynd thame and boyle them in gude vynegar, and quhen it is cauld put into ane sponefull of hony and ane saucer of mustarde, and medle them weill togither and hauld theirof in thy mouth ane sponfull at once as long as ane man may say two creeds and then spit it out into ane vessell and tak more ...

Clearly, the length of time here was thought to be important, and how better to indicate this than to specify an activity which would be well known and understood by all with no need for access to watches or clocks.

OUT OF TOWN – FOLK HEALERS, QUACKS AND WITCHES

Although a major focus of this chapter has been the trend towards formalisation and institutionalisation of the urban, educated elements of medical and surgical practice, the sixteenth, seventeenth and early-eighteenth centuries continued to be characterised by a wide variety of 'alternative' medical practices. The process of urbanisation had not yet resulted in any large-scale displacement or relocation of the population, the vast majority of which continued to live as it had always done. Perhaps the main difference by this time was that most Scots who lived in Scotland would not now describe themselves by a regional loyalty or designation. The same forces of season, hierarchical society and the protestant church directed their daily lives in a variety of forms.

Towards the end of this period, society and economy had changed to the effect that the feudal system was no longer the dominant social pattern. By 1750 urbanisation was progressing, the mercantile outlook was strong, although political power was still vested to a great extent in the land. The effects of all of these on medicine and surgery are difficult to assess. Certainly, urban growth required more medical and other practitioners, while educational opportunities and the growth of schools and universities facilitated entry to all of the learned professions, not just the medical profession. It was also more acceptable for a son of an aristocratic house to go into medicine, although such individuals had done so in Scotland for a considerable time. Indeed, some early masters of the Edinburgh Incorporation of Surgeons were fairly substantial landowners, such as Archibald Pennycuik and Gilbert Primrose, both prominent sixteenth-century surgeons.

Just as town had a symbiotic relationship with country, so lay and professional medicine continued to share many elements. As mentioned above, trained physicians were beginning to question the old philosophical orthodoxy about the structure and functions of the body. This did not mean that these particular individuals immediately started to practise a new or alternative form of medicine. Archibald Pitcairne may have fallen out with his fellow Fellows of the Royal College of Physicians of Edinburgh over the iatromechanical or iatrochemical debate, he may have corresponded regularly with erudite colleagues on anatomical and surgical matters; however the experiences of his patients were in many respects much the same as the experiences of patients in remote localities who were treated by a wise woman, minister or itinerant practitioner.

The types of lay treatments outlined in the previous chapters changed relatively little in the light of social and economic change. A major problem was still the difficulties involved in travel or communication over long distances. The ongoing push towards universal education and literacy meant that more people could read and write, but few of those people at lower levels of society used these skills to write to physicians for advice. Financial and social barriers saw to that. There were, though, perhaps two significant new strands to this aspect of medical practice in its very broadest sense. These were, firstly, the appearance of the itinerant 'quacks', who travelled at least the accessible parts of lowland Scotland, promising miracle cures for all sorts of diseases and conditions;[41] and secondly, the overt politicisation of witchcraft, which had implications for local healers and charmers, whose activities were particularly susceptible to accusations of witchcraft.

In terms of the remoter areas of the highlands, lay medicine continued much as it had done for centuries, and much as it was doing in lowland Scotland, with local and regional variations of the standard cures. The ritualistic, seasonal and superstitious elements were regionalised, but the underlying beliefs and aims were similar. In terms of potential healing abilities, here such individuals as the seventh son of a seventh son bore added influence. Evidence from the late seventeenth century comes from the writings of Martin Martin, who journeyed extensively in these parts. On the Isle of Skye a prevalent cure for 'twisting of the guts' was by 'drinking a draught of cold water, with a little oatmeal in it, and then hanging the patient by the heels for some time', while 'a larger handful of the sea-plant dulse, being applied outwardly ... takes away the after-birth with great ease and safety'.[42] The role of healing places was still important, with inhabitants visiting the Loch Siant Well, in search of cures for a variety of afflictions, including 'stitches, headaches, stone, consumption, migraine'.

Unlike the situation in the lowlands, the division between professional and lay medicine in the highlands was not characterised by urban institutions or universities. Those who practised medicine after having been educated to do so had been trained in a very different way from their lowland urban counterparts. There is apparently no instance of a university-educated physician practising in the Gaelic-speaking areas of Scotland during the seventeenth century, although a few individuals who had achieved an MA degree would have acquired a little medical knowledge in the course of their studies.[43] What was more generally the case with learned Gaelic medicine (which was focused on Gaelic transla-tions of the classical authors, including Hippocrates, Galen and Avicenna), was that medicine was the province of family dynasties, such as the Beatons, who were perhaps the most prominent Gaelic medical group during the early-modern period. The knowledge was passed on from father to son, by an apprenticeship system not unlike that in operation for urban surgeons. These medical men led an itinerant life, consulting at various locations in the highlands and islands, and their medicine was based very much on the same literature as was available to their lowland colleagues.

One other difference between highland and lowland medicine was that there seems to have been at that time no distinction between physician and surgeon. The Beatons practised both, and the major division seems to have been between the members of the hereditary medical families and others who practised one or the other branch at a lower level of compet-ence. The division therefore, was not one of urban, university-educated and rural folk medicine, but rather between dynastic and non-dynastic practitioners. Here as elsewhere, though, all of this took place against the broad backcloth of folk medicine, healing and superstition.

This period saw the politicisation of witchcraft, and a number of concentrated phases of political persecution of witches.[44] This has the advantage of bringing into the public record some evidence of the practices of which witches were accused. There were fine distinctions here between the background activities of charming and witchcraft as part of the general cosmology of healing. Individuals accused of being witches, and particularly those accused of diabolic pact, were singled out for many reasons, partly of course because most of the accused were women of relatively modest means. Although the accusations and rumours were probably highly embellished, the trials give a flavour of healing activities involving both humans and animals, and also accusations of infliction of disease or ulterior motive on the part of the accused. The following is an extract from a case brought to the Justiciary Court in Edinburgh in 1622. Margaret Wallace had been accused of a number of acts of witchcraft and sorcery:

> Is and hes bene thir aucht or nyne yeiris bygane, ane cowmoun consulter with witches ... and ane seiker of help and responssis of thame, alsweil for hir awin cure and releif of dyverse seiknesses and diseassis quhairwith sche has bene uset, as for the cure and help of hir friendes in their seiknesses and diseasses; as also, for the overthrow and distruction of dyverse persones, men, wemen, and bairnes, be Sorcerie, Witchcraft, Charmeing and incantatioun and uther devillish and unlauchfull meanis ...[45]

This extract displays most of the major aspects of witchcraft and healing. The accused was said to offer cures, but also to inflict disease and to consult with witches and, by implication, the devil. It is very clear from this sort of case how fragile the boundaries and interfaces between local folk healing, healing accompanied by ritual or incantation, and the darker side of witchcraft involving infliction of disease and the diabolic pact were – the latter aspects creating the justification for persecution of many of these individuals.[46]

Although men were also accused of witchcraft and healing, the primary focus was on women, and this is not surprising, given their central role in family as well as healing, particularly in the rural areas. The role of women in medicine through the ages was shaped by many factors, not just a gender bias. In earlier periods, everyone, regardless of education, location or gender could practise medicine to a certain extent. The medieval period saw the control of medicine being taken by the church and the religious orders, particularly the male orders and monasteries, preventing secular society from increasing its knowledge or practice, and also serving to remove women in some areas from their central role. Once the process of secularisation of medicine and medical training began to take place, the institutions began to evolve, and these were male institutions. By that time the official sphere excluded not only women, but also men who could not attain the qualifications necessary to become a member of the inner sphere. This in itself produced a rural–urban barrier.

In rural areas the official knowledge was often in the hands of the minister, and women were generally able to operate as they always had done, particularly in periods of war or other conflict, when local societies were left to the women in the absence of men serving in the armed forces. The Enlightenment period would emphasise these differences.

THE SHAPING OF AN ORTHODOXY – WHEN THE ORTHODOX BECAME THE ALTERNATIVE?

Writing on the approaches taken over the centuries by historians of medicine, Burnham has identified a number of stages or particular foci of attention. In the early centuries when accounts were written, the 'profession' was deemed to be the body of knowledge possessed by individuals who practised medicine. There were no professional institutions to supervise practitioners. What separated them from others was, quite simply, their knowledge. In the Greek and Roman eras knowledge of the body and its systems and functions – as far as these could be determined – was possessed by a few individuals, and the very possession of that knowledge served to set them apart from other members of society. As time went on, and by the early-modern period, when there were sufficient numbers of practitioners to warrant a group with common aims and objectives, the profession was not only the knowledge but also its individual holders. Subsequently, by the eighteenth century and the Enlightenment period, historians looked at progress in the professionalisation of medicine very much in terms of the 'great doctors' and their achievements.[47]

In this early-modern period, what seems to have happened was that in Scotland small groups of physicians and surgeons decided that what they had and practised was the orthodoxy, despite the fact that they were very much in the minority, and that what the vast majority of the population experienced was different and, by implication, inferior. In other words, general experience and practice could not define the orthodoxy any longer. Not only did early-modern Scottish physicians and surgeons wish to take custody of what medical and surgical knowledge was within reach, but they strove to define it as the orthodoxy. The majority of the population would continue to experience medicine as they had always known it; and those who experienced 'professional' medicine received something not very different at all, but which, helped by the apparent gravitas of an institution, however imperfect, lent the air of authority or orthodoxy to the situation.

What was this 'orthodoxy' which was created? It came from a mixture of classical, European, Scottish and other beliefs, knowledge and traditions.

The identity of early-modern Scottish medicine was just as complex as that of early-modern Scotland. By the end of the seventeenth century Scotland had passed, with considerable difficulty, through not only the Reformation but also the Renaissance, not to mention civil war, union with another country and a great deal of restructuring of society and economy. Although Glasgow would begin to flourish during the early part of the eighteenth century – as the focus of Scottish trade began to change towards the west and the smoke signals sent out by American tobacco – Edinburgh was still the magnetic and dominant focus of Scottish life, intellect, politics and professions. So, the orthodoxy of society, not only of medicine, became an increasingly lowland urban orthodoxy, at least in terms of national government and religion, in addition to medicine. However, for some considerable time yet, the localities would be in many ways just as important as they had always been. The more restricted sphere of enforced medical orthodoxy was as yet ill-defined and depended on external forces just as much as on any advances in scientific or medical knowledge.

THE STATE OF MEDICINE AND NATION AT THE 'END OF THE BEGINNING'

The transition from medieval, to early-modern, to 'modern' medicine was shaped by many interacting factors. Although it is dangerous to look too closely for cause and effect, provided that the language and context of the various periods are taken into account, there is nothing wrong in trying to account for and explain developments, however tentatively. In terms of interacting spheres of influence and the construction of a new orthodoxy at the expense of derision of the old orthodoxy and the creation of mechanisms whereby the new orthodoxy might be promoted and protected, the early-modern period was crucial. It was crucial for itself, in that considerable and influential progress was made in beginning to set up the conditions which would allow the body to become familiar; for secular practitioners to receive appropriate training; and for medical and surgical organisations to take control of practice. The stage which had been reached in Scottish society was one where the social hierarchy was changing; where urban and rural societies were a little more different than they had been in the earlier periods of the developing burgh network. Within urban society, groups of like-minded individuals operated spheres of protectionism. Whether they wished to do so for the same reasons, what happened was that groups of individuals who practised medicine and surgery (with or without a vocation or altruistic intent) also formed themselves into self-controlling and self-perpetuating bodies.

Town Councils in the larger burghs were drawn from small pools of available merchant and, later, craft talent, and it is clear that society – urban society – operated on the basis of the many being brought under the control of the few.

What is less clear is the legacy of the period in terms of the location of the increasingly rationally derived medical orthodoxy within the broad, amorphous range of beliefs about God, man and society. It is worth reiterating that at this time many of the prominent individuals who were creating the medical and surgical orthodoxies were doing so in spite of their continuing belief in the supernatural, the unknown or unexplainable in the world. It is assumed wrongly that whenever a group of individuals acquired the external trappings of what would now be described as an academic, rational body, the members of the group immediately abandoned beliefs which could not be explained rationally or empirically. It is precisely this complex and interesting interface which characterises the early-modern period. Isaac Newton did not abandon his alchemy; Archibald Pitcairne did not dispose of his astrological charts; Robert Sibbald did not suddenly give up prophylactic bloodletting. As is well known, Newton revolutionised physics, Pitcairne was a leading proponent of new explanations of body structure and function, while Sibbald turned his talents to other matters, including the post of geographer royal and a vain attempt to establish a philosophical society long before the Enlightenment proper. None of these individuals, though, could be translated out of his own time. The image of the body, its structure and functions may have been debated by those who gained knowledge of the new science of the seventeenth century, but this did not mean that they immediately abandoned any or all of their cosmological antecendents.

CONCLUSION

The main characteristics of the early-modern period were the trends towards institutionalisation of professional medicine, and the attempted definition of a medical orthodoxy, though this was in large part a lowland urban orthodoxy. Medicine outside the growing urban sphere continued as it had done for centuries; medicine within the urban sphere was organised very differently but practised in very much the same way. The last major outbreak of plague attacked Scotland in 1645, but other diseases would emerge to take its place. The nation was essentially stable and despite the loss of crown and then parliament, Scotland remained very much a nation seeking to develop. Progress in the period covered by the next chapter confirmed that the foundations established in the early-modern period allowed the 'great doctors' to emerge and influence the Enlightenment period. Much greater strides would be made in terms of elucidating the facts of the human body and its workings, and the Edinburgh Medical School would, for a time at least, draw students from all parts of the world. The period is designated early-modern; there is debate as to what exactly this term might mean, but it was clearly the early phase of the modernisation of the structure, education and practice of urban medicine. There is some justification for the claim that this period was the most significant; but there is equal claim for subsequent centuries. The transition from medieval and feudal to 'modern' and mercantile was not without difficulties and pitfalls. The continued progress from modern and mercantile to enlightened and empire-building was also problematic, but would be another very significant phase in the shaping of the nation itself.

What seemed to be emerging in medicine and in society in general was a series of concentric circles, with the epicentre around Edinburgh. The inner circles contained most of the elements of change, while the outer circles, outer in all senses of the term, were not changing nearly so quickly or decisively. In the early-modern period, all of the circles shared some common characteristics, but the inner sphere contained different elements, and so the social construction of medicine and the medical orthodoxy were increasingly centralised and localised.

NOTES

1. Bannerman, *The Beatons*.
2. Dingwall, *Physicians, Surgeons and Apothecaries*, esp. pp. 34–98.
3. Vesalius, A., *De Humani Corporis Fabrica* (Basel, 1543).
4. Comrie, *History*, i, 346.
5. For a full recent account of Lowe, see Geyer-Kordesch, J. and Macdonald, F., *Physicians and Surgeons in Glasgow. The History of the Royal College of Physicians and Surgeons of Glasgow* (Oxford, 1999), 2–77.
6. See account in Gelfand, T., *Professionalising Modern Medicine. Paris Surgeons and Medical Science Institutions in the Eighteenth Century* (London, 1980).
7. Geyer-Kordesch and Macdonald, *Physicians and Surgeons in Glasgow*, 21–5.
8. Ibid., 117.
9. Hamilton, *Healers*, 32–3.
10. Covered in Lynch, M. (ed.), *The Early Modern Town in Scotland* (Edinburgh, 1987).
11. Brockliss, L. and Jones, C., *The Medical World of Early Modern France* (Oxford, 1997), 8.
12. Gentilcore, D., *Healers and Healing in Early-modern Italy* (Manchester, 1998), 56–95.
13. For a new detailed analysis of court doctors, see Furdell, E. L., *The Royal Doctors 1485–1714. Medical Personnel at the Tudor and Stuart Courts* (Rochester, 2001), though there is little coverage of Scottish royal practitioners.

14. Smout, T. C., ' A Scottish medical student at Leyden and Paris 1724–1726: Part II', *Proc. Roy. Coll. Phys. Ed.*, 24 (2) (1994), 264.

15. Cook, H. J., 'Boerhaave and the flight from reason in medicine', *Bull. Hist. Med.* 74 (2) (2000), 221–40.

16. Clark, G., *A History of the Royal College of Surgeons of London* (London, 1964), 59.

17. Young, S., *Annals of the Barber-Surgeons of London* (London, 1980), 310.

18. MacQueen, J., *Humanism in Renaissance Scotland* (Edinburgh, 1990) gives an erudite account of many of these influences.

19. Examination of the Reims records shows that between 1620 and 1753 some 227 Scots graduated there, as did 115 English and a remarkable 542 Irish medical students. Bibliotheque Carnegie, Reims, Médecins de la Faculté de Reims 1550–1794.

20. Smout, T. C., 'A Scottish medical student at Leyden and Paris 1724–1726: Part III', *Proc. Roy. Coll. Phys. Ed.*, 24 (3) (1994), 430.

21. This particular attempt is covered in MacHarg, J., *In Search of Dr John MakLuire. Pioneer Edinburgh Physician Forgotten for over 300 Years* (Glasgow, 1997).

22. Ouston, 'York in Edinburgh'.

23. Full coverage of the foundation and early progress of the College in Craig, W. S., *History of the Royal College of Physicians of Edinburgh* (Oxford, 1976), and Dingwall, *Physicians, Surgeons and Apothecaries.*

24. Coverage of Edinburgh apothecaries in Dingwall, *Physicians, Surgeons and Apothecaries*, 185–213; also Dingwall, H. M., 'Making up the Medicine. Apothecaries in sixteenth- and seventeenth-century Edinburgh', *Caduceus* 10 (3) (1994), 121–30.

25. Cunningham, A., '"Medicine to calm the mind". Boerhaave's medical system and why it was adopted in Edinburgh', in Cunningham, A. and French, R. A (eds), *The Medical Enlightenment of the Eighteenth Century*, (London 1990), 40–66. Similarly, Schaffer claims that the Leiden model 'provided important new resources for settling sectarian dispute and restraining polemic'. Schaffer, S., 'The Glorious Revolution and medicine in Britain and the Netherlands', *Notes and Records of the Royal Society of London* 43 (1989), 182. This is probably to overstate the case somewhat.

26. For fuller coverage see Dingwall, *Physicians, Surgeons and Apothecaries*, especially ch. 5.

27. Turner, A., *Story of a Great Hospital. The Royal Infirmary of Edinburgh, 1729–1929* (Edinburgh, 1937).

28. Comrie, *History*, i, 343–64; see also Coutts, J., *A History of the University of Glasgow from its Foundation in 1451 to 1909* (Glasgow, 1909).

29. Hamby, *Case Reports*, 74–5.

30. Christopher Lawrence considers the consultation, or 'clinical encounter', to be at the heart of medical change and development in Britain from the early eighteenth century. Lawrence, C., *Medicine in the Making of Modern Britain* (London, 1994), 3.

31. Henry, J., *The Scientific Revolution and the Origins of Modern Science* (Basingstoke, 1997) gives a concise but comprehensive account of the interactions between religion, magic and new science in this period.

32. NAS, Commissary Court CC8/8, 20 October 1642.

33. NLS, Adv. Ms. 80.2.5, 172,174, 177.

34. NLS, Adv. Ms. 33.2.31,173, document dated 18 October 1621.

35. NAS, Clerk of Penicuik Papers, GD2129.

36. Ibid., GD2131.

37. NLS, Adv. Ms. 80.7.2., 57.

38. NLS, Ms. 548.

39. Buchan, W., *Domestic Medicine* (London, 1769).

40. NLS, Ms.165, f58.

41. Porter, R., *Quacks: Fakers and Charlatans in English Medicine* (Stroud, 2000), is a typically comprehensive view, the major elements of which are applicable to Scotland. An older-fashioned account is contained in Thin, R., 'Medical quacks in Edinburgh in the seventeenth and eighteenth centuries', *Book of the Old Edinburgh Club* 22 (1938), 132–60.

42. Martin, M., *A Description of the Western Highlands and Islands of Scotland Circa 1695* (Edinburgh, 1999), 116–17.

43. Bannerman, *The Beatons*, 127.

44. Recent account of the North Berwick witches in Norman, L. and Roberts, G. (eds), *Witchcraft in Early Modern Scotland. James VI's Demonology and the North Berwick Witches* (Exeter, 2000).

45. Pitcairn, R. (ed.), *Ancient Criminal Trials in Scotland*, Vol. III Part II (Edinburgh, 1883), 508–36.

46. Larner, C., *Enemies of God: The Witch Hunt in Scotland* (Edinburgh, 1981).

47. Burnham, J., 'Concept of profession'.

CHAPTER 6

MEDICINE IN ENLIGHTENMENT SCOTLAND

INTRODUCTION

When did Scotland stop being early-modern and become enlightened? Was the nation different, or did it have a different sense of identity or purpose? This chapter will consider in some detail the major processes which took place throughout the eighteenth century and early nineteenth century, in terms of the significant changes brought about by the advent of home-based university medical training, together with the intellectual thrust of the Enlightenment and its effects on medicine, medical training, medical men and medical treatment. The period began with the tentative steps taken by Edinburgh Town Council, stimulated by the foundation of the Royal College of Physicians in 1681, in the appointment of three physicians, Sibbald, Halket and Pitcairne, to teach medicine on behalf of the Town Council. There is no evidence that they did any medical teaching at all, but it was the beginning of a trend which would grow, firstly in Edinburgh and, with the customary lag period, throughout Scotland, culminating in the eventual consolidation of medical training in Aberdeen in the early decades of the nineteenth century; this latter process delayed considerably by the internecine disputes between the two university colleges. The ongoing friction between the medical institutions and the University hindered progress in Glasgow, however, there were cross-currents. Both Joseph Black and William Cullen started their academic careers in Glasgow, before being head-hunted by Edinburgh University, and the so-called father of the Scottish Enlightenment, Francis Hutcheson, was a professor of philosophy at Glasgow University. So, the major processes affecting the development of medicine in Scotland were not confined exclusively to the capital. Edinburgh came to the fore because of a unique combination of circumstances, the combined effects of which resulted in the much more rapid progress which characterised Edinburgh medicine and brought it to fame as a world leader by the end of the century. The subsequent decline in university standards in the early part of the nineteenth century, though, was both the end of the ascent and the beginning of new directions for medical education in Scotland and elsewhere.

The establishment and consolidation of the Edinburgh Medical School was a major factor in setting up Enlightenment Edinburgh or, at least, the possibilities of practical application of enlightened thought in relation to medical science and practice. While the founders of the medical school agreed that hospital medicine and clinical training were essential elements of good practice, the medicine that was taught and administered to the patients was hardly enlightened, although certainly well-intentioned and based on beliefs which were held sincerely. The caring ethos was there, whether or not the knowledge was based on erroneous beliefs about the structure, function, decay and repair of the human body. The later eighteenth century would see what has become known by the rather clichéd expression 'the flowering of the intellectual life of Edinburgh' and Scotland. There is no doubt that the literati made a significant contribution, both directly in their philosophical discussions and published treatises, and indirectly in the freedom of individuals to pursue thoughts and ideas which may not have been drawn from long tradition or from the tenets of the Christian faith. It may be, indeed, that the later eighteenth century saw the real secularisation of medical philosophy and training, although religious influences on the acceptance of new medical treatments would continue. The release of the mind – which may be an alternative definition of 'enlightening' – which was achieved by the acceptance of new thought by the very institutions which had long guarded the souls and consciences of the nation, was a stimulus to medical progress just as important as the creation of medical institutions in the past, or of the development of anaesthetics and antiseptics in the future.

In terms of the totality of man, medicine and society, it is clear that the period was still one in which a holistic view was taken about the role of medicine and how phenomena might be explained. New science, including Newtonian physics, brought new and provable knowledge, but much of that knowledge was still seen in terms of its place in a larger scheme of things. There are a number of potential models which can be used here, but one which has been discussed is the image of the family, or, as Jordanova describes it, a modular approach.[1] A family consists of members interacting on a number of levels, held together by its head. Medicine, philosophy and chemistry, for example, were all modules of the larger module, or members of the 'body' of knowledge. So, it is important to remember that Enlightenment medicine and Enlightened society did not abandon a 'total' view of medicine as part of a much larger whole, from which it could not or should not be isolated.

This was certainly the age of the 'great doctors'. The Enlightenment, almost by definition, was an individual, as well as corporate or institutional, experience or process. The Scottishness of the Scottish Enlightenment was very much the result of the desire and ability for the effects of this new thought to be disseminated downwards throughout the whole of Scottish society, and, in particular, through the major institutions of church, university and legal profession (which was strongly political and influential). This view was in contrast to the Enlightenment period in other countries, where enlightening had to take place in the shadow of the major institutions, and where new thought tended to be viewed as insurrection rather than inspirational.[2] While there may appear to be little connection between the highly charged atmosphere of late-eighteenth century Edinburgh and the medical treatment received by patients in the outer isles, or in a country village, or, even, in Mussel-burgh, it is possible to see long-term influences from this period, long though they may have taken to become plain.

While a significant part of the discussion in this chapter relates to the Enlightenment, there is not enough space to enter into the debate on Enlightenment philosophy in great depth. The 'Further Reading' section includes suggestions for wider reading on these aspects. This chapter is concerned with medicine as practised and experienced in eighteenth-century and early nineteenth-century Scotland. The intellectual context was important but was not the only factor which shaped both the context and the construction of medicine. What happened in Edinburgh, Glasgow or Aberdeen may have happened differently from events or influences in the remoter parts of the kingdom, but rural medicine was just as important – and to more of the population – as localised, elite, urban medicine. Other factors which shaped the construction of medicine in this period included urbanisation, demographic realignment, politics, religious dissent and the beginnings of industrialisation. In terms of concentric circles, Edinburgh may have been at the centre, and medicine may have been much slower to change in the outermost circles, but these areas were part of the whole and need to be considered. Further justi-fication for assessing the more practical aspects of the Enlightenment in this context comes from the more revisionist view of the intellectual process, which claims that it was natural philosophy and, importantly, its application in medicine and science which gave a major stimulus to the particular version of the Enlightenment in Scotland.[3] Here, the Habermas spheres theory is appropriate also, given the wider access to debate and knowledge and the proliferation of clubs, societies and institutions.

THE INSTITUTIONS AND THE ENLIGHTENMENT
– THE CREATIVE DIALECTIC?

In terms of the grander scheme of progress in nation and medicine, the Enlightenment period demonstrated a number of very specific features, not all of which were connected either backwards or forwards historically, but which did combine to heighten the atmosphere of competitiveness, protectionism and, ultimately, progress. The major national institution of government was now located a week's journey away by stagecoach; the royal court was similarly distant. It was left to the remaining and new institutions to promote themselves and, almost as a by-product, help to stimulate the intellect and organisations within this 'new' nation. Scotland was in effect governed by a very few dominant individuals. The institutions of the intellect were, for the moment, centred in a few places, but these places were extremely important. The effect in medical terms was something of a creative dialectic within the changing spheres and shifting orthodoxies.

By the middle of the eighteenth century the older established institutions of Scotland were undergoing considerable change. The national church was in a process of fragmentation and polarisation, and was in some ways less of an influence on the lives of the nation and Scottish people. Scots law, on the other hand, was flourishing, particularly since the publication in the 'golden' year of 1681 of Stair's *Institutions of the Law of Scotland*, which was followed by a steady stream of publications seeking to codify and set down the fundamental principles of Scots law. To help the lawyers, the Advocate's Library, also a product of the golden year, was building up its stocks and would eventually become the National Library of Scotland. The medical and surgical institutions were consolidating. The Surgeons of Edinburgh gained a royal charter in 1778 and continued their determined efforts to transform their organisation from craft to 'learned and flourishing society'. The Physicians of Edinburgh were collegiate from 1681 under a royal charter granted by Charles II, and were helped along the way by Charles's brother James, Duke of York. The University of Edinburgh (and also those in other parts of Scotland) was going through a period of transformation and development. Two major influences in Edinburgh were particularly significant for the future of academic life as a whole. Firstly, stimulated by the then principal, William Carstares, the historic regenting system began to be phased out in 1708. This shift allowed the more specialised teaching of a much wider variety of academic subjects at a higher level than had before been possible. The emergence of a teaching professoriate was crucial. Secondly, as has been outlined in detail already, the foundation of the first real medical school at Edinburgh in 1726, followed by the provision of a teaching hospital, cannot be underestimated in terms of its importance for the future of medicine and medical training in Scotland.

Singly, each of these factors was important; taken together they were even more important. What followed was competition, healthy or otherwise, among these institutions. The universities offered medical degrees, the physicians' colleges did not, but they became increasingly influential in what was taught at the medical schools and who the teachers were. It became very clear, again as has been mentioned, that these competing institutions in their quest to attract students had to improve themselves and their product in order to compete in the increasingly wide global market for students. So, the product of the dialectic was, for example, the development of clear and enforced medical and surgical curricula; more rigorous enforcement of regulations; more careful examination of candidates; and, thus, the production of physicians and surgeons who had knowledge as well as access to patronage. These were the aims and intentions; the reality was not so positive, but at least circumstances had produced change.

THE INNER CIRCLE – HOW IMPORTANT WERE THE 'GREAT DOCTORS'?

In terms of assessment of the professionalisation of medicine, the 'great doctors' period has been identified as a phase through which historians of an earlier period went in their attempts to account for the process of transformation of groups of individual practitioners into an exclusive professional body, whatever definition of profession is used.[4] In terms of Scotland, the later eighteenth century was certainly a period during which a number of high-profile individuals attempted – and sometimes succeeded – to break out of the confining sphere of ignorance and lack of understanding about the workings and relationships of the various systems of the body. It is clear that any changes in medical treatment and any moves away from holistic, humoral medicine could not have taken place without clear evidence and description of the internal mechanisms and processes of the body. Thus, the contribution of the individual was important, but cannot be assessed properly in isolation. The prevailing and changing social, economic and political background was just as important. In other words, individuals must be assessed in terms of context as well as contribution.

If the sphere of professional medicine and medical training were to be able to justify its exclusivity in the face of ongoing belief in the value of self-treatment and cures offered by the unqualified, then the next milestone had to be the elucidation of the structure of the body and the means by which its various systems functioned. In addition, this knowledge required then to be put into practices to which untrained doctors and physicians had no access. So then, while the 'great doctors' theory is perhaps a little old-fashioned and too Whiggish in terms of the debate on the professionalisation of medicine, these individuals must be given some recognition for the contributions which they made as individuals as well as members of medical schools and for the ways they developed the Scottish input to eighteenth-century medicine.

In eighteenth-century Edinburgh medicine, which was where change tended to happen first, several names spring readily into the consciousness of the historian. The following brief mention of a number of these men is of necessity superficial – much fuller details of their lives can be found elsewhere – but the purpose here is to demonstrate the sheer variety of skills and knowledge which these men brought to the age of the Enlightenment, and to point up the discourse of the individual as a key element in eighteenth-century Scottish medicine and society.[5] The great doctors were certainly not the only factor here, and indeed the very designation of 'great' may be called into question, but assessment of them as individuals will give some sense of their corporate influence within and furth of Scotland. If one part of the defining characteristics of this period was the role of institutions, then the individual contributors to these institutions must be given some mention, if only to restate the degree of their importance.

The anatomists perhaps deserve pride of place, and there was no prouder than the powerful dynasty of Alexander Monros, the first of whom, Alexander *primus* (1697–1767), had been prepared very carefully, both medically and politically, by his father, surgeon John Monro (1670–1740), to dominate the teaching and practice of anatomy – the fundamental knowledge base of the physician as well as the surgeon. He is, rightly, famous for his work in the early decades of the existence of the medical school, though his initial appointment as professor of anatomy was gained by somewhat dubious political means. Once in post, though, the senior Alexander established Edinburgh anatomy on the strong foundations on which it would flourish, at least until the appearance of his grandson, Alexander *tertius*, the proverbial wastrel and family black sheep. In terms of the sheer advance of knowledge of the body, though, the second Alexander, *secundus* (1733–1817), perhaps outdid the achievements of his famous father. Alexander the second is credited with major advances in anatomical knowledge. He elucidated the lymphatic system, crucial for the progress of physiology as well as anatomy (although William Hunter disputed his contribution). He wrote widely on the structure and functions of the muscular system, as well as describing what became an eponymous hole in the head – the foramen of Monro, which forms the connection between the ventricles of the brain. He also dabbled in comparative anatomy, an area which would become more and more significant.

For the time being, an important link between knowledge and its application comes with the dominance and good reputation of Edinburgh anatomy as taught by the Monros, though this would change by the end of the century. Student numbers continued to rise rapidly during this period, helped by the combination of famous teachers and the advent of clinical training in the second building of the Royal Infirmary. It is too simple, though, to attribute this rise solely to the reputation of the Monros. As demonstrated by Rosner, students chose to study at Edinburgh for many other reasons, including the lack of entrance requirements, the lack of religious barriers, the fact that Edinburgh was being built up as a major, cosmopolitan city to which the upwardly mobile would be attracted, and because the freedom of access and choice was attractive to those who may not have intended to pursue a full medical course but who would appreciate the status to be gained by designation as a medical student.[6] The reputation of the anatomical Monros would, however, take a severe downturn with the accession to the anatomical throne of *tertius* (1773–1859). Alexander the third apparently shared little of the dedication, ambition and hard work of his father or grandfather, although this may be too harsh an assessment as the situation was rather more complex. *Tertius* had to compete in a more open market than his father or grandfather. By that time there were extra-mural classes on offer, while anatomical instruction was available and growing in other cities, including London and Dublin. Indeed, it has been shown that in terms of raw numbers, *Tertius*'s audience was relatively similar to his father's.[7] Whatever the case, by the beginning of the nineteenth century, Edinburgh anatomy had lost its intra-mural reputation to the extra-mural teachers, whose classes were becoming increasingly popular, more relevant to the needs of medicine and surgery by that point and, consequently, more marketable. *Tertius* held the chair of anatomy for sixty-three years, but merits, perhaps unfairly in the light of recent work, a single sentence in Comrie's history. Comrie is grounded in the 'names and places' approach, which is restricted and outdated, but still useful prosopographically.

The apparently reactionary nature of teaching at Edinburgh was not the only reason for the decline in popularity of that institution. In this age of free market and as other institutions began to catch up with Edinburgh, there was greater choice available to the students. As the universities began to acquire dominance over primary medical education, the medical students perhaps had less incentive to study at Edinburgh. The apparent decline in the reputation of Edinburgh University has been reassessed in recent times by Jacyna and others, who remind us that universities cannot be assessed out of context, and that the fortunes of Edinburgh University in particular were to a great extent dependent on the complex network of patronage and politics, of which the University was an integral part.[8] This was the age of Whig ascendancy and a general desire for reform of government and local government. Since university chairs were decidedly political appointments, a period of growing general political turmoil would certainly affect institutions which had close ties of patronage. So, it is perhaps not surprising that the older generation, which had received almost unstinting patronage and support from the Town Council, had to give way at times to a younger generation, but one which, perhaps, had to struggle harder for patronage in a period of considerable flux in the country at large. The moderate churchmen, the Dundas ascendancy, the rumblings of Revolution from France and America, and the growing call for reform at home all had their effect on what was happening in the field of academic medical education.

As this period progressed, individuals of high status such as the Bell brothers began to take anatomy out of the mists and mysteries of the past. What was required, if medical practice were to benefit substantially from the theoretical and practical fruits of the Enlightenment, was progression and modernisation of the approach to teaching one of the core subjects of the medical and, particularly, surgical curriculum. The reluctance of the Monros to begin to offer a more enlightened and relevant anatomy has been cited as a major reason why extra-mural anatomical teaching flourished towards the end of the eighteenth century and continued into the early decades of the nineteenth century.[9] It was realised by those who were outwith the walls of the university and, therefore, outwith the political clutches and anatomical conservatism of the Monros, that anatomy would have to be taught as relevant to 'modern', experimental and practical approaches to surgery. It would no longer be enough just to expound historical principles without making the course of instruction relevant to surgery and include a considerable practical element of dissection by the students.

John Bell (1763–1820) and Charles Bell (1774–1842) were prime movers in the teaching of extra-mural anatomy, and one of their major contributions was in the area of accurate anatomical illustrations and engravings. The Bells taught extra-murally and also were pioneers in surgical anatomy rather than classical anatomy described for its own sake. Till then, anatomical teaching had been formulaic and almost ritualised, as was the case with the legacy of humoral medicine which still dominated medical practice, despite all of the advances which were taking place in the period. John Bell, though, fell foul of medical politics and was hounded out of teaching by the entrenched establishment which still held political sway in the University. He was succeeded by his brother Charles, who made significant contributions to knowledge of the functions – as opposed to structure – of the nervous system. He too encountered the opposition of the medical establishment and eventually moved to London in 1804 to continue his work there. The work of John Barclay (1758–1826), a major pioneer of comparative anatomy, was also of considerable significance in the longer term.

One major problem in bringing about any real modernisation of anatomical teaching was the patchy and infrequent supply of anatomical subjects. The only legitimate source of bodies was from executed criminals. It is clear from newspaper reports that corpses came to Edinburgh and, presumably, to Glasgow, from considerable distances. The fact that these events were considered worthy of reporting in the press is interesting in itself. There had been a brief grave-robbing scandal in the early 1720s, just before the final establishment of the Edinburgh Medical School. This scandal did not stimulate sustained debate, though, and the situation remained unchanged until the passage of the Anatomy Act of 1832 in the wake of the much more famous and considerable Burke and Hare scandal.

By that time the extra-mural schools in Edinburgh and Glasgow were offering better – or more marketable – teaching than the intra-mural anatomists. It should be remembered, also, that all of this was taking place against a background of increasing prescription of medical and surgical training, in terms of more and more detailed and comprehensive curricula and examination regulations. It was reasonable that the supply of anatomical subjects should be similarly formalised.

What seemed to be happening with anatomy, perhaps more than with other areas of medical training, was that the pressure for progress was hampered within the walls of Edinburgh University, at least by the continued monopoly held by the Monros. This is a little paradoxical. At the beginning of the eighteenth century, progress depended largely on the efforts of the Monros and their political allies. By the end of the century, the medical school was consolidated and operating efficiently, but the influence of the Monros was by now more negative than positive; a good illustration of the effects of change in the wider context being resisted in the narrower sphere of individuals who had built up a tradition of significance, despite doubts as to the competence of successive members of the dynasty. It may be enough to cite the apparent failings of Monro *tertius* as a teacher; it may not. Whatever the case, the Monros became in effect the reactionaries, forcing the more progressive anatomists to abandon conventional academia for the other side of the wall. When the Monros began their control of anatomical teaching in Edinburgh, their intervention and actions were welcome and had a significant influence on the progress of the medical school and the raising of teaching standards. By the end of the eighteenth century, however, their continued anatomical and political dominance meant that what was being taught to the medical students was becoming more and more old-fashioned and inappropriate for a period during which some of the Monros themselves, as well as others, had made considerable strides in the elucidation, definition and redefinition of body structures and functions. From being the pioneers, the Monros became the reactionaries. This was mirrored to a great extent by the moderate wing of the Scottish church which, by the end of the century, had been rendered more and more reactionary because of its close ties to the politics and influence of Dundas.

However, just as it has been demonstrated that the attraction of Edinburgh University for medical students was not simply that of good anatomical teaching, the decline of Edinburgh – however temporarily – cannot be attributed to this single cause. By the turn of the nineteenth century a relatively free market was still in operation, and there were other options, not least from the Royal College of Surgeons, and from other British universities and medical institutions. This again demonstrates the problems with Comrie's 'great doctors and medical places' approach. The wider context is crucial, particularly when examining the innermost of the concentric circles of eighteenth-century Scottish medicine.

The great doctors were not all anatomists. Those who talk about eighteenth-century Scottish medicine will also breathe the name of William Cullen with a certain degree of reverence – though perhaps also with a hint of ridicule enabled by hindsight. Cullen was a chemist who had been head-hunted from Glasgow by Edinburgh University in the 1770s.[10] There, he made desperate efforts to reduce anatomical and physiological chaos to an orderly system of classification of body structures, functions and diseases along botanical lines. Cullen's nosology (published in 1769, coincidentally the year in which Buchan's famous *Domestic Medicine* appeared) was proved to be erroneous, but he cannot easily be criticised for making the effort. Cullen was just as much a part of the Edinburgh Enlightenment, its spirit of enquiry and the need to reduce problems to reasoned solutions. In the longer term, William Cullen may not have made discoveries which had lasting effects on medicine but he deserves to be included in the list of key players. He did at least try to rationalise the disease process, however misguided his work, and was just as noteworthy as Robert Sibbald or Archibald Pitcairne, who had disagreed half a century before on the question of mechanical or chemical explanations for the structure and function of the body, neither of which was accurate or comprehensive.

Cullen was not the only individual who was trying to make sense of the disease process. One of his contemporaries, with whom he had an acrimonious relationship was John Brown (1736–88), whose theory, known as Brunonianism, attributed diseases not to humoral, mechanical or chemical dysfunction, but to a greater or lesser degree of excitability of the tissues. This was beautifully simple in terms of treatment, which would be either soothing or stimulating, depending on the state of excitability. Unfortunately, Brown perished as a result of treating himself along these lines. He did, though, promote an alternative to the more conventional philosophies being taught at the University and it is likely that his views were widely known within the medical world at the time, being part of the more open forum of debate in the period.[11]

Another non-anatomical 'great doctor', and one who started his medical and scientific career in Glasgow, was Joseph Black (1728–99), discoverer of carbon dioxide. Black also contributed significantly to the common pot of knowledge in the period, and though he did not leave an important legacy to anatomy, his pioneering chemical work (and his links with industry) was important. He is most famous for his scientific rather than specifically medical discoveries, but he also undertook research into the problem of urinary calculi, a major scourge of the Scots for centuries. Medical students studied chemistry, and the link is clear and unambiguous. There was also the important link to, and influence of, the background context of industrialisation and urbanisation.

Other 'great doctors' are remembered for contributions in a variety of medical and scientific areas. These individuals include Benjamin Bell (1749–1806), credited with being the first of a new breed of 'scientific surgeon'; Robert Whytt (1714–66), a true medical researcher in the modern sense of the word, in such areas as the reflexes, elucidation of nervous diseases and the ubiquitous problem of bladder stones; and Thomas Young, appointed to the chair of Midwifery in Edinburgh in 1756, and succeeded by his son Alexander Young. Among the notables in Glasgow were Robert, Thomas and William Hamilton, who oversaw the teaching of anatomy and botany for several decades, and, of course, the Hunter brothers, who had close connections with Glasgow but who made most of their careers in London.[12]

One individual who did contribute much to medical training, if not directly to the furtherance of medical knowledge itself, was John Rutherford, Edinburgh physician and maternal grandfather of Sir Walter Scott. He is perhaps not fêted quite so much as the founding fathers of the Edinburgh Medical School and may have been eclipsed historically by his more famous grandson, but John Rutherford deserves high status in terms of his contribution to the pursuit of the Edinburgh medical ideal. One of the main planks of the 'Leiden system', and one which formed an integral part of the original grand Edinburgh scheme, was bedside teaching in a hospital. This came to fruition in Edinburgh, initially in 1729, in a tiny building with six beds in Robertson's Close. It very quickly became clear, however, that this hospital was wholly inadequate, and progress towards a larger replacement was made fairly quickly thereafter, the Royal Charter being granted in 1738 and the new hospital opening its doors to patients in 1741. Thereafter, much better facilities were available for pursuing the goals of clinical teaching and empirical observation. The next step was clearly to formalise this clinical teaching, and in 1748 John Rutherford announced that he was going to do just that. He stated that his intention was to 'examine every patient appearing before you. I shall give you the history of the disease, enquire into the cause of it, give you my opinion as to how it will terminate, lay down the indications of cure which will arise or, if any new symptoms happen, acquaint you of them that you may see how I vary my prescriptions'.[13] Beds were allocated to him for the purpose and his clinical sessions rapidly became extremely popular with the medical students. Before long, clinical training was a compulsory and integral part of the medical school.

Although Rutherford was one of the first to teach in English rather than Latin, that is not to say, however, that he was 'modern' in the totality of his medical outlook. This was still a period when the superstitious could walk hand-in-hand with the empirically proven and minutely observed aspects of medical knowledge and medical treatment. Rutherford was, apparently, still willing to embrace some of the more outlandish aspects of medical practice which had not yet been completely relegated to the periphery of the medical sphere. One of the most notable quacks of the time, James Graham, is a good example of how practitioners could also become a little schizophrenic in their activities. Graham had apparently had a little formal medical training though he did not qualify. He then went to America, met Benjamin Franklin and became very interested in electrical things (not to mention his celestial bed, guaranteed to cure infertility – at a substantial cost). On his return, Graham came to Edinburgh and was allowed to use his electrical equipment in a vain attempt to cure the weakness in the young Walter Scott's leg with, apparently, the full knowledge and consent of Rutherford, one of the most eminent physicians in Scotland.[14]

The great doctors who influenced medicine did not always do so exclusively in Scotland. Part of the great significance of Scottish medicine in this period was the export of Scottish-trained medical talent south over the border and overseas. Prominent among these were the Hunter brothers, who came from a modest west of Scotland background and became leaders in the London anatomical circle. William Smellie (1697–1763), who hailed from Lanarkshire, was a gynaecologist who also found fame and fortune in London.[15] Although Glasgow lagged a little behind Edinburgh in the area of medical education, there is no doubt that considerable progress was being made there too during the Enlightenment period. It may be that the major thrust of progress was towards shaping and improving the rapidly growing commercial and economic dominance of the town, rather than the more abstract factors in Edinburgh and elsewhere, but physicians and surgeons were also contributing to the pool of knowledge and practice in the west of Scotland. The Hunterian Museum in Glasgow is still one of the major sources for scholars and historians of medicine.

When professional medicine reached the shores of the New World, it was often Scots doctors who led the way. The first medical school in the United States of America was modelled on Edinburgh lines. The first major hospital in America, in Pennsylvania, was also built along the lines of the Edinburgh Infirmary. So once it became possible for students to learn medicine in their own country, the links with, and influence of, Scotland remained strong, and would last for some time to come.[16] All of these trends are, perhaps, not so surprising, given the traditional Scottish regard for education and its availability to all who could benefit from it, and also the pre-medical school links made from Scotland to many parts of the globe through the extensive and longstanding trade networks.

The common characteristics shared by these individuals must, though, be assessed beyond Comrie's 'people and places' approach. Each of them contributed differently, but most made their contribution within the general sphere of the Enlightenment, so that practice was combined with publication, observation and debate. They were typical examples of the product of the interacting forces of the Enlightenment and their contributions were part of this complex web of stimuli and opportunity. In an earlier period their role may have been very different.

What bound all of these 'great doctors' together was that their individual contribution was applied corporately to the teaching of medicine in Edinburgh, Glasgow and elsewhere, with the result that during the Enlightenment period at least, Edinburgh medical students could choose from a wide variety of options and teachers. Enlightenment medicine, though, as experienced by Enlightenment patients, wherever they happened to be, was not recognisably or significantly different from what had gone before. The lymphatic system may have been described by

Monro *secundus*;[17] he may have provided the most detailed elucidation of the musculo-skeletal system to date; clinical medicine may have been introduced into the medical school curriculum; however, the treatments which were offered and consumed were little changed. This is not surprising. Internal medicines were beginning to contain chemical substances,[18] but herbal remedies predominated. Surgeons may have known much more about the structure of the body, but they could not alleviate many surgical conditions until the advent of anaesthetics.

Another important factor which must be considered here, in terms of the characteristics of the period as a whole, is that all of these 'great doctors' published. Many of their predecessors had also done so, but they all did much more of it, and what they published was possibly more significant because of the sheer confluence of new thoughts. They published treatises on their specialties and were, in some cases, pioneers in what would now be regarded as medical science.[19] This was complemented by what was going on in the hospitals. The general culture of print which engulfed at least lowland Scotland by the mid-eighteenth century enabled the medical men to pool and discuss their knowledge, and their own efforts went some considerable way towards confirming the scientific and intellectual necessity of print as well as discussion and informal observation of phenomena. A key theme, then, is the creative and sustaining effects of the printed word. The obverse of this was that the culture of newspaper print also allowed medical men and laymen alike to use the medium to air personal or political grudges, and for the wider public to participate in the debates.

THE OUTER SHELL OF THE INNER CORE – THE MEDICAL INSTITUTIONS

The progress of Scotland through the age of Enlightenment also saw the slow but steady inclusion of more of the geographical area of Scotland into the realms of medical education and hospital medicine. The long eighteenth century saw the foundation of the reputation of the Edinburgh Medical School; by the end of the first quarter of the nineteenth century, organised and increasingly reputable medical education was available to students in Glasgow, Aberdeen and St Andrews, as well as in a clutch of extra-mural institutions in Edinburgh and Glasgow, and the medical and surgical colleges of these two major Scottish towns. The concomitant steady progress in the foundation – for many reasons – of hospitals, particularly voluntary hospitals, meant that the sphere of training and observable practice was enlarged. However, this was not yet the day of the specialist. The medical and surgical graduates and diplomates were still very much in the mould of the general practitioner. So, another trend may be identified in this transitional period – in medical terms at least, the majority of the population had at least the possibility of access to qualified and hospital medicine, although of course large areas of the highlands, islands and remoter parts of the lowlands were still peripheral to this ever-consolidating mainstream of Scottish medicine.

In terms of the foundation of hospitals, which were the core of clinical instruction, the later part of the century saw the numbers rising gradually, with infirmaries at Dumfries, Glasgow, Aberdeen and elsewhere joining the network of institutions. Medical schools were also in the process of formation outwith Edinburgh, though not without considerable problems. In Glasgow the major difficulties centred on the longstanding friction between the medical and surgical faculty and the university (there was less of such trouble in Edinburgh), while in Aberdeen the friction was within the university, between King's College and Marischal College, so that the medical school was not finally set up in a recognisable or reliable form until the early nineteenth century.

If, as Habermas and others have claimed, the late eighteenth century saw the gradual shift in the location of knowledge, helped by increasing literacy levels and the development of the newspaper and periodical press, this is one very useful explanation for the fairly rapid developments which took place within the educational institutions of Scotland at the time. By the early decades of the nineteenth century, the situation in medical education was by no means ideal, but had moved considerably towards at least individual internal standardisation of training, examination practices and standards. When the Edinburgh Medical School was established in 1726, there was still no concept of supervision of training all the way through. Medical students opted to study at Edinburgh or one of the other available centres, and then chose to present themselves for final examination perhaps at an institution at which they had not studied at all. This seems to the modern eye to be at best unfortunate and at worst positively negligent. However, when looked at in the context of the period, it is much more easily understood. The universities themselves were developing their curricula and the whole period can be characterised as one of transition, not, perhaps from ancient to modern, but from early modern to more modern. Most of the changes which took place, though, occurred not because of some elegant long-term master plan for medical education. It was clearly still a period of change enforced by current circumstance or the actions of perhaps one individual or one institution. The result, however, was the gradual introduction of change which brought about a much more rigidly defined path to a medical or surgical career.

It would be almost a further century before these standards could be agreed and enforced on a nationwide basis. However, steps were taken, not always for the best of reasons, to show to the medical and wider public that Scottish medical and surgical training was based on the highest possible standards. The Royal College of Surgeons of Edinburgh is a useful case study to illustrate these developments, which were mirrored to a greater or lesser extent elsewhere in Scotland and south of the border. Many of the steps taken by the Edinburgh surgeons were very similar to developments within the Medical School and repay detailed observation.

Real progress started from relatively inauspicious beginnings in March 1757, when a short but ultimately significant letter was delivered to the Incorporation from the War Office in London.[20] This letter asked the Incorporation to 'try the qualifications' of one Mr John McLean, who had applied for a post as surgeon to Lt Col. Fraser's battalion of highlanders. Nothing is recorded as to the content or standard of the examination in comparison to the standard entry tests for master surgeons, but the diploma which was subsequently awarded to McLean was the first of many. The diploma evolved from this quiet start to become a widely sought after subordinate qualification. Regulations for master surgeons continued relatively unchanged, and for the moment the diplomas were awarded only to country surgeons and to the occasional military candidate. It may be that the Incorporation would of its own volition have introduced a diploma in due course, but a scrap of military notepaper sent from London produced a fairly portentous response in the longer term.

A link with the Edinburgh Medical School was established when, in 1777, two medical students presented themselves for the Incorporation's diploma examination and were awarded diplomas on payment of a fee of two guineas.[21] They were followed by increasing numbers of medical students who wished to add a surgical diploma to their medical degree. By 1778 (the year in which the Incorporation achieved Collegiate status), it was becoming apparent that the diploma rules would have to be reconsidered and refined. A two-tier system was introduced to cover military candidates separately from the general diploma.

Once the College diploma was accepted as qualification for surgeons' mates in the navy, further demarcations were necessary, as the certificates awarded to these candidates had to be categorised as to the type of ship aboard which the individual was deemed competent to serve. In May 1797 a list of ship ratings and numbers of surgeons' mates who should serve on each type of ship was sent from the Navy Board.[22] By 1815 the separate military and naval diplomas were discontinued, and the full diploma taken by all candidates, and by the following year all diplomates were designated licentiates of the College.[23]

At this time there was no formal connection between the diploma and the examination for resident membership of the College, for which a full examination had to be undertaken and passed, though apprentices began to appear as diploma candidates increasingly frequently. A development which would affect aspirants to all qualifications, and one which fits neatly into both long-term aims and objectives, and to more immediate external influences, was the increasing awareness that if diplomas and membership qualifications offered by the College of Surgeons were to have credibility both at home and abroad, the College would not only have to examine rigorously but also impose minimum curriculum requirements. Although the 1505 Seal of Cause had sensibly – and far-sightedly – encouraged the pursuit of strictly supervised apprenticeships, it was not specific as to exactly what experience the apprentice should have gained, or the knowledge he should have acquired before presenting himself for examination and subsequent entry into the medical market place. By the end of the eighteenth century, though, steps had to be taken to present a credible product, and the College resolved that 'in order to prevent candidates who have not received a regular education from coming forward to be examined, no person shall be admitted as a candidate for the full diploma unless he produce certificates of his having studied at least two sessions in the University of Edinburgh or some other school of medicine'.[24] There is clear evidence that substantial numbers of surgical apprentices were enrolled on medical courses at Edinburgh University. Between 1763 and 1826, some 84 per cent of surgical apprentices attended lectures in anatomy and surgery.[25] It is clear also that in Glasgow from the early part of the eighteenth century, surgical apprentices were encouraged to attend university classes, which were taught by fellows of the FPSG.[26]

Over the next thirty years several changes were made, the most significant of which were as follows:

1798   All diploma candidates to attend a course of anatomy lectures and demonstrations, and should attend at a public hospital for one year. Knowledge of pharmacy to be demonstrated.

1806   Candidates who had not served an apprenticeship (often medical students) must attend three sessions of classes, together with classes on pharmacy and *Materia Medica*.

1808   Candidates who had not served an apprenticeship must have attended classes on anatomy, chemistry, botany, institutions and theory of medicine, practice of medicine, principles and practice of surgery, clinical surgery, midwifery and *Materia Medica*, together with hospital attendance. Apprentices had to attend similar courses, but for two years only.

1822   The main College entrance (by now known as Fellowship) examination was reduced to three days, comprising general anatomy and surgery, *Materia Medica*, pharmacy and prescriptions, and a final test on the subject of the candidate's pre-circulated probationary essay.

1822   All diploma candidates now had to provide proof of attendance at classes for three sessions.

1828   All candidates had to produce evidence that they had participated in dissection of the human body.[27]

As a result of these decisions, both apprentices for the full freedom and candidates for the diploma spent a fair proportion of their training attending formal academic classes at the University or extra-mural school. Thus the surgeons reacted to circumstance. They realised the importance of a curriculum, and when efforts to ensure surgical teaching in the University failed, took the logical step of setting up their own extra-mural courses.

Care was taken, though, to ensure that the work of potential College Fellows or Licentiates did not cause offence in high places. The content of some probationary essays was questioned, and several candidates were asked to alter or remove certain passages before final acceptance of the work. One such candidate was John McIntosh, examined in 1823. He had submitted a probationary essay on childbirth, making reference to the recent death in childbirth of Princess Charlotte. The following was noted in the College minute books:

> Dr Hay moved that previous to Dr McIntosh's being received on trial on the subject of his Essay, he should be desired to cancel certain passages therein viz. 1. The following passage occurring on page 6th. 'It is now well known that to this last cause the death of the Princess Charlotte is to be ascribed – an event which no human foresight could have anticipated; an event which is not more to be deplored from the national calamity it inflicted, than from the disgraceful feelings it produced in the minds of some accoucheurs which led them into an unjust persecution of the amiable and distinguished individual who had the principal charge on that interesting occasion – a persecution which has not even ceased with the life of him who fell a victim to its virulency – a persecution which I shall never cease to hold up as scandalous and infamous, because it was gratuitous as well as unjust and unworthy of a liberal profession.'[28]

The College was clearly very wary of appearing to endorse inflammatory or political statements, and after discussion the candidate was persuaded to remove the offending passages. The Enlightenment certainly did not mean full freedom of speech or opinion.

During the early decades of the nineteenth century the curriculum was steadily broadened, and the list of pre-examination requirements became ever longer and much more recognisably akin to that of the Edinburgh University Medical School:

Four winter sessions, including courses on:
Institutes of Medicine or Physiology
Practical Anatomy (five months)
Practical Chemistry (three months)
Clinical Surgery (five months)
Clinical Medicine (five months)
Surgery (two winter sessions, or one session and one on military surgery)
Eighteen months attendance at an approved hospital
Midwifery (five months)

Candidates were also required to provide certification that they had received instruction in Latin, mathematics and mechanical philosophy. Latin standards had been criticised by the Army Medical Board in 1813; it being claimed that a number of Edinburgh-qualified surgical assistants had been unable to read prescriptions.[29] As a result of this criticism, an advertisement was inserted in the press to the effect that parents or guardians of potential students should ensure that they had received a good basic education, including Latin.

Thus, the Edinburgh Medical School and medical institutions provided the ideal; it was left to the other medical schools and universities in Scotland to try to catch up with what was going on elsewhere. The University of Edinburgh had tightened its regulations considerably in the *Statuta Solenna* issued by the Senatus in 1763. The steps taken meant that the expectations and examinations held by the University, The Royal College of Surgeons and Royal College of Physicians of Edinburgh were all quite similar in scope and format (the physicians had ruled in 1763 that Licenciateship of the College would be a prerequisite to Fellowship, although this was discontinued in 1829 because of taxation anomalies). The situation in Glasgow was rather different, and that at Aberdeen and St Andrews even more so. The Scottish universities, and in particular Glasgow and Aberdeen, had gained a reputation for awarding degrees of very doubtful provenance or quality, to the extent that many of the degrees awarded by St Andrews were gained in absentia. One candidate resident in Botany Bay was granted an M.D. in 1796 purely on the strength of two letters of recommendation.[30]

The particular problems faced by St Andrews were in part historical and in part because of the isolated location of the town, which was not large enough or near enough the centre of progress, to have a hospital. Thus, there was no access to clinical training, a crucial element in the 'modernisation' of medical teaching. Despite some attempts to improve the situation, relatively little changed before the early 1800s and the setting up of the Commission of Enquiry into Universities. By 1811 the view was being expressed that the Chandos professor of medicine should do some teaching, but it was only by 1825 that there were clearer indications of the realisation that things would have to change if medicine were to continue to be offered by St Andrews. The reputation of antiquity and tradition would no longer suffice.

In Glasgow, the Faculty of Physicians and Surgeons had, for most of the eighteenth century, been making use of lecture courses and other facilities from the University, while managing to maintain dominance over the licensing of surgeons to practise in the West of Scotland. The unique nature of the Faculty perhaps ensured that, from a relatively weaker position than Edinburgh vis a vis relations with Town Council and University, it was able to dominate the medical scene at least until the latter part of the eighteenth century when, as elsewhere, the slow trend towards the M.D. degree as the main qualification began.[31]

The formalisation of teaching in Glasgow University can be dated to the appointment in 1714 of Dr John Johnston as Professor of Medicine, although, as had been the case in Edinburgh in 1685, there is no real evidence that he carried out any sort of systematic teaching at all. By the mid-1740s William Cullen had managed to persuade the university authorities to provide a chemistry laboratory, and he also instituted teaching in *materia medica* and botany – in effect a one-man proto-medical school. Following Cullen's departure east, Joseph Black was the incumbent until 1766 when he too migrated eastwards to the capital. The teaching of chemistry and *materia medica* continued thereafter, and by the 1760s medicine had been separated from chemistry and became a university subject in its own right. This, coupled with the opening of the Glasgow Royal Infirmary in 1794, and the consolidation of teaching in midwifery meant that by the turn of the nineteenth century the University could boast teaching in theory and practice of medicine, anatomy, surgery, botany, chemistry, *materia medica* and midwifery. Thus, there was in place at least the framework for a fully functioning school of medicine, to which went students who would subsequently apply for entry to the Faculty of Physicians and Surgeons, and also provide medical and surgical staff for the new Infirmary and subsequent fever hospitals.

The first quarter of the nineteenth century saw much friction between the University and Faculty, centred on the question of which body should have the powers to license surgeons to practise. In 1815 the Faculty gained a decree from the Court of Session that the M.D. degree was not an automatic entitlement to practise surgery – thus ensuring that the Faculty would have jurisdiction. In response, though, the University promptly instituted the degree of Master of Surgery. There were recurrent bouts of litigation on this point until the issue was resolved finally by the passing of the Medical Act of 1858. Whatever the situation, though, it is clear that Glasgow did acquire a set-up very similar to that of Edinburgh, at a lag of some two decades.

In Aberdeen, the situation took even longer to resolve into a recognisable medical school. There had been a 'mediciner' on the staff since the establishment of the University in 1494, but these individuals did little teaching and the other main requirements of a medical school were certainly not to be found. By the early eighteenth century, the Aberdeen medical degree had becoming something of a joke, and could, as in St Andrews, be had on the strength of the flimsiest of evidence. In 1712, Patrick Blair, an apothecary in Cupar, was granted an M.D. degree because he had been 'recommended by the bishop of Aberdeen and severall eminent physicians in Angus'.[32]

The role of the mediciner became a little more respectable by the early-Enlightenment period, when a succession of the Gregorys took up the appointment. The Gregorys were in some respects the Aberdeen equivalent of the Edinburgh Monros, and indeed several became prominent in the intellectual life of the capital. John Gregory, who succeeded his brother to the mediciner post in 1755 had studied medicine in Leiden, and contributed to the medical literature with works on medical practice. An attempt was made to establish a more formal system of medical education in 1786, by William Ogilvie, who put forward the view that amalgamation of the two colleges would be most desirable. The moves were supported by the intellectual establishment of Aberdeen, as well as by the Town Council, but came to nothing, and subsequently each of the Colleges tried to set up an independent medical school. It was ultimately, though, the efforts of medical students which stimulated progress. Their Medical Society was formed in 1789 and gradually, with the support of the professor of medicine at Marischal College, William Livingston, began to organise a system of medical education. It seems to have been this impetus from the student body which brought about teaching in several medical subjects, and in 1818 a joint system of medical education was formed, with equal contributions made by both colleges. The opening of the Aberdeen Infirmary in the early 1740s had already provided the essential clinical training opportunity.

So, what seems to have happened during the Enlightenment period was that medical education evolved in different parts of the country at different times and for different reasons. It does, though, seem legitimate to claim, as has been done recently, a 'Scottish model' of medical education.[33] Several factors were common: high regard for education in general; the influence of the presbyterian tradition; the very strong European connections; the intellectual climate of the Enlightenment and the wish to develop medical education in Scotland; as well as the social and economic restructuring that was underway.[34] The ways in which this was achieved were very different in Edinburgh, Glasgow, Aberdeen and St Andrews, where individual, local factors played an important part. Whatever the situation, it is clear that by 1820 a great deal had been achieved, whether or not by primary intent, in terms of the availability and standards of medical training in Scotland; still more required to be done, and this would await the enforced stimulus of nationwide legislation and the beginnings of standardisation. The extent to which the new science of the Enlightenment had a central role is perhaps debatable, and the receivers of medical care may not have noticed too much change.

HOSPITAL MEDICINE IN THE INNER CORE

As the Enlightenment period continued and steps were taken to ensure that the custody of the increasingly public body of medical knowledge was in the right hands, one area which made significant contributions was that of clinical and hospital medicine and medical training. At the core of hospital medicine, and its significance for medical training, was the means to carry out detailed, repeated and long-term observations of the patients, their conditions and their reactions to treatment. It is evident from surviving casebooks and hospital ledgers that great care was taken to record minute details of patients and their treatments.[35] This level of detail could only have been good for the future of medicine. Indeed, the case histories as written down in the eighteenth century set the template or benchmarks for modern case histories, and the very process of teaching observation was of fundamental importance as a solid basis on which to build medical care and teaching in future periods when treatments would be very different.

Although eighteenth-century medical pioneers were able to demonstrate how newly discovered body systems were structured and functioned, a very important aspect of medicine in hospitals was the ability to carry out detailed observation and recording of symptoms and the results of treatments over long periods. There was something old-fashioned about this approach, but at the same time something very new and significant. The origins of Western (and Scottish) medicine were in the mists of ancient Greece and Rome. The core of Hippocratic medicine was the assembly of a detailed picture of the patient's symptoms, appearance and lifestyle. Treatment was of a holistic nature, based on a holistic view of the patient within his or her environment. Hospital medicine in eighteenth-century Edinburgh would appear at first sight to be very different. It was, certainly, different in two major respects. Firstly, the supernatural or unexplainable aspects of the environment were largely eliminated. No longer did the physician look to the patient's astrological chart as a primary element of the diagnostic process. That is not to say that aspects of medical treatment which would nowadays be regarded as mere superstition were not still included as part of the overall package of treatment (at the beginning of the century no less a personage than Archibald Pitcairne was not at all reticent in advising the application of live doves to the soles of the feet of a patient *in extremis*). Secondly, the eighteenth century, in the context of increasingly available education and knowledge and, of course, literacy, meant that, in effect, written down Hippocratic medicine was possible. Hippocrates had advocated careful observation; eighteenth-century Edinburgh hospitals advocated the writing down of these observations.

This latter point, which at first sight may seem peripheral or trivial, is perhaps one of the most significant aspects of medical development. The custody of knowledge, though increasingly in the hands of individuals selected by training, could be communal within that restricted sphere, and could be shared, compared and analysed in as scientific a manner as was possible in the period. This was the period where scientific method was emerging, or at least the means to disseminate the results of experiments in the flourishing culture of print. This culture of print in turn was key to progress in most aspects of Scottish intellectual, social and economic life. This was particularly true of science and medicine, and new discovery in these fields.

What was of crucial significance for clinical medicine and, in particular, hospital medicine, was that records could be written down and kept over long periods. The records of the Royal Infirmary of Edinburgh and other hospitals are fruitful in elucidating the mechanisms of care and treatment, precisely because case records survive in significant numbers to allow this to be done with some degree of confidence. The major academic figure in recent years to utilise these case records is Guenter Risse. His two major, indeed magisterial, monographs have provided seminal insights into this aspect of the progress of medicine both in Scotland and in the wider, global context. His earlier book, *Hospital Life in Enlightenment Edinburgh: Care and Teaching at the Edinburgh Royal Infirmary* gives a number of detailed case histories and a useful index of the commonly prescribed drugs, in addition to a judicial analysis and assessment of the role of the hospital in the medicine of the Scottish

Enlightenment. Together with Rosner's equally important work on medical training in the period, it lit the torch as far as the historiography of eighteenth-century medicine was concerned. If Risse's first contribution were not enough, he has recently produced a massive work on worldwide hospitals and the evolution of hospital treatment.[36] It helps to contextualise Scotland in the global context, and is just as important to the historian of Scottish medicine – not the least because the Scottish hospital model was used as a model in many parts of the world, particularly in the New World and Australia, from the later eighteenth century.

So, the hospitals of eighteenth-century Scotland, led by Edinburgh and followed at some distance by Glasgow (1794), Aberdeen (1742) and the other major towns, offered a new dimension to the sphere of medical knowledge, medical treatment and the experience of the patients. The careful recording of observations did not mean that patients could be cured more quickly. The records show that most patients spent some considerable time as in-patients. Their symptoms were recorded, often several times a day, as were the treatments. However, despite the strides being taken in advancing medical knowledge, there was the inevitable lag between discovery and new treatments. In effect, then, the hospitals still offered largely humorally derived treatments, including bloodletting, purging and a variety of diets to suit particular diseases and conditions.[37] Surgical possibilities were extremely limited and would remain so until the middle of the nineteenth century, as they awaited the dual stimuli of anaesthetics and the means to control infection, which had, till then, restricted surgical opportunities severely. It matters not that the observation and recording of the minute details of patients' conditions did not – immediately – result in the advent of new treatments or new explanations for these conditions. What was important and of great significance for the future was that the habit of recording and consideration of long-term observation was combined with the historic Hippocratic habit of taking a detailed history.

The following extract from the history of a patient in the Glasgow Infirmary in 1799, as noted in the dresser's diary is typical:

13 November
Face is flushed and he appears languid and oppressed. Pulse 112, skin warm, tongue white and moist. [treated with enema and tincture for cough] The stupor having increased three leeches were applied to his temples and though very little blood was taken away the pain in the head and insensibility seems to be diminished.
15 November
The leeches were applied to his temples and about three ounces of blood taken away. The breathing continuing laborious, the blister was applied, since which he

breathes with more freedom. Pulse 84, still full. Tongue furred in the middle and skin very hot. Cough and headache abated.

16 November

The head having again become painful and face flushed, four leeches were applied and he was again relieved. Pulse at present 84, full but sluggish and compressible. Tongue uncommonly foul and slaked. Cough less troublesome but from the sound of his respiration the bronchial tubes seem gorged with mucus. [treated with ipecacuhana].

17 November

Cough is abated and breathing easier. Pulse at present 72, full, sluggish and somewhat hard. Tongue excessively foul. Breathing regular, skin moderate, in heat very high.

18 November

Rested well and sweated profusely. Pulse 68, full and less sluggish. Breathing and cough relieved.[38]

This is a typical account, and one which demonstrates the transition between full-scale humoral medicine and a more 'scientific' approach, in terms of monitoring pulse and breathing. Typically also, no specific diagnosis is given. In terms of the practicalities of hospitals and the practical application of Enlightenment principles a recent, detailed account of the Infirmary attached to the Glasgow Town's Hospital (opened in 1733) indicates that not only was observation the central core of practice, but also that nurses were increasingly required to participate in the observation process.[39]

As time went on, other factors began to influence the minds of those who had it in their power to found hospitals. It was not just the necessity as part of a coherent medical school; nor the need to care for troops wounded in the Jacobite campaigns; nor to keep infected individuals in isolation. Some of the late eighteenth-century hospitals bore witness to two other factors, which would become of more and more import once the twin processes of industrialisation and big civic government would exert their pincer grip on urban Scotland in the first half of the nineteenth century. Big civic government meant big civic pride. Industrialisation necessitated a working population fit to work. Civic pride included philanthropy. All of these factors combined, particularly in Glasgow, in the latter decades of the eighteenth century, a period when 'the prosperity of the nation was dependent upon the size and health of the population'.[40]

DENTISTRY

Until the middle of the eighteenth century medical or surgical specialties were not a feature of legitimate medicine and surgery. Ironically, it was often the 'alternative practitioners' who claimed specialist knowledge.

From the itinerant lithotomists of the seventeenth century, to the oculists and cataract operators of the early eighteenth century, to the electrical wizardry of John Graham in the late eighteenth century, individuals who claimed to be expert at a specific procedure were generally to be found on the fringes of orthodox medicine. It may be, of course, that the fact that they concentrated on a single procedure did make them better at it than those who offered a more general service. This is a factor which began to affect legitimate medicine more and more, particularly towards the end of the second millennium, when the totality of medical knowledge was too great to be absorbed by individuals, and when procedures developed to the point where generalists could not be expected to perform wide ranges of tasks.

One area which did begin to emerge as a discrete, specialist area fairly early on was dentistry. The pulling of teeth had long been part of the lay medical sphere, but had also drawn the interest of kings. James IV was known to indulge in a little surgery and dentistry, and the royal accounts of 1503 include the cost of 'an irn to byrn sair teeth'. By the eighteenth century in Edinburgh, the Monros were including dental matters in their lectures, but the individual generally credited as being the first specialist practitioner in Scotland was James Rae, a Fellow of The Royal College of Surgeons of Edinburgh. In the 1770s he began to offer a course of lectures, which he advertised in the local press, covering 'diseases dependent on the teeth'. He also offered a service as a dental practitioner, claiming to be able to cure all sorts of dental ailments and to produce high quality false teeth. From these small beginnings dentistry began gradually to emerge as a separate branch of the medical profession, although the Edinburgh and Glasgow Dental Hospitals and Schools would not be established until the later part of the nineteenth century. Nowadays there is a hierarchy of higher dental examinations, degrees and diplomas, in parallel with those for medicine and surgery, and dentistry is a completely separate area of the medical sphere. 'Quacks' still pulled teeth in the towns as well as the country in Enlightenment Scotland, but the long-term effects of the Enlightenment ethos would see the channelling of knowledge into specialist areas and its application at least in the urban setting. It has been claimed that the generation of Milton and Newton in the seventeenth century was the last period when it was possible, at least theoretically, for one individual to know everything. Certainly, by the turn of the nineteenth century this was not possible, and, more importantly perhaps, not necessarily desirable.

THE SPHERE OF THE MIND – CARE OF THE MENTALLY ILL

Nowadays, attitudes to, and treatment of, patients with conditions of a non-organic nature are complex. Ironically, perhaps, things were much simpler in earlier periods in which the cosmology was complex, but where 'madness' was regarded rather differently. Madness, or its manifestations, was a state, not a disease, and thus individuals who were afflicted were not necessarily thought to be ill. The wide spectrum from mild eccentricity to overt madness was not separated into areas where the cause was an illness or a personality disorder or dysfunction. Consequently, the mentally ill were not deemed to require different sorts of treatment or to be isolated from their communities. Indeed, care in the community can be said to be a feature of early periods and not an invention of twentieth-century professionals much given to theorising and societal models.

Till the mid-eighteenth century then, madness was a state of being, not necessarily a state of ill health. There were close connections here with manifestations of witchcraft and the activities of healers and charmers. Any treatments given would be in the form of attempts to palliate the symptoms (as was the case with organic disease), or to prevent the individual concerned from doing harm to himself or others. That is not to say, however, that the treatments themselves were not often as bizarre as the symptoms they were intended to treat.

The separation of mental from bodily illness was an important process. The realisation that madness could be due to an illness or condition of the mind, as opposed to an unfortunate state of being which could only be contained rather than cured, produced separate institutions. These institutions were often referred to as asylums, or places of safety, again implying that containment was the major aim. As time went on, mad people were seen increasingly as both a threat and an embarrassment to 'normal', 'civilised' people, and it may be claimed, cynically, that progress in the treatment of mental illnesses owed a fair amount to the rejection of these individuals from the public sphere rather than a simple realisation that diseases of the mind perhaps required different treatment from diseases of the body.

As with many aspects of the evolution and development of Scottish medicine, it would take the efforts of pioneering individuals to begin to deal with these problems. In relation to the treatment of mental illness the name of Andrew Duncan immediately comes to mind. Clues to notable individuals can often be found in eponymous buildings or institutions, and the Andrew Duncan Clinic would, for many decades, be the focus of the treatment of mental illness in the Edinburgh area.

The history of mental illness or incapacity and its treatment is at a relatively early stage in relation to Scotland. The difficulty is that, before the advent of asylums or hospitals built for the purpose, and, indeed, before hospitals of any sort were a feature of the medical sphere, it is extremely difficult to gather any sort of quantitative, or even reliable qualitative, information. A major step forward in this direction came with Roy Porter's study *Mind Forg'd Manacles*, which addressed the topic of madness in England.

A recent detailed study of eighteenth-century Scotland by Houston is focused on the 'social construction' of madness, principally in terms of litigation concerning the acquisition of power of attorney by the relatives of those thought to be mad.[41] Although based on a narrow cohort of source material, which tends to render the conclusions less than unequivocal, it provides useful insights and rich primary source material. The work is concerned with court cases brought by the relatives of individuals perceived to be mad or 'furious', with the intent of having them declared incapable of managing their lives and, in particular, their assets. So, what we are given is an account of court cases and an analysis of the perceptions and discourse of madness, at least at the level of society where there was the possibility and, indeed, the need, to try to gain control of the assets of a relative. We cannot be sure about the accuracy of the reported evidence, given that the pursuers in most of the instances covered would gain financially, should their litigation prove to be successful. However, what is illustrated very usefully is a new angle to the more common discussions on mad people and their gradual removal from their communities.

Further work by Houston has also added usefully to the interaction among professionals in the area of mental illness. He concludes that although, apparently, the numbers of medical men serving on juries in cases relating to mental capacity declined, medical men and lawyers seemed to have come to a general agreement about the role of medical men in the definition of insanity. While doctors were becoming more interested in the definition or delineation of madness, they were, apparently, content, for example, to allow institutions to be run by laymen and lawyers to state the legal case.[42] This would certainly fit in with other evidence of the ways in which the norms of social and medical conditions were constructed by a combination of general influences and the particular expertise relevant to the specific situation or condition.

In terms of the progress of institutional medicine and the treatment of madness or mental handicap, whether permanent or temporary, the trend was clearly one from acceptance or toleration of the mad or mentally deranged within their communities, to the incarceration of these individuals and their consequent separation from society. It is difficult to analyse the processes leading to this trend. Were the mad or mentally ill separated from their communities because of increasing fear or embarrassment caused by their apparently threatening or illogical behaviour? Or were they treated thus purely in line with other trends in the institutionalisation of medicine? The general background emphasis on rationality and politeness may also be important. By the end of the eighteenth century more people were treated in hospital for 'ordinary' illnesses, thus separating the sane from their communities and relatives during the period of treatment. Indeed, the plans for the new Edinburgh Infirmary (opened in 1741) included a section with cells for the restraint of the insane, which was the first part of the hospital to be finished.[43] Was it the case that the slowly expanding corpus of medical knowledge, coupled with better medical training and the availability of hospitalisation facilities, extended quite naturally to the care of the mad? There was an extremely complex network of factors and influences at play here, and the combination of medical men with an interest in madness and the increasing institutionalisation of medical treatment were two important factors. In addition, analysts and philosophers who debate the influences on social progress in terms of aspects of power and control might consider the increasing interest in removing the mad from their communities in terms of Foucault and his ideas of social control through policing and the institutions of incarceration and punishment,[44] as well as the middle-class ideas of civility and polite behaviour. In some ways, Enlightenment resulted in the emergence of increasingly strict parameters of acceptable behaviour, despite the liberating aspects of intellectual freedom.

Whatever the case, the trend in this period, which would become much more formally organised and legislated in the Victorian period, was towards regarding the mentally ill as different from the physically ill and, therefore, requiring similar separation from society but perhaps different methods of treatment or restraint once they had been so isolated. As mentioned, a name that comes readily to mind in the annals of mental institutions is that of Andrew Duncan senior (1744–1828). Duncan was elected President of the Royal College of Physicians of Edinburgh in 1790, and shortly afterwards succeeded Dr James Gregory to the chair of the Institutes of Medicine. In 1792 Duncan set out proposals for the foundation of a public asylum for lunatics, which resulted eventually in the establishment of such an institution at Morningside in 1807.[45] This was the start; from then the trend would be to isolate the mentally ill or mentally insufficient. The title usually given to these institutions was asylum – but for the safety of the patient or the public?

As time went on, and the age of the asylum dawned in Scotland, the term itself perhaps became less and less appropriate. If the word 'asylum' signifies safety, then its usefulness is questionable, given the increasingly draconian treatments meted out to the patients. It was one thing to take mad people off the streets and keep them safe from danger, but it was quite another to impose régimes which did little to attempt to find a cure with any prospect of returning the individual to society. Conditions and attitudes within these institutions gradually worsened as Scotland entered the industrial age of civic pride and thrusting government. The age of the state hospital was yet to come, but the groundwork was being done. A further distinction and division would come between the treatment of and attitudes to the insane who had committed crimes. So, in this period of apparent Enlightenment, the medical establishment and probably the public were becoming less tolerant of the mad, less liberal in their approach and more draconian in their treatment of these individuals. It would take another century before the notion of care in the community, as a replacement for the large institution, would again come to the forefront of medical thinking on mental illness and disability.

By the early decades of the nineteenth century a number of asylums were operating in Scottish towns such as Montrose, Aberdeen and Glasgow, and by 1815 legislation required these institutions to be licensed and inspected. From the middle of the eighteenth century institutions to treat, incarcerate or punish the insane were appearing. Edinburgh's Charity Workhouse opened its doors in 1743, and by 1749 the institution contained nineteen lunatics.[46] This was followed by the establishment of an asylum at Montrose in the early 1780s, which was the first purpose-built institution of this sort. These asylums were in some ways a curious mixture of social levels and practices. Fees were charged, and by 1820 the Dundee asylum had six different categories of patient, charged between 7 and 63 shillings per week – not inconsiderable sums.[47] Different institutions had different methods for confining and treating their patients, but from that point the large institution became the currency of the care of the mentally incapacitated until the end of the twentieth century. In terms of comparison with the situation in England, it is claimed that the voluntary principle was more apparent in Scotland and that, despite the predominance of Scots-trained medical practitioners in Britain, England led the way in pioneering the so-called 'moral' approach to the treatment of inmates.[48]

WIDER CIRCLES – INOCULATION AND VACCINATION

As well as the considerable effects of the Enlightenment and the general progress of intellectual Scotland, against the background of continuing adjustment to the effects of the union of 1707, medicine in Scotland began to see what has been referred to by one historian of medicine as the 'entry of the state'.[49] The involvement of the state in terms of national legislation, and the attempts to introduce prophylaxis rather than merely reaction to circumstance, would be difficult and opposed by some surprising sections of the community. The first tentative steps towards this general state intervention can be traced back deep into the early eighteenth century, although at the time this would not have been admitted as a possibility.

One of the major scourges for several centuries had been recurrent visitations of smallpox, which had both individual and collective debilitating effects, from the perspective of the household right through the gamut of ability to wage war or develop the economy. The recurrent episodes of the disease had long been considered to be the wages of sin and, consequently, little attempt was made to alter circumstances to try to prevent the disease. Rather, what happened was reaction to outbreaks, mainly the attempt to isolate infected individuals in order to protect the rest of the community. Any medical interference was seen in many quarters to be going against the will of God – this despite centuries-long belief in the prophylactic effects of seasonal bloodletting or the use of scurvy grass. The Enlightenment was beginning to take religion out of its former location at the core of intellectual debate on Man and the universe, but God could not be easily extracted from the historical package of explanations of misfortune.

The eighteenth century is, perhaps, just as interesting for its juxtaposition of the very old and the very new. Ancient beliefs persisted, new beliefs were superimposed, but the new beliefs and opinions took time both to translate into medical practice and to disseminate that practice, not to mention achieve acceptance as the new orthodoxy. Medicine without religion was just as difficult to achieve as reason without the inexplicable, particularly in the more remote corners of the realm, where life moved at a slower pace and beliefs were harder to change.

The prevention of smallpox is a very useful case study to illustrate some of these paradoxes, which are entirely rational and reasonable within the context of the discourse of the time. Inoculation had been available in Scotland from the early decades of the eighteenth century. As with a number of significant medical developments, its application and use were, in the beginning, confined to the drawing rooms of the élite, who made use of the technique as a sort of after-dinner entertainment. It would take several decades before the 'authorities' began to consider that mass inoculation of the population might be of significant economic as well as physical benefit. In order for the technique to be used, of course, it was necessary to have at least one current sufferer from the disease. Matter from a pustule could be then transferred to a non-sufferer in an attempt to create immunity. Gradually, the technique became more widely used. This created at least three problems. Firstly, the practice was completely unregulated and rarely carried out by qualified medical practitioners. Secondly, there were strenuous objections that such artificial transfer of the potential to kill was, in fact, acting against the will of God. The simple belief, as with many other visitations and misfortunes, was that any affliction was incurred as the result of some sort of individual or collective sin, or that it was merely God's will that a certain individual should not only contract a disease but die of it. Thirdly, and a problem that would occupy the energies of local authorities increasingly, was the implications and consequences of compulsion if it were decreed that everyone should be inoculated. This controversy may be seen in a very similar light to the current debates and anxieties surrounding the MMR vaccination against measles, mumps and rubella.

Despite all of these problems, as the century of the Enlightenment progressed, more and more people were inoculated. The practice was sporadic and localised, and depended on a number of very local factors, not on any central wish or decree. In smaller, rural communities, the frequency and level of uptake of inoculation depended on the frequency of smallpox outbreaks, the belief system or cosmological focus of the area, and the presence or absence of an individual or individuals prepared to carry out the technique. These individuals were mostly lay, and included ministers and farmers, as well as a particular character in the Shetlands, known as Camphor Johnnie, who apparently operated as an inoculator for many years.[50] Once it began to be realised that there were positive benefits to be gained, and that the wrath of God did not seem to be descending on individuals or communities who participated in the practice, it was encouraged as a good thing to do. The medical and surgical colleges began to endorse the practice actively, making good use of the increasingly widely available medium of the advertisement columns of the newspapers.[51] In rare instances of co-operation, for example, the Incorporation of Surgeons and Royal College of Physicians of Edinburgh inserted regular joint exhortations to partake of the opportunity of gratis inoculation. However, these institutions were not unanimously in favour, and one of the main objections put forward related to the element of compulsion and possible punishment for non-compliance that would be involved. One of the leading Edinburgh surgeons wrote to his colleagues in these terms, expressing strong opposition to compulsion, in spite of the growing evidence that inoculation seemed to work. William Brown hoped that 'the great cause of vaccination will be promoted by a legislative measure which will not needlessly interfere with individual liberty'.[52]

A very wide variety of opinions on the topic is contained in the reports of all the parishes of Scotland collected by Sir John Sinclair in the 1790s, in a series of volumes entitled *The Statistical Account of Scotland*.[53] These reports were compiled by the parish ministers and are certainly not remotely objective or statistically accurate. They do, though, give a useful insight into how varied were the practices and opinions on the principle of inoculation, and also into the current and equally varied notions as to the fundamental causes of the spread of diseases among the population.

The pattern of prejudice or acceptance was varied throughout the country, and the following samples from the *Statistical Account* illustrate the situation well. It was reported from the parish of Carmunnock that 'the small pox returns very often, and the distemper is never alleviated, as the people from a sort of blind fatality, will not hear of inoculation, though attempts have often been made to remove their scruples on this subject', while in Hamilton 'inoculation for the small-pox is practised, but the common people are not reconciled to it'; though some headway was apparently being made in Monklands, where 'prejudices against inoculation, though not entirely eradicated, are gradually wearing out'. Further afield, in Thurso, it was stated that 'we have it [remedy] in inoculation, and yet the ancient fatal superstition is so little overcome'; while in Lerwick it was claimed that 'for some years past inoculation has been practised among all ranks, with very remarkable success'; and in Dumfries it was reported that 'most of the country people still entertain strong prejudices against inoculation, though not so great as formerly'.

There is some debate among demographic historians nowadays about precisely how much of an effect the process of inoculation (by direct transfer from a sufferer) and vaccination (by cultured cowpox vaccine) had on the demographic map of Scotland.[54] It is claimed that these measures had, at best, limited and patchy effects on mortality statistics in the longer term, and that other factors, such as improving diet and better awareness of public health matters were more important. There is, though, no doubt that inoculation and vaccination were procedures which could, and did, save many lives. Vaccination was not made compulsory until 1863 with the eventual passing of the Scottish Vaccination Act, a measure which had had a long and difficult gestation period, facing opposition from within the ranks of the medical profession itself, mostly in relation to the element of compulsion and the proposals to introduce specialist vaccinators. Medical practitioners were wary always of any of their number being perceived to be *primus inter pares*.

THE OUTER CIRCLE – TOWN AND COUNTRY, RICH AND POOR, MALE AND FEMALE

Although the demarcations between the lifestyle, political activity and access to medical care in town and country had become sharpened during the seventeenth and early eighteenth centuries, it was towards the end of the Enlightenment period that these differences became increasingly marked. Locality has been a crucial feature in all aspects of the history of Scotland and the experiences of the Scots through the ages; however, the later part of the eighteenth century was perhaps the time when locality was more crucial than it had been before or would be thereafter (the advent of the railway, for example, would alter the dynamics of locality significantly, as would subsequent progress in road, sea and air travel). General Wade's roads were meant to help the government to tame the highlanders – they also made general travel easier.

Scots who lived within easy contact distance of the growing urban centres had potential access to most things that were new, in terms of intellectual progress, social interaction, the culture of print, education and the latest ideas in medicine and medical treatment. It was also generally the case that individuals at the highest levels of society, wherever they lived, had fairly ready access to most of these things. They could and did contact their legal and political friends and, importantly, their medical practitioners by letter. They could also afford to do this and were at the core of the disseminated network of patronage which kept the sphere of the upper stratum of society relatively intact. Urbanisation and manufacturing wealth had not yet begun to displace the power of land in Scotland. High status physicians travelled long distances to see high status patients and would continue to do so for some time to come.

Those at the middle economic levels were able to a slightly lesser extent to 'move with the times'. Their influence, by the nature of their economic activity, was confined in the main to the lowland and eastern part of Scotland – including the important mercantile centre of Aberdeen. Their access to qualified medicine was relatively easy within the urban setting, although their influence in the patronage stakes was not as forceful as those above them in social and landed rank. In contrast, the poorest levels of society seem to have fared relatively similarly, whatever their geographical location. It did not really matter whether the poor lived next door to the flourishing medical school or in the wilds of the remotest island community; there would be little or no chance of access to any sort of qualified medical practitioner (apart from those who worked as domestic or other servants, when their employers often paid for medical attention from their own attendants). Perhaps the main difference caused by distance was that in the far-flung parts of the country the superstitious or ritualised elements of medical care might have survived longer than in the more concentrated population of the urban lowlands.

Certainly, in the highlands many of the long-held beliefs and practices of herbal treatments continued. It was reported in 1777, for example, that 'the Highlanders have a great esteem for the tubercles of the roots [vetch] ... and affirm them to be good for most diseases of the thorax'; while well into the nineteenth century plantain leaves were considered to be very effective for the treatment of wounds and abrasions, and poultices made of oatmeal and urine were applied to boils with apparent success.[55] The skin of a hare applied to the chest was thought to assist in the cure of asthma (the long-winded animal and the short-winded patient); while seaweed poultices were used to counteract rheumatism.[56]

The experiences of both gender groups can also be usefully compared and contrasted, in terms of the practice and receipt of medical care. The latter is the easier aspect. At all levels of society the access to medical opinion and treatment seems to have been relatively similar for men, women and children, depending on social level and economic circumstances. Aristocratic women consulted the best physicians, middle-rank women were able to consult as much or as little as their husbands could, while all people at the lower poorer end of society had an equal struggle to regain or maintain a state of health adequate to allow them to continue to do manual work in field or manufactory. Any gender difference would come from the influence of separate spheres of work, particularly in the case of men who served in the armed forces. Here, at least, surgery was available, however primitive, and performed by qualified surgeons. Sanitary conditions in barracks or crowded ships, though, brought about epidemics of very similar diseases to those which could be found in civilian life.

Where the stark gender difference appears is within the sphere of the practice of professional medicine. In terms of the activities of folk healers, wise women, charmers and, indeed, witches, the role of the female continued much as it had done for many centuries. Poor women were treated by poor women; middle-rank women were perhaps less likely to practise medicine, but there were instances, even of the wives of eminent physicians acting as amateur medical advisers. Aristocratic women, too, did not indulge to any great extent in the hands-on practice of medicine. What they did do, though, was participate in a network of recipe circulation. The latest fashionable cure taken by one household would soon appear in the commonplace books of many other households. This communication of cures took place alongside the increasing publication of 'Poor Man's Guides', which also contained much of the same sort of advice.

The key contrast, though, lies in the professional sphere of medicine, but some of the factors which prevented women from becoming practitioners also proved to be a barrier to men (such as illiterate or poor men who could not attend university or gain any sort of qualification). There is a view that by the end of the eighteenth century women had been effectively eclipsed from economic activity at the middle and upper levels of society.[57] This may well be the case, but the point must be remembered that many men also found it difficult to progress. Women could not matriculate at universities, therefore they could not enter the increasingly lucrative area of the professions. Women could not take up surgical apprenticeships, therefore they could not become surgeons. A further significant factor is the stifling effect on middle-rank women, who were the most likely to want to enter the learned professions, engendered by the gradual realignment of the social structure with the emergence of the middle class, the more marked demarcation of the working class, and the dilution of responsibility between and among socio-economic groups. It is not quite clear how the stereotype of the middle-class woman emerged or was created by society at large. What is undeniably clear, though, is that the role and activities of middle-class women would become restricted, prescriptive and to an extent ritualised. If the Enlightenment in Scotland and elsewhere gave intellectual freedom, the appearance of social class did little for the women of Scotland. This is not to claim that all middle-class women felt repressed or restricted in their role. It is, though, a key factor in the exclusion of women from the professionalising process and the increasingly exclusive sphere of the professions.

There is also the cultural, aesthetic element to the gender account. In a study of the female image within the confines of the elite medical sphere, it is claimed that the female body was portrayed in ways which reinforced the very obvious differences between male and female anatomy, and this in part helped to maintain the attitude held by the male medical profession that women were biologically unsuited to professional medicine.[58] This problem would become much more acute in the nineteenth century (see next chapter).

It has been claimed that one of the major characteristics of the Enlightenment period in Scotland was that the effects of the process filtered down to all levels of society in all corners of the country. This conclusion is a little more difficult to justify in relation to formal, increasingly orthodox, medicine. There may have been a medical school in Edinburgh, Glasgow or Aberdeen; there may have been teaching hospitals in these places and elsewhere. What difference, however, was experienced by the sick in Elgin, Eyemouth or Ecclefechan? More of the worthy citizens of these airts may have been able to read; their journeys along new turnpike roads may have been a little easier; they may have been inoculated against smallpox. But where were their hospitals, their qualified physicians or surgeons? The short answer is that there were none, or very few. Rural, remote medicine remained outwith the sphere of the new orthodoxy and, in fact, it is perhaps possible to claim that there were still dual orthodoxies or, at least, longer survival of the old. It is a little too simple to claim an urban and a rural orthodoxy. Many larger towns also had little or no access to qualified medicine.

The observant reader will remember, however, that the very first listed patient in the new first Infirmary (opened in Edinburgh in 1727) came from Caithness. This is a timely reminder that clear-cut cases are meant to be challenged. It is still the case, though, that in general, the concentric circles emanating from the central belt contained progressively less of the new, the further away from the core they were traced. True, General Wade may have provided the means for rural or remote patients to travel to the urban centres, but this was the exception rather than the norm.

It was in these areas that the influence of folk medicine held sway. Legend and oral tradition informed medical practice to a much greater extent than in the increasingly sophisticated urban setting, although orthodox medicine was by no means dominant in the largest towns. Any 'enlightenment' gained in rural areas was slow and patchy. The increasingly available 'Poor Man's Guides' were perhaps the only orthodox medical publications to reach remoter parts, but their contents were certainly not at the cutting edge of medical advances. Plant-based treatments were of necessity the core of drug treatment, and it cannot be claimed that they were any less effective or helpful than the latest chemical compound manufactured in the laboratory at Glasgow University.

THE INTELLECTUAL ORTHODOXY – DEFENCE AGAINST THE PUBLIC?

Many theories have been expounded about how societies developed intellectually during the second half of the eighteenth century, in the period known by repute as the Enlightenment. If it is accepted, though, that 'enlightenment' does not necessarily mean solely the illumination of the intellect through freedom of thought, reasoned and empirical investigation, and the acquisition of new knowledge freed from the bounds of a religious orthodoxy, it is possible to argue that the discourse of pre-institutional medicine was no less enlightening. However 'amateur' or unproven many of its tenets were, and however much it would be derided in later periods by those who claimed intellectual property of knowledge and declared it to be the orthodoxy, it is possible to argue that in its rationale and practical applications, it was just as culturally important in its own time.

In terms of the consolidation of professional medical and surgical practitioners as the sole custodians of knowledge, the Enlightenment period was one of the crucial periods in which medical and surgical institutions realised that they had to prove themselves worthy of being appointed custodians of knowledge by others who had access to the same knowledge. The Habermas theory is one quite useful method of explaining some of the events of the period, particularly the moves taken by medical and surgical institutions and the universities to show their worth.

One of the main ways in which these bodies tried to show that they were now at the centre of the medical and surgical orthodoxy was by introducing more detailed and comprehensive rules and regulations. It was felt that by demonstrating that diplomates and graduates had not only been tested on their knowledge, but that they had also pursued a rigorous programme of training and experience before taking their final examinations, it would be clear that these individuals deserved sole rights of application of their knowledge in society. The need for royal commissions and enquiries in the next century, though, would show that real progress was slow to achieve.

It is difficult to underestimate the importance of print in these middle centuries of the second millennium in Scottish history. The first printing press was set up in Edinburgh in 1507. From small and relatively inauspicious beginnings, the culture of print, including the newspaper press, would be of crucial – though perhaps not at first sight – importance to the professionalisation process and to the shaping of the profession and its custody of the knowledge.[59] Print was a means whereby knowledge could be disseminated to the far corners of the country. It was also a medium of debate, controversy and advertising. Print was, perhaps, the essential core of the public sphere. Anyone who could read was a potential contributor to the ever increasing pool of knowledge. The Habermas theory focuses specifically on the public sphere between the private sphere of the household and the administrative sphere of the state. In relation to medicine, and in terms of the approaches taken by historians of medicine, the profession being the custodians of the knowledge was no longer enough. Other people had access to the same knowledge. How, then, were those Scottish physicians, surgeons and university professors who had come to the forefront and were in the vanguard of the professionalisation of medicine and the pushing back of the boundaries of knowledge, going to ensure that they were still the major players?

CONCLUSION

The key themes to emerge from this chapter are those of the individual, the intellect and the institution. The paradox was that the more freedom and enlightenment there was, the more it was channelled through and into institutions which became more and more exclusive, dominant and prescriptive in their actions. In a number of ways this was unique to Scotland, where the potent combination of education, presbyterian religion, tightly controlled government, individual brilliance and scientific discovery created a situation in which freedom could not grow unless and until it was controlled and institutionalised. This may be a reason why Scotland progressed so rapidly in these areas. The changing general background is also important. Industrialisation, urbanisation, population growth and demographic realignment all helped to shaped Scottish society and, consequently, Scottish medicine.

A similar pattern can, in some ways, be identified for the nation as a whole. The period from the mid–eighteenth century to the early decades of the nineteenth witnessed an equally complex combination of circum-stances and trends. The individual continued to dominate politics, with Henry Dundas still able to control Scotland to a considerable extent, although after his final demise from office it was less easy for Westminster to wield a similar level of control. The intellect was certainly there, with the giants of the non-medical Enlightenment. With the gestation of Empire, Adam Smith's political economy was food for thought, while the debates engendered by philosophers, artists and poets shaped Scotland's cultural life in a unique way. The church was becoming less able to maintain its position and political role; the nation was becoming accustomed to the effects of the union of 1707; and by the early 1800s was fully occupied with the process of industrialisation and empire building. So, the transition phase from the relatively underdeveloped state of early-eighteenth century Scotland to industrial world leader a century later was characterised, perhaps, by a subordination of national and medical identity to the larger identity of Britain and certainly by a realignment of the socio-economic profile of the country. There is little doubt that this relatively short period was crucial to both medicine and society.

NOTES

1. Jordanova, L., *Nature Displayed. Gender, Science and Medicine 1760–1820* (London, 1999).
2. The literature on the Enlightenment is immense and growing. See 'Further Reading'.
3. Wood, P., 'Dugald Stewart and the invention of the Scottish Enlightenment', in Wood, P. (ed.), *The Scottish Enlightenment. Essays in Reinterpretation* (Rochester, 2000), 19–20.
4. Burnham, 'Concept of profession'.
5. Biographical details of most of the individuals mentioned can be found in the *Dictionary of National Biography* and also in general works such as Comrie, *History* and Hamilton, *Healers*. (See 'Further Reading' and 'Select Bibliography' for other specific items.)
6. See Rosner, L., *Medical Education in the Age of Improvement* (Edinburgh, 1991), 11–24.
7. Rosner, *Medical Education*, 49.
8. Jacyna, S., *Philosophic Whigs. Medicine, Science and Citizenship in Edinburgh, 1789–1848* (London, 1994).
9. Lawrence, C., 'The Edinburgh Medical School and the end of the "Old thing" 1790–1830', *History of Universities 7* (1988), 259–86.
10. See Doig, A., Ferguson, J. P. S., Milne, I. A. and Passmore, R. (eds), *William Cullen and the Eighteenth-century Medical World* (Edinburgh, 1993).
11. For a full and scholarly account of the Brunonian controversy, see Barfoot, M., 'Brunonianism under the bed: an alternative to university medicine in Edinburgh in the 1780s', *Med. Hist.* Supplement No. 8 (1988), 22–45.
12. Full recent account of these and other individuals in Geyer-Kordesch and Macdonald, *Physicians and Surgeons in Glasgow*, chs 5–6.
13. Turner, *Story of a Great Hospital*, 133.
14. Dingwall, H. M., '"To be insert in the mercury". Medical practitioners and the press in eighteenth-century Edinburgh', *Soc. Hist. Med.* 13 (1) (2000), 42.
15. For a factual account of these individuals see Comrie, *History*, ii, chs xvi and xvii.
16. See Rosner, L., 'Thistle on the Delaware: Edinburgh Medical education and Philadelphia practice, 1800–1825', *Soc. Hist. Med.* 5 (1) (1992), 19–42, for fuller account of these connections and influences.
17. Kaufman, M. H. and Best, J. J. K., 'Monro *secundus* and 18th-century lymphangiography', *Proc. Roy. Coll. Phys. Ed.* 26 (1) (1996), 75–90.
18. For reasons which are not altogether clear, the introduction and use of chemically based treatments was much slower in Scotland than in England, where by the mid-seventeenth century a Society of Chymical Physicians had been established.
19. Among the many publications of the 'great doctors' were: William Cullen, *First Lines on the Practice of Physic* (1776–84); Alexander Hamilton, *Elements of the Practice of Midwifery* (1755); Alexander Monro *Secundus*, *Observations on the Nervous System* (1783); *Treatise on the Brain, the Eye and the Ear* (1797); Robert Whytt, *Physiological*

Essays (1755). A useful and more detailed list of books published by Scottish authors from 1746–1800 may be found in Sher, R. B., 'Science and medicine in the Scottish Enlightenment', in Wood (ed.), *The Scottish Enlightenment*, 114–23.

20. RCOSEd, Minutes, 2 March 1757.

21. Ibid., 1 May 1777. A further sum of 100 merks was payable by any individual who chose to settle and practise in the local area.

22. Ibid., 15 May 1797.

23. Ibid., 15 May 1816. The matter had been considered in 1805, but the title of licentiate rejected on that occasion. Ibid., 19 February 1805. Curriculum requirements in Glasgow developed along similar lines. See Geyer-Kordesch and Macdonald, *Physicians and Surgeons in Glasgow*, 342–44.

24. Ibid., 11 September 1794. Candidates for diplomas as surgeons' mates were required to attend one session only.

25. Rosner, *Medical Education*, 96.

26. Geyer-Kordesch and Macdonald, *Physicians and Surgeons in Glasgow*, 214.

27. RCOSEd, Minutes, 1 August 1798; 3 February 1806; 15 March 1808; 15 October and 11 November 1822; 1 April 1828. Nowadays, medical students in Edinburgh do not dissect at all, a development which would have horrified the early masters of the Incorporation.

28. Ibid., 4 July 1823; Rosner, *Medical Education*, 101–2.

29. RCOSEd, Minutes, 7 May 1813. The Army Board complained that a number of candidates had appeared who 'are very young and very indifferently qualified being so destitute of a due degree of preliminary education as to be unable to translate the Pharmacopoeia or to read the Latin directions to prescriptions'.

30. Blair, J. S. G., *History of Medicine in the University of St Andrews* (Edinburgh, 1987), 30.

31. Full coverage in Geyer-Kordesch and Macdonald, *Physicians and Surgeons in Glasgow*, ch. 5.

32. Comrie, *History*, i., 369.

33. Geyer-Kordesch and Macdonald, *Physicians and Surgeons in Glasgow*, 154.

34. Ibid., 154–91.

35. A particularly good example of this is Risse, G., *Hospital Life in Enlightenment Scotland. Care and Teaching at the Edinburgh Infirmary* (Cambridge, 1986). See also Risse, G., 'Hysteria at the Edinburgh infirmary: the construction and treatment of a disease, 1770–1800', *Med. Hist.* 32 (1) (1988), 1–22, which covers the description of hysteria as a specific disease susceptible to specific treatments.

36. Risse, G., *Mending Bodies, Saving Souls. A History of Hospitals* (Oxford, 1999).

37. Ibid., 243–73 covers the general aspects of in-patient management at this time.

38. NLS, Ms. 8922, ff1–17.

39. Macdonald, F., 'The Infirmary of the Glasgow Town's Hospital: patient care, 1733–1800', in Wood (ed.), *The Scottish Enlightenment*, 199–238.

40. Jenkinson, J. L. M., Moss, M. and Russell, I., *The Royal. The History of the Glasgow Royal Infirmary 1794–1994* (Glasgow, 1994), 13.

41. Porter, R., *Mind Forg'd Manacles. A History of Madness in England from the Restoration to the Regency* (London, 1990); Houston, R. A., *Madness and Society in Eighteenth-century Scotland* (Oxford, 2000) – though much of its statistical detail is in fact drawn from the early decades of the nineteenth century.

42. Houston, R. A., 'Professions and the identification of mental incapacity in eighteenth-century Scotland', *Journal of Historical Sociology* 14 (4) (2001), 441–66.

43. Craig, *Physicians*, 487.
44. For a detailed discussion of the philosophies of Foucault, see M. Foucault, *Madness and Civilization. A History of Insanity in the Age of Reason*, trans. Howard, R. (London, 1971); Gordon, G., '*Histoire de la Folie*. An unknown book by Michel Foucault', *History of the Human Sciences* 3 (1) (1990), 1–26.
45. Henderson, D. K., *The Evolution of Psychiatry in Scotland* (Edinburgh, 1964). Duncan's own account is set out in Duncan, A., *Short Account of the Rise, Progress and Present State of the Lunatic Asylum at Edinburgh* (Edinburgh, 1812). Duncan had been stimulated to pursue the matter in the first instance, it is claimed, because of his distress at the state in which the poet Robert Fergusson had been kept before his death in the Town Bedlam.
46. Houston, R. A., 'Institutional care for the insane and idiots in Scotland before 1820: Part I', *History of Psychiatry* 12 (2001), 12.
47. Houston, R. A., 'Institutional care for the insane and idiots in Scotland before 1820: Part II', *History of Psychiatry* 12 (2001), 177. This article gives a detailed account of conditions and treatment in Scottish asylums.
48. Ibid., 195–6.
49. Hamilton, *Healers*, 196–234.
50. Smith, B., 'Camphor, cabbage leaves and vaccination: the career of Johnnie "Notions" Williamson, of Hamnavoe, Eshaness, Shetland', *Proc. Roy. Coll. Phys. Ed.* 28 (1998). 395–406.
51. See account and examples in Dingwall, 'To be insert in the mercury'.
52. RCOSEd, Minutes, 28 March 1863.
53. Sinclair, J. (ed.) *The Statistical Account of Scotland* (Edinburgh, 1791–99).
54. Brunton, D., 'Smallpox inoculation and demographic trends in eighteenth-century Scotland', *Med. Hist.* 36 (4) (1992), 403–29.
55. Beith, *Healing Threads*, 248, 233, 187.
56. Buchan, *Folk Tradition and Folk Medicine*, 103, 106.
57. This view was expressed originally in Clark, A., *Working Life of Women in the Seventeenth Century* (London, 1919).
58. Jordanova, L., *Sexual Visions. Images of Gender in Science and Medicine between the Eighteenth and Twentieth Centuries* (London, 1989).
59. Harris, R., *Politics and the Rise of the Press 1620–1800* (London, 1996), includes coverage of the eighteenth-century Scottish press.

PART THREE

A NATION ECLIPSED?

Medicine in Scotland from c. 1800 to 2000

CHAPTER 7

SCOTLAND AND SCOTS IN MODERN SCOTLAND

In terms of the evolution of the nation, the close of the eighteenth century saw Scotland in a strong position in global, national and medical spheres. The fruits of the Enlightenment afforded the small nation considerable intellectual status; the early process of industrialisation drove Scotland into the vanguard of the industrialising world; Scots built the ships and railways of Empire, but Scots also travelled in these ships to transport themselves and their talents to all parts of the globe. Industrialisation would bring problems as well as benefits, though; problems which would occupy the minds and energies of medical men as well as those involved in local and national government.

Increasingly, this period saw Scots involved in a succession of wars and conflicts of a rather different sort from the religious conflicts and wars of the seventeenth century or, indeed the long-distant Wars of Independence. The Crimean and Boer wars proved to be something in the nature of warm-up sessions for the two devastating global conflicts in the first half of the last century. Since then, Scotland and Scots have been involved in a seemingly never-ending series of wars and conflicts, from Aden and Korea to the Falklands, from the Gulf to Bosnia, and Kosovo to Afghanistan; not to mention the continuing and seemingly intractable problem of Northern Ireland. Scots have historically provided recruits to the armed forces in considerably higher proportion to the relative size of the constituent parts of Britain, which has meant that Scots have been closely involved in conflict as a nation, as an army, and as medical personnel.

In the second half of the twentieth century, Scotland witnessed many changes which have had direct effects, both on the character of the nation and on its medical services. The almost complete demise of coal mining, for example, has reduced the potential numbers of individuals suffering from the diseases associated with that economic and industrial sphere. Asbestos has been removed from most buildings, again preventing further occupational disease from that cause, though the aftermath of that particularly toxic material is still a concern to victims, as well as to the medical profession. Service industries and technological production have replaced heavy industry. Silicon Glen produces very different medical problems from the now redundant coal mines. The ailments suffered by the modern workforce are more likely to be those of repetitive strain injury or psychological stress in its many forms. In this sense, then, the industrial decline and subsequent economic redefinition of the nation have altered both the lives of the people in general and the nature of their medical complaints. This has, of course, necessitated concomitant changes in the organisation and provision of health care.

In earlier ages, Scotland looked very much towards Europe rather than south to England. As part of Britain, Scotland is now once again connected to Europe but in very different circumstances. This makes the recent re-establishment of a Scottish parliament problematic in any assessment of Scottishness, either re-invented or resurrected. The relationship between Scotland and Brussels is certainly not the same as that between Scotland and the Low Countries, or between Scotland and France in earlier times. These old ties had helped to maintain not only pan-European contacts and influences, but also in some ways had helped Scotland to remain Scottish, whereas nowadays the connections are less distinctive and often resented.

The Victorian period is characterised not only by the influence of the Hanoverian monarchies on Scotland, Britain and the expansion of the Empire, but also in the effects of the Enlightenment. Whether or not this was a process unique to Scotland, or whether what happened in Scotland was similar to what was happening in other countries, there is no doubt that Scotland contributed to the intellectual world in a measure out of all proportion to its size.[1] By the middle of the eighteenth century Scotland was firmly part of Britain, for better or worse, and also a major part of intellectual Europe and beyond. It is difficult to account for the position in which Scotland found herself. The postmodernist view would no doubt be that it was merely the coincidental concurrence of intellect; more orthodox historians might conclude that the combination of elements which made Scotland 'Scottish' played a part, not least the development of institutions and the historic importance given to education in all its aspects. Whatever the causal factors, the result was that while political Scotland may have been subordinated to political England, and managed on behalf of London by a few individuals, in other spheres Scotland was certainly not the weaker partner.[2]

However, although the eighteenth century is regarded as the period of high intellectual development, the consolidation of Edinburgh and the gradual acclimatisation of the Scots to absentee government as well as absentee monarchy, recent work has shown that Scotland was not quite as calm and settled as has been assumed previously. Whatley's recent book demonstrates convincingly that at the 'grass roots' level, Scots were in many ways just as rebellious, disruptive and disgruntled (often for very good reasons) as they had always been.[3] So, the approach to industrialisation and empire was not quite one of political calm or meek acceptance of the domination of Scotland by Westminster. The first agitation for political reform in the 1790s may have been short-lived, and it would take another three decades for legislation to extend the franchise, but Scotland was changing.

Late eighteenth-century Scotland had demonstrated many divisions and difficulties, which would help to shape the nineteenth century and beyond. Communication between highlands and lowlands may have already been made a little easier, courtesy of General Wade, during the period of the Jacobite campaigns, but highland and lowland cultures and lifestyles were still very different. This would, of course, have implications for the development of any sort of united concept of Scottish national identity and, indeed, for Scottish medicine. It seems that by the turn of the nineteenth century, at least in the view of those who accepted the concept of North Britain, that it was perfectly possible, and not at all contradictory, for an individual to be a loyal Briton and a patriotic Scot.[4] By the end of the twentieth century, this was no longer the case, or is deemed not to be possible by those who wish Scotland to be not only devolved from the British sphere, but to return to a wholly separate sphere, whatever the advantages or disadvantages of this might be.

VICTORIAN SCOTLAND

The nineteenth century dawned with Scotland more adjusted to, or at least resigned to, the long-term consequences of the act of union passed almost a century previously. Large-scale electoral reform was still some three decades in the future; politics were much as they had been, with a pitifully small electorate of around 4,200 serving only to reinforce the political status quo, though this period is also noted as being the beginning of the end of the political, social and economic domination of the landed gentry. Industrialisation was proceeding apace; the population was ever more mobile in order to make use of new employment opportunities – and indeed disease opportunities in the larger towns; the universities were offering more and more specialised curricula; big local government was looming; and in the warm afterglow of the Enlightenment, Scotland was confident, as part of both a confident Britain and a confidently embryonic British Empire,[5] or as a confident part of both of these. Those in control of the public sphere took greater charge of public affairs and public health. Great interest was expressed in just how industrial change affected those at lower ends of the socio-economic scale. The Scottish presbyterian church, long an important and defining characteristic of a separate Scotland within Britain, was becoming ever more fragmented and quarrelsome, and in 1843 a deep fissure brought about irreversible division.[6] Many of the dispersed fragments re-amalgamated in 1929, but it could never again be claimed that the Church of Scotland was the church which represented all of the people of Scotland. It had, indeed, never been quite able to claim universal influence, but by the middle of the nineteenth century any lingering hopes of universality were dashed. The removal of responsibility for education and the operation of the Poor Law in the mid-Victorian period denoted the effective end of the parish state and the global influence of the state church.

Perhaps the major characteristic of this period was the very rapid economic development which took place, particularly in the changes brought by the industrialising process and the advent of the first areas of heavy industry. By the turn of the nineteenth century, cotton had replaced linen as the pioneer of industry. It is the view of some economic and industrial historians that cotton was somehow the bridge between large-scale, but largely domestic-based, linen production and the might of heavy industry and the height of the phase of empire-building for Scotland and Britain as a whole.[7] The transition in industry had not yet, however, reached the point where town and country had become completely separated or alienated from each other. Iron was coming, but for the moment cotton was still king. Once the iron smelters took over as the industrial furnaces of the country, the town and country divisions were clearer. By 1850 over 25 per cent of Scots lived in Glasgow, Edinburgh, Dundee or Aberdeen, and by the turn of the twentieth century over half were urban dwellers.[8]

By the third quarter of the nineteenth century the demographic map of Scotland had changed significantly. Glasgow was by far the dominant and most rapidly expanding urban area, and provided a microcosm of 'modern' Scotland and all the problems that this brought along with the benefits. The boost to Glasgow had come initially with the important, though temporary, effects of the tobacco trade with North America. Glasgow's Tobacco Lords were at the pinnacle of entrepreneurial pursuits and achievements. Their profits did much to lay the foundations for the flourishing of Glasgow.[9] The ancient medieval burgh was transformed out of all recognition. Suburbs sprang up rapidly, and the more unscrupulous landlords literally made a killing out of their minutely sub-divided and seriously overcrowded, disease-ridden and insanitary properties.

Much of the historically constructed identity of Scotland relates to what happened in the highlands at the end of the eighteenth century and the first part of the nineteenth century. The population was becoming more concentrated in lowland areas, but before this process had got fully underway there were, quite simply, too many people in the highlands to be sustained by the land, which although vast, was often impossible to make productive in any meaningful way. There has been in recent times a great deal of attention paid by historians to the problem of explaining the notorious highland clearances, next only to the Jacobite episodes in the list of oppressions meted out in that area. There is no doubt that a great deal of suffering was caused to a great many people, but the matter was complex, and not just centred on the desire of a few landlords to replace their tenants with sheep for reasons of greed and lack of concern with the culture of the highlands.[10] For a complicated set of reasons, people from the highlands were 'encouraged' to leave their homes and travel either to the lowland areas to help swell the population of the industrial towns, or to acquire a one-way ticket to the alleged utopia of the New World. By the middle of the nineteenth century the devastation of the potato famine was yet another factor in a difficult equation. The result of it all was to write another emotive chapter in Scottish history and to alter permanently the demographic configuration of the nation. Increasingly the population was concentrated in the central belt, and the highlands became progressively depopulated. The plight of the highlander served to intensify the tartan romantic image of Scotland, centred on its rugged and emotive landscape. This image was sustained by the growing interest displayed by royalty, so that for much of this period, the Scottish landscape was, it is claimed, an 'icon of identity'.[11]

In order to service the rapidly growing industrial base the major resource was, of course, labour. At this point the population of Scotland began to rise much more rapidly, and this was boosted by immigrants from Ireland, particularly towards the middle of the nineteenth century when the lethal scourge of the potato famine drove many to make the short sea crossing to apparent safety, nutrition, housing, health and work in the industrial hotbed of Glasgow and its environs. By the beginning of the 1830s it is estimated that individuals of Irish origin made up some 17 per cent of the population of that area. At this time also, and entirely uncontroversial, at least for the moment, was the widescale use of child labour to keep the machines in the cotton factories operating, or to work in coal mines, or crush iron ore. Adult women, of course, made up a significant proportion of factory and mining labour.[12]

In terms of the gender balance of labour, this evolving system changed the situation at the lower levels very little. Women had always taken an equal role in domestic-based manufacturing and agricultural pursuits. Higher up, though, middle-class and upper-class women found themselves more and more restricted as to what sort of occupations were considered to be suitable for the so-called weaker sex. In this respect Scotland was no different from the rest of Great Britain. Middle-class women did charitable work or taught in genteel private schools for the most part. They were expected to be decorative and passive, rather than create economic wealth or take up paid employment. In the context of this particular work, this gradual isolation of most, but not all, middle-class women from the centres of economic activity would prove to be extremely problematical for two groups of women: those who wished to become doctors and others who saw the need for hospitals to be staffed by trained, educated and intelligent nurses.

Once the class system was consolidated, each sector sought to maintain its interests as a group, rather than through the still hierarchical but more complex system of social ranks which had persisted for many centuries before. Working-class individuals wished for a say in the political process; members of the middle class demonstrated the desire to move upwards to join the ranks of at least the lower levels of the upper class. There were a number of ways in which these could be achieved. Scottish workers began to combine, firstly in the form of friendly societies and then in trade unions, which would fight long and hard for the rights of their members. Middle-class men and some women were able to take part in the increasingly complex and large-scale area of local government, while the landed aristocracy did what they had always done. It was, though, the security of the latter group which became threatened as the nineteenth century wore on and the sphere of wealth passed from the land into the factory or shipyard in the industrial central and west of Scotland.

Agitation for political reform had begun in the last decade of the eighteenth century in the heady atmosphere of the American and French Revolutions. By the 1790s more organised protest was beginning to take place, and Societies of the Friends of the People were set up in most large towns. These Societies were composed mostly of middle-class, not working-class, members, and their major aim was to achieve electoral and political reform by constitutional means, certainly not by violence.[13] This early movement was crushed relatively easily by the government, which used the effective tactic of accusing the Friends of being revolutionaries, an accusation which quickly eclipsed the activities of all but a few. It took little more than a few exemplary deportations and threats against social progress for the middle-class supporters to take their carefully prepared statistical evidence and other publications, and retire from the conflict. At no point, though, had these groups advocated universal franchise.

By the 1820s the movement for reform had risen from the ashes, but the phoenix bore a rather different plumage. The combined consequences of the severe economic downturn, particularly in the fortunes of the over-manned handloom weaving industry, and the end of the Napoleonic wars, which saw the return to Scotland of thousands of demobbed troops looking for work in a shrinking, mechanised market place, brought about renewed and more active, violent protest for change. It is debatable whether the Radical War of 1820 can be called a war or even particularly radical, but it did have the effect of stimulating debate, and by 1832 the so-called Great Reform Act extended the franchise in a modest way, giving the vote to around one in eight adult males, compared to the previous ratio of one in 125.

As the nineteenth century moved on, a number of areas of society began to take on the shape which they would maintain well into the next century. A millennium previously, the whole aspect, cosmology and characteristics of the Scots and their nation had been bound up in matters of religion in its very broadest sense. The medieval church dominated society, influenced politics and provided direction to all Scots, this including, of course, the provision of medical care and treatment within the compass of biblical christianity. A thousand years later, the church was still important to many Scots, but was not a single all-inclusive church. Politics and religion together had defined the nation and shaped its early progress, but early in the eighteenth century cracks had begun to appear at the edges of state religion. Secession after secession punctuated the state church, and this culminated in the famous Disruption of 1843, when the state church was finally riven asunder. The splits and conflicts were centred, as they had been for over a century, on the nature of the relationship between church and state, and the extent to which the state church would tolerate secular influence, or, in other words, just how Erastian it was permissible to be. The details of these events are outwith the brief compass of this chapter, but the result was that henceforth the state church represented only a minority of the citizens of Scotland in a religious sense.[14] This brought problems, of course, as matters of poor relief and education were still the responsibility of the church. However, in terms of the evolution of the nation and the definition of its character, the Church of Scotland – by law established and still holding to its principal subordinate standard as defined in the Westminster Confession of 1644 – was by now playing rather less of a character-forming role. By 1829 Roman Catholics had been relieved of their disabilities and could thenceforth take a fuller role in secular society. The legacy of this is still to be found, particularly in the west of Scotland and the highlands and islands, notoriously on the field of sport, but also, and increasingly controversially, in the area of separate denominational education. Religion may not now be a major force in the shaping of the nation, but its long shadow penetrates many secular spheres. The religious map of Scotland has also been redefined more recently in terms of the 'multi-faith' composition of the community, and in consequence of different patterns of immigration and emigration. Scots have left Scotland in large numbers, not least on the £10 tickets to Australia, but they have been replaced by individuals from all over the globe.

What was also an important factor in this period was the rather artificial creation of Scottishness in terms of the 'tartanisation' of the Scottish national character. The definition of Scottishness appeared to take on the symbols of the oppressed and suppressed aspects of the nation. The highlander, the tartan and the legend were increasingly the image of Scotland portrayed furth of the nation.[15] When Cook's tours came to Scotland, they came to the highlands, not the towns. Royalty became increasingly 'tartanised' and royals took to making lengthy visits to Scotland, but to the highlands and not to the urbanised, industrialising lowlands. It is interesting and, perhaps a little ironic, that the image of the Scot and the Scottish nation by the middle of the nineteenth century was focused on an imagined reality, which may be related to Anderson's view on national identity being constructed in terms of imagined communities.[16] This may have been quite simply an attempt to rescue Scotland's past and shape its future. What it did produce, though, was a relatively schizophrenic picture of a nation which was at the same time individual, part of Great Britain and an active participant in the process of empire.

THE LAST CENTURY OF THE SECOND MILLENNIUM

The closing century of the second millennium has also seen significant change, but also the continuity of problems. War can be a stimulus for change in many areas, and the Great War was no less of a catalyst, though the conflict had been fought on foreign shores. The results of the loss of some 110,000 men had considerable implications for the development of industry and the shaping of society. Industrial Scotland had been boosted by the requirements of war; Scottish women had been involved in occupations alien to their normal spheres of home and work; and Scotland had taken part in the great conflict as a matter of course, there being no real political drive on the part of Scottish radical politics against it. The effects of the Second World War were also important on many aspects of Scotland and the lives of the Scots. Scotland shared in the optimism and also the monochrome dreariness of the early post-war period, but a number of the measures taken to provide medical care to the population as a whole during the war were adapted or modified to form elements of the National Health Service. As will be discussed in subsequent chapters, the consequences of wars on shaping not just the medicine of war but also the medicine of peace time were key elements in the construction of Scottish and British medicine. For example, surgical techniques developed in wartime have been applied to the general population, particularly in plastic surgery and the development of artificial limbs. Hospitals built as temporary structures to house war casualties remained for decades as district general hospitals. The prefabricated housing provided as a temporary measure to house families made homeless by war also survived well beyond their project lifetimes, and, indeed, became something of an icon or symbol of the problems and characteristics of this time.

Scots experienced deprivation and unemployment during the period of the Depression, and the decline of the shipbuilding industry was a particularly hard blow. Whether or not Red Clydeside was a real political threat to the stability of Scotland, the Home Rule movement saw little success, perhaps because of common economic difficulties. What characterised particularly post-1945 Scotland was the great speed of economic change and the technology of economic change. Economic change saw the decline of many of the heavy industries which had helped to shape the identity of Victorian Scotland. Coal, steel and shipbuilding have largely gone, to be replaced by service industries and new technology. The economy seems nowadays to be built largely on virtual trade and industry, rather than physical trade and industry. This has not, though, resulted in economic advancement for all, and some of the old problems remain, particularly in the areas of urban poverty, poor housing and crime. The slums may have gone, but urban ghettos have replaced them and perpetuated the problems, made worse perhaps by the high levels of rented housing in Scotland.[17]

Political change was rather slower to come, although the Scottish National Party (SNP) had been in existence since 1934. There had been some political concessions since the 1880s, with the re-establishment in 1885 of the post of Scottish Secretary, a post which had been phased out in the 1720s. At first cosmetic rather than practical, the post took on more significance from 1926, when it was given full Secretaryship of Scotland status. The input of influential individuals, as always, would boost the political status of this office and a key figure in wartime politics and

post-war industrial development was Tom Johnson, who was also prominent in the drive towards improved health policy.

The political face of Scotland in the 1930s was rather similar to the
political countenance of Britain as a whole. This may have been helped
by the gradual and piecemeal devolution to Scotland of parts of the
government's administrative apparatus, so that by the 1950s, if visual
symbolism still mattered – and it seems that it did – there was at least
some semblance of 'independence' of the physical or material trappings
of government, if not of real power. It was not until the 1960s that the
political map of Scotland began to differ to any real extent from that
south of the border.[18] Following the nationwide demise of Liberalism
(Scots had voted Liberal in all but one of the general elections between
1832 and 1918), and the emergence of a different two-party structure,
Conservative and Labour, Scottish politics mirrored British party politics
to a great extent. During the 1960s Conservative fortunes declined, and
Winnie Ewing won a famous by-election for the SNP at Hamilton in
1967. From that point the Labour party has dominated Scottish politics,
although the SNP by the turn of the millennium has become a
considerable force. Since the reconstitution of the Scottish parliament in
1999, the SNP has been able to strengthen and attempt to prove itself as
a credible force in national government; its effectiveness has still to be
measured.[19] The independence of Scottish or British government is
nowadays constrained to a considerable extent by the tentacles of Brussels,
which penetrate the minutiae of legislation, so that at least one symbol of
Scottishness, the haggis, may well find itself redefined in the cumber-
some and bureaucratic jargon of European 'standardisation'.

The effects of devolution have yet to be assessed. The Scottish
Executive claims to have health as an important priority and has outlined
ambitious targets for reduction in the incidence of some of the most
socially-destructive health problems facing Scotland in the twenty-first
century. Ambitious targets have been set for dealing with many of the
social, economic and health problems faced by modern Scotland, but the
devolved administration faces many problems. Whether this devolution
alters significantly the identity of the modern Scot is also imponderable
for the present. In terms of the creation or evolution of a new national or
medical identity for post-devolution Scotland, a verdict based on rigorous
historical analysis must be withheld for some time. Many factors have
influenced the evolution of Scotland as a political, social, economic and
indeed medical entity. Many things have changed since 1800; other things
have not. What is not yet clear, though, is whether it is possible, or indeed
desirable, for historians to try to redefine post-devolution Scottishness in
political, social or cultural terms. In her recent book *Scotland. A History*,

Fiona Watson has entitled the final chapter 'Scotland Renewed'. The question is, what has been renewed? And had it ever really been lost?

The two main chapters in this section will consider, firstly, the complex network of factors and influences which shaped the construction of Scottish society and its medicine in the period c. 1830–1918, and, secondly, the equally significant but very different forces which were brought to bear on medicine in an age of technology and global communication.

NOTES

1. The literature on the Enlightenment is immense. For general coverage and views on the distinctiveness of the process in Scotland, see Allan, D., *Virtue, Learning and the Scottish Enlightenment* (Edinburgh, 1993); Campbell, R. H. and Skinner, A. S. (eds), *The Origins and Nature of the Scottish Enlightenment* (Edinburgh, 1982); Chitnis, A. C., *The Scottish Enlightenment. A Social History* (London, 1976). See also 'Further Reading' section.

2. For a new account of politics in the period, see Shaw, J. S., *The Politics of Eighteenth-century Scotland* (London, 1999).

3. Whatley, C.A., *Scottish Society 1707–1830* (Manchester, 2000).

4. Finlay, R. J., 'Caledonia or North Britain? Scottish Identity in the Eighteenth Century', in Broun, Finlay and Lynch (eds), *Image and Identity*, 143–56.

5. See extensive analysis in Fry, M., *The Scottish Empire*, (East Linton, 2001).

6. Brown, *Religion and Society in Scotland.*

7. Lenman, B., *An Economic History of Modern Scotland* (London, 1977).

8. Devine, *Scotland*, 140–1.

9. Devine, T. M., *The Tobacco Lords: A Study of the Tobacco Merchants of Glasgow and their Trading Activities c. 1740–90* (Edinburgh, 1990).

10. Recent opinion in Cameron, E .A., *Land for the People. The British Government and the Scottish Highlands c. 1880–1925* (East Linton, 1996). See also Richards, E., *The Highland Clearances. People, Landlords and Rural Turmoil* (Edinburgh, 2000).

11. Watson, F., *Scotland, A History* (Stroud, 2001), 193.

12. Whatley, C. A., 'Women and the economic transformation of Scotland c. 1740–1830', *Scottish Economic and Social History* 14 (1994), 19–40.

13. Nenadic, S., 'Political reform and the ordering of middle-class protest', in Devine, T. M. (ed.), *Conflict and Stability in Scottish Society 1708—1850*, (Edinburgh, 1990), 65–82.

14. See *Religion and Society in Scotland.*

15. See Cameron, E. A., 'Embracing the past. The highlands in nineteenth-century Scotland', in Brown, Finlay and Lynch (eds), *Image and Identity*, 195–219.

16. Anderson, B. R. O., *Imagined Communities: Reflections on the Origins and Spread of Nationalism* (London, 1991).

17. Rodger, R., *Scottish Housing in the Twentieth Century* (Leicester, 1989).

18. For a concise and masterly account of politics in the recent past, see Hutchison, I. G. C., *Scottish Politics in the Twentieth Century* (Basingstoke, 2001).

19. Account of rise of the Scottish National Party in Finlay, R., *Independent and Free. Scottish Politics and the Origins of the Scottish National Party 1918-1945* (Edinburgh, 1994).

CHAPTER 8

PUBLIC MEDICINE IN PUBLIC SCOTLAND

INTRODUCTION

As the nineteenth century wore on, and as the machinery of big government, particularly in the large cities, became less ad hoc and reactive, the effects were to be felt by both the givers and receivers of Scottish medicine. The point was being reached where it may be questionable to maintain the distinction between Scottish medicine in Britain and British medicine in Scotland. Once the effects of the 1858 Medical Act began to filter down from the rarefied heights of the newly formed but still relatively toothless General Medical Council, medical and surgical practitioners found increasingly that they were obliged to follow rather than lead in the development of criteria for licensing and the particular courses of study that had to be followed in order to achieve medical qualification.

This period can be characterised by a considerable strengthening of the public sphere of government, legislation and social control. The rise of the city, epitomised by Glasgow, at least in terms of the scale of the problems, had the result of concentrating ills and diseases in small crowded areas. In order to cope with epidemic and endemic diseases, the public sphere and the medical sphere were forced perhaps more than ever before to co-operate, legislate, enforce and enable. Medical practitioners were pulled in many directions: by the increasing length and scope of their training; by the growing centralisation of administration, registration and supervision of their subsequent careers; by the needs and aims of their professional body; and by the needs and aims of their local situation, central government and nation, not to mention the consumers of medical care, to whom they gave their services.

Parallel to this were the giant leaps in Victorian and early-twentieth century medicine, particularly in the two most obvious areas of anaesthetics and infection control. Although medical training had developed and improved almost out of all recognition, the experiences of the patients and the ability of their medical attendants to cure their ills took somewhat longer to develop. Major advances in anaesthetics were furthered by the work of one famous Scot, James Young Simpson, with a little encouragement from the willingness of the monarch to accept anaesthesia during her later confinements. Progress in the theory and practice of infection control came from a number of sources, but in both acute medicine and public health the work of pioneers such as Semmelweiss and Pasteur left a much more lasting and practical legacy than perhaps Cullen or Black, though in their own spheres the latter two individuals had outranked most of their contemporaries. Scotland was very much part of the growing imperial sphere, both as part of the larger nation and as a Scottish entity.

This concentrated period of industrialisation and empire building brought Scotland into the world in a more direct and positive way than before. Scots built the ships of empire, but once they had been launched, Scots sailed in them to claim the empire. Scots had always been international, particularly European, in outlook but by the mid-nineteenth century the horizons had been expanded markedly. Scots doctors took their skills to all corners of the globe and Scottish medical expertise was exported freely.

Scotland the nation experienced many changes. Urbanisation and industrialisation altered not only the settlement patterns of the population, but also created the circumstances which produced condition-induced or environmentally induced diseases and injuries. This was the time of the major epidemics of cholera, typhus, measles and other potentially deadly diseases. Although these diseases did not confine their fury to the towns, it was in the large urban conurbations that their devastating effects were felt the most. It was also the large urban areas which came to the attention of those who were interested in how the people lived in the vast sphere of unprivileged labour. Edwin Chadwick, Thomas Chalmers and others represented the social conscience of the few (though they disagreed as to the nature of the problems and, in particular, how to deal with them); those who ran large-scale municipal governments operated by gift of a few electors but were forced to bring in large-scale measures and social policing in order to control a precarious general situation.

The *Report on the Sanitary Condition of the Labouring Population of Scotland*, published in 1842 and undertaken at the request of the Poor Law Commissioners, makes harrowing reading, and would have done without the devastation wrought by the major cholera outbreaks. One or two examples are sufficient to illustrate the conditions under which many of the poorest lived in early Victorian Scotland. The following describes conditions in Greenock, typical of many other places:

> The great proportion of the dwellings of the poor are situated in very narrow and confined closes or alleys leading from the main streets. I might almost say there are no drains in any of these closes, for where I have noticed sewers, they are in such a filthy and obstructed state, that they create more nuisance than if they never existed. In those closes where there is no dunghill, the excrementitious and other offensive matter is thrown into the gutter before the door, or carried out and put in the street ... There is one poor man who was in my care in the hospital with asthma for six months, he was dismissed as incurable, and is now living with his wife and seven children in a dark room on the ground-floor, more fit for a coal-cellar than a human being; it is lighted by a fixed window about two feet square; the breadth of the room is only four feet, and the length eight. There is only one bed for the whole family, and yet the rent of this hole is 5l.[1]

The limitations of current legislation are pointed out in the report from Stirling:

> The powers of the municipal authorities of Stirling are not sufficient for the purposes of a medical police. They do not, for example, possess the power of entering private property, and removing therefrom nuisances injurious to health. This was serious felt immediately before the invasion of the cholera in 1832.[2]

The first devastating outbreak of cholera struck Scotland in 1832 and there would be several subsequent attacks. For much of the first part of the century at least, government, both national and local, tended to react to events rather than try to prevent them. Improving housing, providing clean water supplies, initiating vaccination programmes and other public health measures was expensive, and although the Samuel Smiles philosophy may not have informed and driven the actions of all, many of the attitudes held and expressed were related to the views that self-help should be at the core of social progress. The public sphere was also changing, insofar as the social hierarchy was in the process of rearranging itself from a pattern of ranks and stations to a simpler, but much more heavily meaningful division into the three main classes, upper, middle, and lower, with all their consequent socio-political implications.

This chapter will consider the major continuing processes of interaction among spheres of medical and other influences, and will assess the new trends towards large-scale, pro-active government, medical advances, medical reform, wartime medicine, the opening skirmishes in the conflict between women and the medical establishment, and the changing experiences of the patients. The social construction of medicine in this period was very much the construction of legislation and the influence of national and local government, as well as voluntary agencies.

PUBLIC HEALTH – THE VERY PUBLIC FACE OF OFFICIAL MEDICINE

There had always been endemic and epidemic diseases. In earlier times bubonic and pneumonic plagues devastated Scotland; fevers caused widespread debilitation; harvest failures caused malnutrition; the injuries and mutilations caused by war, bloodfeud or other violent encounters reduced the capacity of the combatants to cultivate their crops or buy food for themselves and their families. By the early nineteenth century, while the notion of the divine retributive purpose of these visitations had perhaps been eclipsed a little, plagues of a different sort afflicted a population which was becoming geographically much less evenly distributed. This demographic realignment had considerable effects on the spread of epidemic disease, endemic illness and undernourishment. In the large towns, particularly Glasgow, with their densely packed populations forced to live in often wholly insanitary conditions, there was thus a proportionately increased potential for the spread and devastating effects of virulent disease.

The first major outbreak of cholera struck Scotland in 1832. There would be several further outbreaks, and these had to be dealt with in conjunction with the ongoing though less headline-making problems of fevers of all sorts, measles, rickets, high rates of maternal and infant death, and industrial injuries. The ways in which Scottish medicine approached these problems were very much informed by the prevailing attitudes of the day. Government acted to combat the spread of epidemics; civic pride prodded town councils into looking at schemes to improve conditions, at least in the better parts of these towns; medical men argued over the rival contagion and miasma theories; but it still seemed impossible to agree on sensible immediate or forward plans to deal with these recurrent problems. If the nature and mechanisms of transfer of diseases were not known, or agreed, then no matter how much it was desired to alleviate the situation for whatever reason, altruistic or not, it was very difficult to convince the majority of those in the sphere of power that one or other viewpoint or explanation was the most likely to be accurate.

The views of Edwin Chadwick and William Pultney Alison have come to characterise the opposing views on the nature and transmission of diseases. Chadwick was a keen proponent of the miasma theory. If diseases were transmitted through miasmic forces, then there was not so much point in, for example, ordering the enforced isolation of those infected with any particular disease. The foul miasma could only be improved by large-scale measures, such as improving water supplies, sanitation, nourishment and enforcing building regulations in the cramped urban centres. In the view of Alison, on the other hand, contagion theory, which involved the direct transmission of disease by contact, required strictly enforced isolation and quarantine to deal with infectious disease. The state, in the form of large-scale central and local government measures, was only too anxious to improve the health, if not the housing or wages, of the labourers who built the Empire and to glorify urban centres with impressive buildings; the intent, though, was not always sufficient, and until public health and epidemiology were focused on the same causal relationships, progress would be of necessity patchy and slow.

Whatever the precise disease of the moment, the various fevers and recurrent epidemics put further pressure on the already cramped and inadequate hospitals and their management. Eventually purpose-built fever hospitals would be provided in the major towns (or their outskirts) but pragmatism still needed to play a part. In Glasgow, for example, in 1819 two wards at the Royal were designated as fever wards. The subsequent effects on the capacity of the hospital to treat other patients were such that by 1825 discussions were afoot on the possibility of constructing a separate hospital to house fever patients. This was eventually achieved in 1829, but would not prove adequate for long, particularly once the scourge of cholera began to hit Scotland, and temporary fever sheds had to be constructed at various times during the epidemics in order to cope with the situation.[3] Although Glasgow was hardest hit by these problems, they were mirrored in most of the other large towns. There is some debate as to the extent to which cholera was the catalyst for sanitary reform in general,[4] but there is no doubt that the outbreaks concentrated the minds of those who wished to promote urban health as well as individual health. The concentration of cases in confined urban areas was perhaps more of a catalyst for the introduction of permanent measures than the more sporadic and less devastating outbreaks in rural areas.

PUBLIC HEALTH – THE 'SANITATION' APPROACH

In terms of the organisation and direction of public health on behalf of the government, this period saw the introduction of public health committees and the appointment of medical men as Medical Officers of Health (MOH) in the larger burghs. Their task was to oversee measures introduced to improve the sanitary condition of the population and to deal with epidemics as they arose. The increasingly public face of Scotland necessitated an increasingly public and co-ordinated approach to matters of health which affected the public. After many delays the Public Health (Scotland) Act was at last added to the statute book in 1867, and this placed on a legal footing many of the ad hoc, piecemeal trends which had characterised the first half of the nineteenth century. After this point the Medical Officers of Health and their departments were able to wield some considerable power over actions and methods. The first incumbent of such a post in Scotland was Sir Henry Littlejohn, who, in line with the now established need for key figures to publish in their fields, wrote the influential *Report on the Sanitary Condition of the City of Edinburgh*, published in 1865, some two years before the definitive legislation mentioned above. Against considerable opposition from the medical establishment, he was the instigator of disease notification, a practice which would have important effects on the control and mapping of the patterns of infectious diseases, particularly during times of epidemic. In Glasgow, following initial work carried out by John Ure, Chairman of the Sanitary Committee, and William Tennant Gairdner, who occupied the post of MOH part-time but achieved a great deal, the post was taken up in 1871 by one of the most notable officers, Dr James Burn Russell, who served the people of Glasgow for a quarter of a century.[5] During this time, records indicate that the crude death rate in Glasgow was reduced from twenty-nine to twenty-one per thousand, this against the background of steadily increasing population, with consequent worsening of social conditions. Russell was, unlike some of his equally notable colleagues in other cities (Henry Littlejohn in Edinburgh, or John McVail in Stirling), a full-time MOH and did not combine these duties with academic or other medical practice. Russell gathered statistics assiduously in order to demonstrate the full horror of the problems of urban overcrowding, stating bitterly that 'we choke and hustle each other out of existence'.[6] As with most developmental processes, there is some debate as to exactly how much of the progress was due solely to the efforts of Russell and his counterparts in other large Scottish towns. The supply of clean water from Loch Katrine in the 1850s must have played some part, as must the gradually improving standards of nutrition and better control of infectious diseases. There is little doubt, though, that in locations where civic action took place for whatever reason, the effects seem to have been significant. The MOH was an individual with unique opportunities to shape both the medical and social parameters of the burgh for which he was responsible.

Town councils had considerable powers to introduce local policing legislation, and in some cases this provided the basis for general nation-wide measures. For example, Henry Littlejohn, MOH in Edinburgh, introduced the compulsory notification of infectious diseases in 1880, while the ticketing system introduced in Glasgow gave sweeping powers to the MOH to set limits on the numbers of inhabitants in any house or room.[7]

Evidence that the growing interest in matters of public health demonstrated in the large cities was being taken seriously by the medical institutions comes from plans drawn up in the late 1880s by The Royal College of Surgeons of Edinburgh to institute a Diploma in Public Health. The scope of the examination demonstrates what was considered to be the most important areas of the subject. There would be no set curriculum, but the examinations would comprise laboratory as well as written work. The examinations would include, firstly, 'chemistry, physics, topographical atmospherics and climatic influences in their relations to disease', and secondly, 'epidemic and endemic diseases, contagion, drainage, water supply and conservancy, construction of public buildings, barracks, hospitals, schools, factories and dwelling houses, establishments connected with food supplies, cemeteries, sanitary science in general and sanitary laws, laws related to the duties of an officer of health in all its departments including vital statistics'.[8] In the practical part of the examination, the students would be expected to demonstrate knowledge of procedures related to the 'examination of water, air, foods, beverages, condiments, sewage, soils, disinfectants and deodorisers, building materials, clothing, bacteriology and examination of water, bread, milk and tea'. This was apparently to be a rigorous and comprehensive examination, and encompassed most of the functions currently undertaken by Health and Safety and Food Standards Officers. While ever mindful of the commercial imperatives of their own institution, the Edinburgh surgeons were clearly trying to ensure that any improvements in public health would be supervised by individuals who were sufficiently well-trained to produce and maintain results.

In rural Scotland the environment was not quite so threatening as it was in the large, crowded and squalid urban conurbations. Disease was not absent here either, though, and the very isolation, while effective perhaps in times of rampant epidemic, was a danger in cases of acute illness which required hospitalisation or specialist medical treatment. Occasionally also, attacks of epidemic disease would prove devastating, precisely because of the lack of immunity in the community

As the Victorian period dawned, so the sphere of officialdom began to make more direct and sustained interventions into the sphere of medicine and its organisation. This came about for several major reasons. Firstly, the growth of urban populations made it increasingly difficult for smaller local authorities to be able to cope with the organisation of hospitals and reaction to epidemic diseases, not to mention coping with recurrent outbreaks of cholera and the endemic illnesses which were exacerbated by the living conditions of many of the urban populations. The middle years of the nineteenth century were a period of increasing centralisation in terms of the passing of legislation to regulate many aspects of life. Laws would be passed to regulate medical training and the subsequent supervision of doctors and their practice; towns would be obliged to institute regulations for the oversight and supervision of public health; individuals would be appointed as custodians of public health – the MOH would become a crucial figure in local government, but local government was, increasingly driven by, and answerable to, the all-powerful sphere of the state.

Once it began to be realised that creating and maintaining a healthy population could no longer be simply a process of reaction to adversity, but necessitated anticipation and permanent change, big government began to be involved in a big way. The Victorian period in Scotland, as in other parts of Great Britain, was shaped and characterised not so much by a developing sense of Scottishness or Britishness, but rather by a combination of factors which mainly affected the urban situation. The rapid growth of the industrial areas, the increasing importance of civic authority, the subsequent fostering of civic pride, the need to do things on a larger scale, the temperance movement, the self-help ethos, the voluntary principle, and perhaps other more amorphous factors, were all part of a complex set of attitudes which combined to produce the new phenomenon of the large, industrialising Scottish Victorian town. One of the main planks of Scottishness, the presbyterian kirk and all it stood for, finally broke down, at least in terms of its role as the all-encompassing state church, with the Disruption of 1843. The results of this event were equally complex and far-reaching in secular as well as in religious terms. The so-called protestant work ethic, coupled with the apparently dour and sober nature of presbyterianism, may have produced a hardworking but fatalistic population, but society was changing. The urban situation had not only produced medical problems; social problems were equally pressing, and exacerbated by unemployment and poor nutrition as well as overcrowding and bad working conditions for those fortunate enough to find work. A few more individuals were enfranchised in 1832, following a period of increasingly loud political protest, in the inaptly named Great Reform Act; the importance of this and other reforms, though, was not in the initial, relatively low numbers involved, but in the fact that any change had taken place at all. A few hundred extra voters in 1832 paved the way, however haltingly, for the eventual advent of universal franchise, which would not be achieved for almost another century, and considerably longer for women.

What seems to have been happening in Scotland in the first half of the nineteenth century was a redefinition and reinforcement of the increasingly stark contrasts between the urban and rural parts of the country – which itself had effects on the shaping of the nation and its identity. What was taking place during the eighteenth and early nineteenth centuries was a blurring of the distinctions between highland and lowland, and urban and rural. The considerable and ongoing redistribution of the demographic map of Scotland during the eighteenth century, helped in the nineteenth by the expansion of the rail network, not to mention the lack of war on the British mainland, had perhaps meant for the first and only time that Scots had the opportunity to experience something of a common experience. That is not to claim that the highland identity or way of life had gone entirely, or that the rural lowlands were just like the rural highlands. What does seem to have been the case, though, is that even with the rapid urbanisation and industrialisation processes which were underway for much of the eighteenth century, the nation was brought together to a greater degree than before or since. By the middle decades of the nineteenth century the highland/lowland and urban/rural differences were once more re-emphasised, as the large cities became even larger and even more industrialised. The close ties of industry with the local countryside began to be loosened, and since that time it is possible to claim that Scotland has been divided physically and economically once more.

These characteristics can certainly be seen in the realms of Scottish medicine. The later part of the seventeenth century and all of the eighteenth century may be seen as a period of transition. During this time professional medicine and professional medical and surgical training developed fairly rapidly. The knowledge upon which the training was based may not have changed greatly, but by the end of the eighteenth century medical training in universities and the medical and surgical colleges was on a relatively sounder footing. Standards were set and curricula defined, although their enforcement and consistency are difficult to establish with any degree of confidence. The quality of the teaching and, indeed, of the graduates, was difficult to assess, but none the less medical and surgical training were much more organised and controlled. The Medical Act of 1858 would close one chapter in the long history of the professionalisation of medicine, and at the same time start another, in terms of the organisation, supervision and progress of medicine on a nationwide standard rather than by a proliferation of local standards and qualifications. The increasing influence of big government would continue to affect medicine and medical training for the rest of the millennium and beyond. However, that is not to say that big government itself was better organised or controlled. Measures such as the Medical Act owed their final shape and contents in large part to political bargaining and in-fighting in the manner of politics for several centuries. Party politics in the modern sense was in its early stages of development, and to that extent big government continued to operate on less than solid foundations.

This combination of factors created the circumstances in the early decades of the nineteenth century which stimulated corporate involvement in the health of the people. In the industrialising cities, particularly Glasgow, conditions could no longer be ignored, and could no longer be dealt with purely at a local level. The motivations for intervention may not always have been the most altruistic, but at least some consideration was being given to the circumstances and health of the industrial working population. Just as Victorian society was characterised by the twin strands of government intervention and philanthropic activities, so progress in medical care and public health was affected by these same factors. A more revisionist perspective, though, characterises the role of central government as enabling rather than enforcing, and claims that many of the legislative measures came about as a result of change, rather than being the cause of it. What was enabled was not so much government intervention as a combination of central and local legislation, combined with an important philanthropic and voluntary aspect.[9] It is claimed that for much of the Victorian period there was a broad framework of increasingly active central government, but one which enabled the localities to act independently and the voluntary sector to continue to operate – described as 'firmly governing an unequal but stable society through a process of negotiation among the major social factions'.[10] By the outbreak of the First World War, though, this system had become pressurised and would be forced to change. Industrial magnates and entrepreneurs perhaps had the most selfish of motives behind the drive towards improving the health of the industrial workforce. They wished to make profits, and could only do so if the workers were capable of working at full capacity. A sickly workforce, as a sickly army, could do little good for the general health of the nation. Similarly, the motives of central government may be cast in a rather less than wholeheartedly altruistic light. Just as individual industrial giants looked to their profits, so government looked to status in the Empire and a healthy balance of payments.

There is, though, evidence that although central government was increasingly active, voluntaryism was still a major – and often essential – feature of the broad sphere and social construction of public medicine. Voluntary hospitals, voluntary societies, charitable organisations and the church (which in Scotland had responsibility for poor relief) all continued to contribute to the 'central fund' of medical and health provision. If, as the more revisionist view would claim, the function of government was more to enable than enforce, then it is not surprising that continuation of the activities of a plethora of voluntary agencies would be a key element. For example, the new Scottish Poor Law Act of 1845 made it more difficult for individuals to meet urban residency requirements for the receipt of relief, and this made charitable organisations even more essential.[11]

At a more individual level, however, people like William Pultney Alison, Thomas Chalmers and Edwin Chadwick demonstrated genuine concern for the condition of industrial society. The solutions they proposed may have differed in some cases, particularly that of Thomas Chalmers, who was very much of the 'charity' school, but they clearly had an impact on government policy and actions. Alison's view was that poverty was the root cause of disease, and was strongly of the view that alleviation of poverty would go far in dealing with the problems of endemic disease. Reform of the Poor Law, for Alison, was the key to change. Chadwick, on the other hand, as a miasmatist, favoured large-scale sanitary improvement schemes. Probably both approaches would have been effective to some degree, but public disagreements could produce hesitancy on the part of those who had the power to implement measures.

PUBLIC HEALTH – THE PROBLEM OF POVERTY

From earliest times there had been some sort of provision of medical treatment for the poorest members of society. Under the Old Scottish Poor Law, which was not replaced until 1845, relief of poverty in general, as well as help with medical treatment in particular, was the province of the kirk and the local parish. This meant that circumstances varied greatly according to geography, degree of urbanisation and economic status. Extra help may have been provided in times of epidemic or other natural disaster, but it was rarely possible to do much more than provide for the most basic of medical treatments. At the start of the period covered by this chapter, then, medical treatment for the poor was funded either by the kirk session or at times by the town council. Larger towns appointed medical staff specifically to treat the poor gratis, and in Glasgow and Edinburgh the major medical and surgical institutions offered free dispensary provision and medical treatment for the poor. The question of admission to hospitals, though, was more problematic, as patients seeking admission required sponsorship, and hospitals were reluctant to admit accident cases, or patients whose prospects of survival or recovery were remote. Statistics were just as important then as now.

By the start of the Victorian period, a number of factors were coalescing within the sphere of public debate which would lead eventually to reform of legislation in Scotland, some years after similar steps had been taken for England. The aftermath of the Napoleonic wars, which ended in 1815, was, by the 1830s, very clear. The war had ended during a period of economic downturn; many demobilised soldiers could not find work; unemployment was rising rapidly; and consequently the problem of poverty, particularly urban poverty, was pressing. The fragmentation of the state church was continuing, and by 1843 it could hardly be said to represent the majority, let alone all of the population. It became increasingly difficult for the 'parish state' to function in a secular sense, particularly in areas such as poor relief, when many of the poor by that time did not adhere to the state church. The secularisation of the parish in administrative terms was becoming inevitable, but the question was in what form the secular parish should operate in these areas.

There were considerable problems in Scotland in providing comprehensive care for the poor. Rural poverty was considerable, particularly in the highland areas and especially in the time of the potato famine of 1845, not to mention the severe economic depression of the early 1840s. The poor relief system in Scotland was based on shaky foundations in comparison to that in England, where a compulsory levy was in operation. Also, the system of Poor Law unions in England could not be reciprocated in Scotland, where the traditional boundaries between parishes meant that co-operation on a large scale was not possible.[12]

Although the question of reform of the Poor Law began with rumblings south of the border against the English Poor Law, the debate in Scotland was stimulated as early as 1815 by a questionnaire issued by Thomas Kennedy of Dunure, a lawyer and would-be MP, enquiring about the nature and levels of support given to the poor by individual parishes. The Kirk then set up various committees and the debate became more and more heated but still centred on opposition to the poor, or at least to the undeserving poor. Added to this were the contributions of key individuals (yet again the familiar combination of general debate and stimulation by the individual within the particular sphere of debate). There is no room here to enter into great detail of the work and influence of Thomas Chalmers, who was resolutely opposed to statutory provision for the poor, or of Kennedy, who brought many bills before parliament, but suffice it to say that by 1830 the arguments over poor relief were very much in the public, political, religious and medical spheres.[13] By that time Scotland had been transformed, or was in the process of being transformed, from an agricultural to an industrial society; and from a society structured on a hierarchy of rank with the remnants of two-way dependence or responsibility, to the class structure which is still in place. By 1840 the old parish structure simply could not cope, and the publicity of poverty brought about by royal commissions and the work of Chadwick and others was to some extent the result of change as much as the proponent of change.

Finally, the sphere of debate on poor relief was entered by W. P. Alison, who set forth stridently his views on the inadequacies of current measures to relieve destitution. To some extent the methods used by Alison to propound his views can be seen as old-fashioned. He published pamphlets. Ever since the advent of easier access to the printing press in Scotland, dissidents of all sorts had utilised the medium to great effect. By the end of the eighteenth century newspapers and magazines were also widely available. The tit-for-tat of the pamphlet exchange still apparently had some currency, and it was largely by this means that the Alison debate raged.

In the medical arena itself, matters were also hotting up. Medical schools were by this time operating in Edinburgh, Glasgow and Aberdeen and, to a lesser extent in St Andrews, not to mention the firmly established extra-mural medical schools in Edinburgh and Glasgow. These institutions were providing more and apparently better-qualified doctors, but the politics of public medicine tended to be focused more within the medical and surgical institutions to which these medical graduates might proceed. Nineteenth-century medical politics, when it applied to practice rather than education, seems to have been influenced more by the colleges, which were at the same time heavily involved in the politics of medical education and its reform – a parallel problem dealt with elsewhere in this chapter. All of these factors came to a head with the severe economic depression of the early 1840s, which proved finally that some sort of legislation and central planning was unavoidable as the rickety old structures could no longer support an increasingly intolerable burden.

Once the new Poor Law entered the statute book in 1845, care of the poor was, at least in terms of central control and legislation, secularised, though the 'parish' remained the focus of organisation. Parochial boards were set up to oversee parish relief, and this relief of necessity involved medical and surgical care to a degree. Overseeing the parochial boards was the Board of Supervision, based in Edinburgh, and, from 1894, the Local Government Board for Scotland. The influence of the Board was such that by 1894, some sort of basic medical provision was offered by all parishes, whereas this had been the case in fewer than half of the parishes at the time of the Board's inception in 1845.[14] The report of the Royal

Commission on the Poor Law which reported in 1844 showed that less than half of the parishes provided medical relief, though the problem was not the lack of doctors, as most of the remotest areas did have a doctor within reasonable reach. As expected, the large cities had the better provision, with, for example, no less than seventeen district medical officers in Glasgow, together with the Town's Hospital and active medical charities.

Once the Poor Law Amendment (Scotland) Act came into effect in 1845, the next half-century saw considerable improvement in the provision of medical relief to the poor in most areas of the country. Although responsibility for implementation of the Act was locally devolved, the central Board of Supervision proved to be relatively efficient in its supervisory and enforcing role. Among the dictates it issued were that parishes should introduce measures to provide emergency medical help, by the appointment of suitable medical practitioners; that rules for medical relief should be observed; that poor houses should provide medical treatment; that there should be trained nurses in poor houses; and that lodgings should be provided for those who were both sick and homeless. (This is reminiscent of the remit of the Glasgow Town's Hospital in the eighteenth century.) The Board also had increased powers to act during epidemics such as cholera. For example, the parish of Methilhill in Fife failed to act on cholera regulations in 1866, and was then the victim of a severe attack of the disease, following which the Board appointed no less a figure than Dr Henry Littlejohn to enquire into the situation.[15]

The Board concerned itself also with matters of poor law hospitals, trained nurses and medical staff (the latter regulated even more closely following the Medical Act of 1858), and this meant that by 1894, when responsibility passed to the new body, the Local Government Board, and responsibility for implementation lay with elected parish councils, systems were in place in all parts of Scotland. These systems were by no means perfect and indeed the state of medical knowledge was not yet advanced enough to provide very different medical or surgical treatment. The setting up of the Board, and its attitudes and influences, had themselves been influenced by changing attitudes towards the causes of poverty, the causes of disease, the extent to which self-help was possible, and the role and responsibilities of central government as opposed to the individual or the locality.[16]

It cannot be claimed, though, that formal provision of poor law medical care had a significant effect on the decline in overall mortality statistics which was a feature of the period. Recent research has indicated that the balance between medical and surgical cases in both voluntary and poor law hospitals became skewed heavily towards surgical cases, whereas the reduction in mortality rates was due to a much greater extent to decline in deaths from respiratory diseases.[17] There is also evidence to confirm that in Glasgow at least, entry to hospital still depended on family and employment connections, so that again the effects of hospitals on improving the health of the sick poor were restricted, though cannot be ignored. Improvements in general health were the result of a combination of factors and influences, and the availability of hospitals was undoubtedly one of these, but by not means the only factor.[18]

HOSPITALS – THE NEW FOCUS OF MEDICAL ADVANCE?

Although there had been hospitals in Scotland in some form from the medieval period, and although the origins of the large voluntary hospitals were in the Enlightenment period, it does seem that as the nineteenth century progressed, the hospital became increasingly important as the focus of professional medicine and surgery, medical and surgical training, and developments in the technology of medicine. The hospital doctor emerged as the élite of the profession, and whereas the great majority of doctors still practised as general practitioners, the focus of prestige, funding, advances and clinical developments was more and more the hospital, and more and more the large voluntary establishment. As with many things, the original purpose of these foundations had been a combination of necessity, socio-economic pressure and charitable intent, by the mid-nineteenth century the hospital was becoming something rather different.

As the Victorian period moved inexorably on into Empire and then successive wars on foreign battlefields, Scotland itself became more and more heavily industrialised, and the contrast between town and country sharpened. In the larger urban centres, the voluntary hospitals became a vital part of the delivery of medical care. They tended to flourish in areas where there were centres of medical education, particularly Edinburgh (1729, 1741), and later Aberdeen (1742) and Glasgow (1794). Together with some local general hospitals funded by local authorities, and the poor houses and workhouses, these ensured that some rudimentary hospital care was available to most, except in the furthest corners of the country, where domiciliary medicine remained the norm for the majority of the population, unless circumstances – and the willingness of a subscriber – allowed complicated cases to be referred to the larger centres. The rationale behind the voluntary hospital movement was complex. It was not just charitable intention; it was not just the need for a fitter workforce and armed services; it was not just the wish of élite physicians and surgeons; it was not just the prevailing ethos of self-help and middle-class values. It was an intricate combination of all of these factors. In some areas of Scotland, it was clearly industrial necessity which was the major driving force. In less industrialised areas it may have been ambitious medical men who sought the prestige attendant on a hospital post. Whatever the case, and however inadequate their provision, the voluntary hospitals lasted until they were transferred to central authority in 1948, and provided a core element in the confirmation of the hospital as the focus of acute medicine and surgery. Statistics show that in Scotland between 1871 and 1938, the voluntary hospitals provided between 0.5 and 1.2 beds per 1000 of the population, and between 2.5 and 19.2 in-patients per thousand persons. These figures may seem at first sight less than impressive, but the trend was upwards.[19]

It was not just large general hospitals which began to appear in this phase of Scotland's health care development. In the second half of the nineteenth century specialist dental hospitals appeared in Edinburgh and Glasgow, together with London, Leeds, Manchester and other larger English towns. The Edinburgh Dental Hospital was established in 1879. As with many similar instances, it took the combined influences of individual ambition and educational improvements to bring about the change. In this case the individual concerned was John Smith, an Edinburgh medical and surgical graduate, who introduced a course of lectures on 'Physiology and Diseases of the Teeth', at Surgeons' Hall in 1856, a time when Syme, Lister and other famous men were at work in Edinburgh. He was not the first to do this – James Rae had provided a similar service in the 1770s. The important connection between theory and practice took place in 1857, when Smith gained an appointment as surgeon dentist to the Royal Public Dispensary. Some years later he tried to interest the Royal College of Surgeons in trying to provide better dental education than by means of the apprenticeship system currently in operation, but without much initial success, and Smith branched out on his own, setting up the Edinburgh Dental Dispensary in 1860. Dentistry was not covered by the Medical Act of 1858 (see below) and the only available qualification was a licence from the Royal College of Surgeons of England. Gradually, and supported by articles in the medical press, and in the light of the provisions for medicine made in the Medical Act, moves towards similar standardisation for dentistry were made, and in 1878 the Dentists Act allowed for much more rapid progress to be made in formalising dental education and examinations. Examinations were arranged by the various colleges, including the Royal College of Surgeons of Edinburgh, and it was clear that there was an urgent need for a dental hospital as part of the overall package of dental education, and the Dental Dispensary was absorbed into the new Dental Hospital. Thus dental education in Edinburgh acquired status and would thenceforth develop academically on the same lines as medicine and surgery. The Glasgow Dental Hospital followed suit and offered similar treatment to patients, together with training for the Licentiate in Dental Surgery of the Glasgow College and subsequently for the university degree in dentistry.

In line with trends which have been identified from the later eighteenth century, not only did dental education begin to become more standardised and reliable, but the qualified dentists felt the need to have an organisation. In some ways the Royal Odonto-Chirurgical Society of Scotland had much in common with the Edinburgh clubs of the Enlightenment period. It was a medical society[20] rather than a professional institution, formed by a group of dentists who wished to further their profession intellectually and, importantly, to encourage the practice of 'ethical dentistry' rather than the previous 'elasticity of ethics' which had allowed a variety of quacks and charlatans to operate relatively freely.[21] Founded in 1867, the members met regularly, heard scientific papers and subscribed to dental journals. Among the topics on which lectures were delivered were 'mechanical dentistry with spiral springs', 'conservative treatment of exposed pulp', 'case of sarcoma of the lower jaw', and, a lecture very peculiarly Scottish, on 'the effects of bagpipe playing on the teeth', delivered by Mr W. Bowman Macleod in March 1890. There is also confirmation that the dentists were considering and applying new developments. Lectures were given on 'nitrous oxide gas' (1868), 'inhalation of gas and ether' (1898) and 'micro-organisms of the mouth and their relationship with disease' (1883). More practical evidence comes also from the minutes of a meeting of the Society held on 13 March 1869, at which 'Mr Visick (of Berwick on Tweed) exhibited the nitrous oxide gas in two cases, both of which were successful'.[22]

It was not just dental hospitals that emerged in this period of specialisation, though. A number of other specialist establishments were founded, including mental hospitals, children's hospitals and cancer hospitals. The Royal Hospital for Sick Children in Edinburgh opened in 1860, followed by a similar institution in Glasgow in 1883. Maternity hospitals had been one of the first separate institutions or separate wards within larger hospitals. The Lying-in hospital was established in Edinburgh in 1791, while specialist units dealing with eye diseases appeared in Glasgow and Edinburgh in 1824 and 1834 respectively. Many of these developments were very much in line with national and international trends but also in tune with the general outlook of Victorian medicine and society where, as Porter states aptly, specialisation 'combined the scientific, the institutional and the therapeutic'.[23] A children's hospital had opened in Paris as early as 1802, and the National Hospital for Sick Children at Great Ormond Street in London dates from1852.[24] The implication is that the progress of specialisation in Scotland was similar to that in operation elsewhere. Here Scottish medicine may have become a follower rather than a leader, but none the less was, in spite of the small size of the nation, keeping up with the international medical view. On the periphery of the prevailing orthodoxy were homeopathic hospitals, one of which was established in Glasgow in this period.

As well as a proliferation of hospitals of all sorts and covering many specialties, this period also saw a trend towards the hospital providing laboratory services, such as pathology. This meant that not only were facilities available to diagnose and treat, but also to research and to offer a twin focus of traditional hospital services and the application of new science. This is a move which would prove to be more and more important, especially in the twentieth century, when medicine is in large part influenced by the laboratory as much as by the clinical consultation.[25]

ANAESTHESIA

Most observers would not hesitate to cite the twin developments of anaesthetics and antiseptics as two of the crowning achievements of nineteenth-century Scottish medical men. There is no doubt whatsoever that until it was possible to operate on an unconscious patient and to ensure that post-operative infection could be controlled, no matter how high were the aims, no matter how well-organised the profession, no matter how much effort was made to develop surgical techniques, medicine and surgery would remain stagnant in practice, if not in theory. Surgery in particular could not progress beyond the 'putting back together' stage, or the rapid amputation of a limb which had considerable potential to be saved, were it not for the few seconds allowed to the surgeons. The possibilities afforded by time meant that some eponymous surgical procedures developed at this time were so successful that they are still performed today. Syme's amputation of the foot is one of these.[26]

For as long as surgeons had been attempting to treat patients by manipulation, excision, ablation or trepanning, there had been endeavours to dull the senses of the patients to try at least to offer some prospect of pain relief. Just as herbs and plants were used as the main ingredients of medicines, so various concoctions, fortified with some alcoholic content, were used to render the patient as close to oblivion as it was possible to get. However knowledgeable surgeons might become, and despite the best efforts of the great men of the eighteenth century to elucidate the structures and workings of the body, no real progress could be made until means were acquired whereby the patient could be rendered unconscious. Matters did not change greatly until the middle of the nineteenth century, and again Scotland was at the forefront.[27] Whatever the reasons, the major development, and one which was pioneered, in perhaps a less than scientific manner, was the elucidation of the anaesthetising properties of chloroform by Edinburgh obstetrician James Young Simpson. When he and some of his friends found themselves rendered insensible and 'under the mahogany' of his drawing room table in Edinburgh in 1847, it had not been Simpson's prime purpose to seek out a universal anaesthetic for surgical procedures. He was an obstetrician and his primary aim was to try to find some means by which the pain of childbirth could be alleviated.

There was some competition at this time from other techniques for dulling the senses, though, and for some time mesmerism was a serious competitor to chemical agents of anaesthesia. Just as nowadays operations are performed, apparently painlessly, under hypnosis or acupuncture, so mesmerism – a subject of great general interest – was considered to be potentially very useful. The debate over the introduction of anaesthesia was set in the context of the need to change attitudes towards pain. With hindsight it seems surprising that any method of relieving pain during surgery would not have been seized on enthusiastically, but the alleviation of this sort of pain had not been a priority in the medical world. The acceptance of any form of general surgical anaesthesia required a change in this outlook, and it may be that the controversies surrounding mesmerism stimulated debate on the whole question of anaesthesia as a means of relieving pain as well as improving surgical techniques. Whatever the case, in the 1840s, mesmeric anaesthetics provided an alternative to chemically induced insensibility, and this was an important aspect of the pain relief discourse. The technique was used in many areas of society, as entertainment as much as pain relief, but should be noted here as an important part of the social as well as medical context of the time.[28]

There is some controversy about just when and where the very first anaesthetic was administered in Britain, and, perhaps surprisingly, Dumfries in the rural south-west of Scotland makes a strong claim. The first successful use of ether appears to have occurred in America, when a dentist, William Morton, anaesthetised a patient at the Massachusetts General Hospital on 16 October 1846. This was followed, apparently, by similar procedures undertaken in London in December of that year. The second of these, on 21 December, was an amputation performed by Robert Liston, another surgeon with strong Scottish connections. However, a rival claim to be the British first came from Dumfries where, it is claimed, Dr William Scott, surgeon, 'operated on a patient whom he had anaesthetized with the vapour of sulphuric ether'.[29] An event of note in the world of veterinary anaesthetics seems to have taken place in Dumfries around the same time, as the local press noted that in March 1847, 'ether was applied to a vicious horse ... whilst about to be shod, an operation which it had been found impossible to perform otherwise'.[30]

As with a number of elements of the construction of Scottish medicine and society through the centuries, though, it took the patronage of the monarch – this time in the most practical of ways – to stimulate further progress. James IV had pulled teeth, and had granted the Incorporation of Surgeons of Edinburgh its first charter; Mary, Queen of Scots gave Scots surgeons permanent exemption from bearing arms or sitting on juries; James VII, before his accession, had patronised the Edinburgh physicians and the intellectual culture of Edinburgh in general. However, it fell to Queen Victoria to stimulate perhaps the most important step in the history of medicine in the nineteenth century. When it became known that the Queen had accepted the administration of chloroform (considered a better and more controllable agent than ether) to deal with the pain attendant on the birth of her eighth child, controversy reigned but progress was made, very slowly indeed, towards the acceptance of what was regarded as alien – alteration of consciousness by unnatural means. It was muttered darkly – probably mostly by men – that this sort of thing was bound to bring down the wrath of God.

Anaesthetics were not greeted with universal approbation. Even in the 1840s long-held beliefs and practices could not be changed easily. This was particularly the case with regard to anaesthetic support to women in labour. There was considerable opposition to the artificial easing of what was regarded as a primary and natural function – 'in sorrow shalt thou bring forth children'. It is claimed that had it not been for the willingness of Queen Victoria to make use of chloroform during the birth of her last two children, it would have taken a great deal longer for anaesthesia to be accepted in obstetrics at least. With the more subjective view of hindsight, it is easy to ridicule or express surprise at the apparent reluctance to adopt new procedures, artificial aids or other means to interfere with the natural reaction of the body to pain or disease. This, though, is to do an injustice to the people of the time, who held beliefs sincerely and had to adapt to very new views of the relationship between disease and its cure or palliative treatment. Reluctance to accept anaesthesia was not just a matter of Victorian stoicism or a desire to appear impervious to pain. In an account of developments in medicine and surgery in the Victorian period Youngson describes the period as one of resistance to new ideas and innovations. His chapters are tellingly entitled 'The *fight* for chloroform', 'The *fight* for antisepsis' (though antisepsis was accepted much more rapidly than anaesthesia) and 'The *fight* for new ideas' (my italics).[31] This aptly describes the very significant dichotomy which seems to have characterised this period. On the one hand there was the recognition on the part of big government and the practitioners themselves that the profession had to be more regulated, and that matters of public health were the province of a pro-active attitude and actions. On the other hand, there was often deeply entrenched opposition to progress in terms of radical change in the ways in which medicine and surgery were practised. It was felt by some surgeons that operating on anaesthetised patients somehow emasculated their work. They had prided themselves for centuries on their surgical speed; now they could slow down and perform more complex surgery, but this had to be rationalised – slowly – by the surgeons, who had to rethink their approach and methods, and accept that speed was not the only criterion of surgical greatness.

The important thing here for any account of Scottish medicine and its influence, though, is that, once again, the widespread use of a procedure evolved from much more narrow intentions at the start. Simpson was not looking for an anaesthetic which could be used in all sorts of surgical procedures; he was, rather, concentrating on his medical specialty and trying to advance that. The modern equivalent is, perhaps, the epidural anaesthetic, used widely in labour but also increasingly in a wide range of surgical procedures. Chloroform is no longer administered, and the side-effects of modern short-acting anaesthetics are much less. Despite the best intentions of the postmodernist or post-structuralist, it is difficult to deny a direct connection between chloroform and modern, complex surgical procedures. For his own part, Simpson was acting very much in the Scots tradition of broad education, broad interests and a keen spirit of enquiry.

ANTISEPTICS – CARBOLIC AND ITS LEGACY, OR THE SANITISATION OF MEDICINE AND SURGERY

In conjunction with the opportunities afforded by the introduction and very gradual acceptance of anaesthesia, the other 'A', and equally important 'A' of antiseptics evolved in the growth spurt of medicine in the prolific Victorian period, though the second 'A' perhaps took longer to gain general credence than the first. Once again, the area of obstetrics and childbirth played a significant part here. It is, perhaps, ironic that two of the major forces towards modern medicine had their shared origins in the sphere of women's natural and necessary functions. Although

Joseph Lister, an Englishman, following in the footsteps of Pasteur was, for Scotland, the pioneer, the important work carried out by Semmelweiss in his attempts to reduce the appalling consequences of childbed fever, must be seen as crucial, if at a distance from Scotland.[32]

It was all very well to discover how to make patients unconscious so that they could tolerate increasingly complex surgical procedures. It was quite another matter, though, to ensure that, providing they had survived the anaesthetic and the surgery, they would not die subsequently as a result of overwhelming systemic infection brought about by the still primitive and less than clean hospital or home environment. A major problem here, and one which affected public health in its widest sense, was that the processes by which infection was acquired and transmitted were not understood. As discussed above, by the early Victorian period, beliefs had evolved into two opposing explanatory theories: the contagion theory and the miasma theory. Each of these, if correct, would require different measures for its control. It is not difficult, therefore, to see why progress in this area was so slow. The contagion theory rested on the assumption that direct contact with a source of infection would result in rapid transmission and proliferation of the infecting agent. The treatment, quite obviously, would be to keep infected patients and infected material away from the non-infected. In other words, isolation and quarantine were the main pillars of treatment and prevention. However, the rival miasma theory postulated that infection came about because of the general miasma of poisonous particles in the atmosphere. The atmosphere was everywhere, thus the isolation of individuals could do little to control the situation. The answer here was to improve the quality of the environment in general.

If the miasma theory were correct, then the fact that surgeons continued to operate in their outdoor clothes and did not trouble to wash their hands before or after surgery, or following post-mortem examinations, was not such a primary cause for concern. On the other hand, if the contagion theory were proved correct, then it was perfectly clear that individual as well as corporate cleanliness was more than desirable.

Just as in the case of anaesthetics, the first major steps were taken in the area of obstetrics, and not by a Scot, but by the Hungarian physician Ignaz Semmelweiss (1818–65). He was concerned at the high incidence of childbed fever among his patients and, suspecting cross-infection, attempted to evaluate this by stipulating that students and physicians should wash their hands after examining each patient.[33] This simple measure resulted in substantial reductions in the incidence of childbed fever and, consequently, in the maternal and neonatal death rates. Not surprisingly, Semmelweiss was regarded with a high degree of scorn by his colleagues but would ultimately be proved to be correct. Important also in this area was the microscopic work carried out by Louis Pasteur (1822–95), in relation to germ theory and the agents of infection, particularly anaerobic bacteria. He strongly advised the boiling of surgical instruments as a means of reducing bacterial infection during surgery.

Once again, Scotland seemed to require an individual pioneer to take an individual step against the general background of a clear need for change yet no agreement as to how that change should be implemented. A Quaker, Joseph Lister (1827–1912), trained in London where, perhaps not surprisingly, many of his teachers at University College Medical School were Scots. After graduation he migrated to Scotland, eventually acquiring the Regius Chair of Surgery at the University of Glasgow in 1859, although the intractable friction between the medical institutions and the University meant that he had to wait until 1861 before being allocated any clinical beds at the Infirmary. Once there, the equally intractable problem of hospital-acquired infection became apparent to him, and he turned his attention to assessing the work of Pasteur. He concluded that a carbolic spray might be the solution to many of the problems which prevented patients surviving the more complex surgical procedures which were now possible. Things did not run altogether smoothly and Lister encountered the same sort of opposition that had been voiced against chloroform, against vaccination and against any major innovation which would artificially try to change nature, or at least the patient's experience of nature in all its forces. Eventually, though, refined versions of carbolic were accepted and death rates from hospitalism began to decline, not only in Scotland but gradually in many areas of Europe.[34] Even at the height of Empire, the Scottish medical profession could still influence and be influenced by events on the continent to which it had been 'attached' for several centuries. Lister went on to occupy the Chair of Clinical Surgery at the University of Edinburgh from 1869 to 1876 and at King's College, London, from 1877 to 1893. Lister himself described the results of his work with antiseptics in a number of surgical areas including compound fractures and abscesses, in his *On the Antiseptic Principle of the Practice of Surgery* (1867), and noted, with a hint of pride that:

> Previously to its [carbolic] introduction the two large wards in which most of my cases of accident and of operation are treated were among the unhealthiest in the whole surgical division of the Glasgow Royal Infirmary ... But since the antiseptic treatment has been brought into full operation, and wounds and abscesses no longer poison the atmosphere with putrid exhalations, my wards, though in other respects under precisely the same circumstances as before, have completely changed their character; so that during the last nine months not a single instance of pyaemia, hospital gangrene, or erysipelas has occurred in them.[35]

Among the surgical procedures which could be performed and survived by the end of the nineteenth century, aided by the combined benefits of anaesthesia and antiseptics were lithotomy (a procedure which had been shunned by earlier surgeons), ovariotomy, fistula surgery, hysterectomy and even attempts to deal with aortic aneurysm. None of this would have been possible without the combination of influences delineated in this chapter: rise of hospitals; problems in hospitals; rise of government; and the key contributions of individuals. Although it can be argued that medicine in Britain could not be characterised by reference to specific parts of the multiple kingdom, it does appear that the Scots, or those who worked in Scotland, were still well to the fore.

As with many individual contributions to medicine and medical progress, the historiography has entered a revisionist phase, and a substantial body of more recent work has begun to question the extent to which Lister was the major pioneer or enabler of antisepsis. The new consensus appears to be that while Lister certainly made a contribution, three major factors should be emphasised. Firstly, it seems clear that his own views on germ theory and the principles of antisepsis changed over time, so that his views in the 1880s were rather different from what they had been in the 1860s. Secondly, his was by no means the only available antiseptic procedure. Thirdly, it is claimed that most of those who adopted or adapted Lister's antiseptic techniques did so because they agreed with the practical methods and did not consider the theoretical basis too extensively.[36] Whether or not Lister's contribution has been overplayed, there is no doubt that he was one of the key figures in the adoption of antiseptic methods in hospitals. In terms of the discourse of the time, he was but one of many voices giving opinions on the nature and course of disease and sepsis. The clamour may have been unorchestrated or unfocused but it was certainly part of the complex web of influences which characterised Victorian medicine in Scotland as elsewhere. In addition, it has been claimed that much of the credit for reduction in infection and sepsis should be given to better levels of nutrition in the population.[37] Whatever the case, the work of Lister and others did a great deal in the cause of antisepsis, asepsis and the ability to prevent or survive infection caused by childbirth, surgery or poor conditions in hospitals. Before Lister, surgery may have been initially successful, but all too often the patients succumbed to overwhelming infection very soon afterwards.

MENTAL HEALTH – COPING WITH THE INSANE OR MENTALLY ILL

As noted in the previous chapter, attitudes towards the care and treatment of the mentally ill were changing. By the end of the eighteenth century, the separation and isolation of those suffering from mental impairment or illness was becoming the norm. The reasons for this were complex, and the situation was affected by the ongoing process of socio-economic, cultural and religious redefinition and realignment of the country. By the 1830s the effects of the class structure, of urbanisation, industrialisation and perhaps most of all the growing strength of the middle class meant that abnormal behaviour was an embarrassment to sane society.

In parallel to this, the medical profession's view of mental illness was also changing. For centuries the mentally ill or mentally deficient had not been treated all that differently, and the sorts of treatments given, particularly in the long heyday of humoral medicine, were very similar to those given for organic disease. By the early years of the Victorian period, medical philosophy had changed to the extent that it was apparent that diseases of the mind could not be treated in the same manner as diseases of the body. The early origins of the psychiatric profession are difficult to establish, and again the eclectic combination of changing discourse, changing socio-economic situation, new class structures, medical advances and the catalyst of the individual resulted in the increasing separation from society of those deemed unfit to belong to it, for whatever reason. By the middle of the nineteenth century the asylum was regarded as the best method of separating and treating affected individuals. One of the earlier and most important of these institutions was the Crichton Royal Hospital, opened in Dumfries in 1839, with the aim of providing humane treatment for its inmates.

In keeping with the developing Enlightenment trend towards the gathering of statistics and the growing imposition of frameworks of health enforcement and classification, the Lunacy Act of 1857 specified that insane patients should be certified. The certificate was to be issued by two doctors, accompanied by a petition from either relatives of the patient or the Inspector of the Poor in the case of paupers. The Lunacy Act also stipulated that each district in Scotland had to provide an asylum for pauper lunatics, and one such institution was the Fife and Kinross District Asylum, which opened its doors in 1857. A recent study of the inmates of this institution between 1874 and 1899 confirms trends which had been identified elsewhere, in that the numbers of admissions rose steadily, and the sex distribution of the inmates was roughly equal.

However, what was also clear from the study was that most of the inmates, though poor, had been in some sort of employment and, contrary to assumptions, were not destitute or admitted merely to rid the area of a problem of vagrants.[38]

The major symptoms demonstrated by patients at Kinross and elsewhere were those of delusions, hallucinations and general paralysis of the insane. Although it is problematic to try to relate these to modern diagnoses, the major afflictions seem to have been schizophrenia, affective illness, some sort of organic disease which produced symptoms of mental illness, or a multiplicity of neuroses. Some insight into the treatments given to patients in these institutions comes from the work of Thomas Clouston, one of the giants of Victorian mental health medicine. At his asylum in Edinburgh, Clouston considered that 'the treatment of mental disease is in many cases a fight against morbid, unsocial ways, degraded tendencies, and idle, selfish, listless, uninterested habits of mind, and we fight these by moral means, by employment, amusement, good food, fresh air, exercise, and good hygienic conditions of life'.[39]

This attitude is very much of its time, let alone its medical time. It encapsulates the core of Victorian views and confirms that at whatever stage, in whatever period, the state of medicine and medical opinion could not be divorced from the discourse of the general context. Some treatments were available which had not been in earlier times, and a more 'moral' approach may have been taken, but none the less the aims and intentions were similar.[40] At the Clouston establishment and, most probably at many of the larger institutions, treatment involved a combination of electrical treatments, head blistering, diet and drugs, although Clouston is noted to have become rather less disposed to the use of drugs. Interestingly, though, among the substances which he did favour were *cannabis indica* and bromides, as well as paraldehyde and hyoscine.[41] In addition to Poor Law or other municipal provision, a number of private asylums were established, quite in line with the multi-faceted nature of medical provision, and boarding out in the community was a further, well-used, means of dealing with the insane.[42]

In many ways the advent of the asylum was inevitable, given the complex of attitudes and problems of the time. Whether or not there was a conscious or subconscious Foucauldian approach, the result was the same. It would take another century before treatment of the mentally ill was relocated in the community. In terms of the general thrust of this chapter and the explanation of medicine in Scotland in the Victorian period, the separation of treatment for the mentally ill can be seen as part of the evolution of medical specialties just as much as in the wider sphere of Victorian morals, industrialisation and middle-class attitudes.

It certainly fits into the ongoing push towards a legislated approach to health in all its aspects.

WAR AND THE MEDICINE AND SURGERY OF WAR

One of the major contributions which had been made by Scots for several centuries was in the area of military medicine and surgery. Scottish surgeons had long been at the forefront of the treatment of the consequences of violence – the major focus of much of the surgical treatment carried out prior to the advent of anaesthesia. This is not to claim any great level of sophistication of technique; what the surgeons developed was twofold: great speed and also considerable experience and expertise in the simplest forms of treatment of the casualties of war and other conflicts, including bloodfeud, duels and the possible victors in mortal combat. Scottish surgeons had enjoyed long and close relationships with successive monarchs and the armies of many countries. From Peter Lowe to George Ballingall and beyond, Scots had proved themselves to be 'experts' in the treatment of casualties from all sides in many wars at home and abroad. Although surgical possibilities were extremely limited, and nothing remotely time-consuming or sophisticated was possible, they were reputedly very good at what they did attempt. They also had to be fairly flexible and to adapt their procedures to the changes in the technology of violence, from the hand-propelled weapon to guns of various sorts and various levels of accuracy. The treatment of a gunshot wound often involved searching the wound for fragments of clothing as well as shot, and the more sophisticated the firearm, the more devastating could be its consequences.

A natural consequence was that, in the climate of increasing professionalisation and standardisation of training, military surgery became a special subject, and included in university teaching. In Edinburgh the first such post was set up in 1806, on the authorisation of George III, but with considerable resentment on the part of the University Senatus, which had not been consulted on the matter. The first incumbent, John Thomson (1765–1846), was succeeded in 1823 by the rather more famous George Ballingall (1780–1855), who held the post until 1855, after which military surgery was not treated as a special subject in the University. Ballingall made a considerable contribution to the theoretical and academic development of military surgery, and his *Outlines of Military Surgery*, first published in 1833, saw a number of subsequent editions. As noted several decades ago by Comrie, this work gave good evidence of the enduring limitations rather than the possibilities of military surgery, particularly in the area of abdominal wounds and their treatment. It was Ballingall's view that 'no man in his senses would think of enlarging the external wound, for the purpose of searching out and sewing up the wounded part of the gut'.[43] This sort of enterprise would have to await anaesthetics and antiseptics.

Scots were also influential in this period in the organisation of medicine and surgery in the armed forces themselves. Here, individuals such as Sir James McGrigor were instrumental in the development of the justly noted Royal Army Medical Corps,[44] while military medicine in Russia owed much to the efforts of Sir James Wylie, and it is claimed that during the nineteenth century the Indian Medical Service was 'full of Scots'.[45] The long tradition of Scots fighting abroad and offering medical services abroad continued, and would continue and develop just as long as conflict continued. Although by the twentieth century and the scourge of the Great War, military medical services were centralised and can perhaps no longer be characterised with any degree of Scottishness, Scots continued to operate in this area with distinction, in field hospitals on the Western Front or dealing with the physical and psychological aftermath of the conflict. Certainly the experience of the First World War influenced medical, surgical and organisational trends in the inter-war period, and also confirmed that general fitness levels in the population as a whole needed to be considered and improved. Although in many aspects of professionalised medicine women had been reduced to a peripheral role, a number of Scottish women were able to come to the fore during the First World War, when the Scottish Women's Medical Service was an important feature of medical and surgical care. A number of hospitals staffed by Scottish women were set up near theatres of war, and provided much needed medical help and expertise during the First World War. Among the more notable of these institutions were hospitals in France and Serbia.[46]

MEDICAL REFORM – STATE CONTROL OF TRAINING AND PRACTICE

During the 'state' phase of the history of medicine in Scotland (or, as put by Roy Porter, 'the enforcement of health'),[47] it was not just urban or national governments which began the progress of standardisation of legislation and measures to improve the general health of the population. In its own turn, the medical profession was greatly in need of under-going some sort of process of standardisation, or at least an attempt to ensure that physicians and surgeons would gain their licence to practice on the basis of some commonly agreed principles and courses of study.

This brought in a more British dimension to the shaping of medicine in Scotland – as it did in England. The problems were similar in both countries. In England the main conflict was between the medical colleges and the ever powerful Society of Apothecaries which, by means of its 1815 Act, had acquired sweeping supervisory powers over medical appointments and practice, and virtually excluded practitioners with Scottish qualifications from practising south of the border. In Scotland there was growing concern and friction between and among the medical and surgical organisations and the universities. Over the latter part of the eighteenth century and the early decades of the nineteenth, moves had taken place to try to deal with irregularities in the universities and to eliminate the possibility of students acquiring medical degrees on the basis of little or no resident or certified training programmes. The reputation of some of the major seats of learning, such as Edinburgh and St Andrews, had diminished since the hotbed days of the Enlightenment period. Politics and dynastic manipulation meant that what was being taught, or not taught, in these establishments was becoming increasingly inadequate for the period. A new century did not bring in its wake instant modernisation of medicine or of medical teaching. Outside the universities, the Scottish medical and surgical colleges were fighting their own territorial wars. The Edinburgh surgeons put forward proposals for there to be a single Royal College of Surgeons of Scotland, with the surgical facet of the Glasgow Faculty acting as a subordinate sub-office (this prospect being met with much resentment on the part of the Glasgow surgeons).[48] The Edinburgh physicians were hampered by their agreement in 1681 not to undertake the teaching or examining of medicine in their own right – perhaps a curious concession but one that was necessary in order for their campaign for a college to be finally successful. So there was, in effect, a collision course in the making between the universities and the colleges.

When faced with most sorts of difficulties, what governments tend to do is to set up a commission of enquiry, and the situation was no different here. The Royal Commission on the State of the Universities in Scotland was set up in 1828, and as a result efforts were made to provide good and consistent teaching in all aspects, including medicine. One of the more anomalous situations in Scotland was that the University of St Andrews continued to award externally examined medical degrees, despite the fact that there was no clinical teaching of any sort available at that university. Given the acceptance that clinical training was crucial to the preparatory experiences of potential physicians and surgeons, the advent of closer controls seems rather urgent. However, within the context and discourse of the period it was possible for the University of St Andrews to refer to its ancient constitution as ample justification for its continuing to award degrees in medicine.[49] Shortly after this, the medical and surgical colleges and institutions began to participate in national discussions regarding possible action to be taken to institute some sort of national controls. This would culminate in the milestone of the Medical Act of 1858, but much ground had to be covered before then.

Progress after the Royal Commission had completed its task would come very slowly and become more and more entangled in British politics, and there are alternative explanations as to why the push for medical reform occurred when it did and took the eventual form that it did. One view is that two different background factors combined to bring about change. One of these was the increasing knowledge of the structure and function of the body as deduced from morbid anatomy and pathology, which enabled more rapid advance in the sphere of science. If medicine and surgery were now able to be more and more scientific, the natural consequence was that medical and surgical education should be equally scientific and comprehensive. However, at the same time, the problem of the sheer proliferation of all sorts of qualified and partly qualified physicians and surgeons meant that if quackery and other peripheral or amateur practice were to be eliminated, then the core institutions must be themselves organised, supervised and standardised in order to justify their continuing and increasingly exclusive custody of both the knowledge and its transfer and application.[50] There were also the more diffuse and amorphous elements of public awareness, altruism and civic pride, not to mention the more collegiate stance taken by groups of practitioners, and the growing influence of medical societies.[51] However, given the general arrangements for governing Scotland by this time, the Scottish medical and surgical colleges and the universities were obliged to shift the focus of their discussions to London and, in particular, to the lobbies of the British parliament. The fate of medical education in Scotland and also the sorts of controls and regulations which might be imposed on Scottish practitioners would, to a considerable extent, be decided by the debating, manipulative and bargaining skills of self-interested Members of Parliament, not by the practitioners them-selves. It would depend to a considerable extent on, firstly, gaining the support of MPs and, importantly, the support of MPs who were highly regarded in Parliament and who were of sufficient national political weight to make a difference. The Edinburgh surgeons had some three centuries of practice in cultivating politicians, and this experience would prove to be of considerable assistance, though the 'London effect' meant that ambitions could not always be fully realised.

From the point of view of individuals in Scotland and England who were undergoing medical or surgical training at whatever institution they had chosen, their major priority was to ensure that, once qualified, their degree or diploma parchment would be a passport to practise in all areas of the country and overseas. Edinburgh surgeons had served on eighteenth-century slave ships as well as in the armed forces of various countries. The East India Company was a lucrative source of medical employment. More recently, the various versions of the Passenger Acts, designed to control the flow of emigrants out of Scotland, required that a surgeon be on board any vessel with fifty or more passengers. This is certainly one area where the general social and economic situation had some impact on medicine. Most of the individuals who boarded emigration ships came from the highlands as a result of the infamous highland clearances, a process brought about partly as a result of the realisation that sheep could be more lucrative than people, together with the very real problems of overpopulation in that area, and also the devastating effects of the potato famine. The increasing involvement of the state in the enforcement of health meant that, in England in particular, there was regular employment to be found as medical officers in poor houses and other such institutions. The power of the London apothecaries was such that only individuals with their licence could be considered for such posts, and it is not difficult to see why a considerable head of resentment was being built up on both sides of the border.

Thus began a process of bargaining and negotiation on a possible solution. Various bills were introduced in successive parliaments and many hours of debate and negotiation took place. The proposals were for a single supervisory body to oversee and regulate the training and post-qualification registration of doctors. The major points of controversy surrounded the degree of prescription which the central body should have and, conversely, the amount of freedom which the institutions would have, as well as the validity of the qualifications offered and the list of such qualifications that would be acceptable to the new registration body.

From Scotland's point of view, it began to appear more and more that the London College of Physicians was pulling all of the political strings. Despite the recurrent meetings organised among the medical colleges of Edinburgh, Glasgow, London and Dublin, there was growing resentment that the views of the London College were taking precedence within the political sphere of influence. There was, on the surface, a fair degree of co-operation and a certain amount of astute political wheeling and dealing. In this, the Edinburgh surgeons' long-fostered connections in high places were of considerable value. As early as the middle of the seventeenth century the Incorporation had realised the value of patronage, either royal or political, and had instituted a system of awarding honorary fellowships to individuals who were deemed to have political potential in assisting the surgeons, initially in their constant skirmishes with the physicians, and later in the broader sphere of medical politics and cross-border difficulties. If nothing else, the Scottish medical bodies, grounded so deeply and necessarily in a culture and tradition of patronage, were able to wield considerable influence on the eventual shape of the legislation, passed after several failed attempts, in 1858. At no time was there a view that reform was not needed; what was in dispute was the way in which reform should be put into practice and the powers of any supervisory body which would be set up as a result of the legislation.

The first gentle excursion down the road of reform took place as early as the 1830s, when proposals were put forward, stimulated in large part by the difficulties caused by the overarching powers which had been acquired by the London apothecaries, who operated what was in effect a closed shop in the area of medical appointments, particularly public medical appointments, in England. This meant that most Scottish-trained or Scottish-certified physicians and surgeons were unable to gain employment south of the border. Negotiations continued during the next two decades, in parallel with the crucial developments in medicine and surgery which have been discussed, and when industrialisation, the empire and university education were themselves consolidating. So, what was happening in medical politics and education was, to a large extent, the almost inevitable consequence of a sort of 'standardisation' which was taking place in many other areas of the nation and its functions. The very advent of big central government and equally big local urban government was also a factor which pushed medicine towards a common framework. The Scottish colleges put considerable time, effort and money into funding their opposition to many of the proposals, principally by means of direct lobbying of MPs at Westminster. The records of the Royal College of Surgeons of Edinburgh contain a note of £150 spent in 1856 'for resisting an invidious measure of proposed legislation which threatened the College with utter extinction'.[52]

From 1840 a number of unsuccessful bills were put to parliament, including those by Warburton and Hawes (1840), Sir James Graham (1841), Lord Palmerston (1854) and by Mr Headlam (1856). After much debate and negotiation, the Medical Act was finally added to the statute book in 1858; its importance and effects on medicine and medical training cannot easily be underestimated.

What this piece of legislation, known simply as the Medical Act (*An Act to Regulate the Qualifications of Practitioners of Medicine and Surgery*, 21 and 22 Victoria c. 90) brought about were the beginnings – but really only the beginnings – of 'state medicine', sanctioned and supervised by the state. The most important practical consequence was the setting up of the General Medical Council (GMC) and the Medical Register. Thenceforth no practitioner could call himself a doctor, be placed on the Medical Register or sue for fees within the British Isles unless he had obtained his qualifications and licence from one of the twenty-two designated awarding bodies, and had his name entered on the register. This would not, of course, produce doctors and surgeons with equal qualifications. The twenty-two institutions licensed to license were not the same, and did not all teach or examine in a similar manner. The group was a mixture of universities and medical colleges, and the time had not yet come when a basic medical degree would be taken at a university by all, or even most, medical students. It was better than nothing, though, and instituted some sort of accountability. It would be easier to remove inadequate physicians or surgeons from a central register than to police them locally or in other ways.

The GMC started as a body very much in line with, and reflecting, the composition of the upper echelons of the medical profession and, at the start, the general practitioner had no role to play. Gradually though, the GMC has established itself as a significant regulatory body for doctors, although in more recent times criticism has been made about its ability and impartiality in dealing with cases of alleged incompetence.[53]

Of similar significance to Scotland was the passing of the Universities (Scotland) Act in the same year. This act appointed commissioners to oversee the structure of medical training. Some semblance of uniformity was created by these measures, but there still remained a considerable degree of flexibility in the requirements. Although the overall trend would be towards the goal of a single portal of entry by means of an MBChB degree, it is clear that in the decades following the passing of these acts the medical students of Scotland were able, and chose to be mobile and selective in their choice of location and programme of study.[54]

1858 – A WATERSHED IN MEDICAL TRAINING OR THE END OF 'SCOTTISH' MEDICINE?

Over the course of the first half of the nineteenth century, considerable progress had been made in the organisation and delivery of medical training in Scotland. A formal medical school was finally established at Aberdeen in 1817 with the ending of hostilities between King's and Marischal Colleges. St Andrews still suffered from the combined effects of geographical isolation, small size and the lack of facilities for clinical training, and the dubious nature of the degrees awarded,[55] although eventually clinical links with the universities of Dundee and Manchester have allowed St Andrews to maintain at least pre-clinical training. This meant that there was some sort of medical teaching available in all of the major Scottish universities.[56] During the early decades of the century steps had been taken, particularly at the University of Edinburgh, to improve the standards of training and examination of candidates for medical degrees. Indeed, a process was underway whereby the transition would be made from a situation where a candidate could merely turn up in Edinburgh (or, indeed, any medical school) and sit the examinations for an MD, to one where not only would a curriculum be imposed and supervised, but a stage would be reached where residence and study at the university of graduation were enforced. As an illustration of the situation shortly before these developments, an analysis of candidates for examinations at the Royal College of Surgeons of Edinburgh carried out at the request of the President's Council showed that of the 157 candidates examined, 74 were trained wholly in Edinburgh and a further 17 partly in Edinburgh, in other words some 40 per cent of the candidates had not received any part of their training in Edinburgh, although they had to produce certificates of attendance at courses given by individual lecturers approved by the College.[57] In the twenty-first century's stifling atmosphere of close academic 'supervision', concern with curriculum control seems hardly surprising; in the nineteenth century, though, it was a bold and considerable step towards the professionalisation and standardisation, as well as quality control, of medical training and, subsequently and consequently, medical practice. Progress would take time, though, and it is clear that even by the 1880s medical students were still gaining medical and surgical qualification by a multiplicity of routes.[58] Rationalisation could not be achieved overnight.

The medical institutions and the universities had thus made considerable progress in the consolidation of medical training, and the Medical Act, which set up registration criteria, was a major step along the road to a single means of initial qualification in medicine, although the colleges continued to offer a primary qualification which was taken by increasingly fewer candidates until its final demise in the early 1970s. One question which may be asked is whether 1858 also marked the beginning of the end of Scottish medicine as a separate sphere within a separate nation. British-wide registration and a British-wide GMC would oversee British-wide doctors and their training and practice. The advent of the GMC did probably alter the focus of Scottish medicine from being more European in sentiment and inclination to a much closer, if forced, co-operation and co-active existence with medicine and medical practitioners south of the border. Gradually the universities would take over as the major, though not as yet the only, entry portal to a basic medical qualification, and concomitantly the medical and surgical colleges evolved into institutions which awarded higher and specialist qualifications, and supervised the necessary training for these awards.

In the more global context, what the Victorian period produced was a template for the methodology of change, which seems to have lasted in recognisable form until the present time. During the nineteenth century the nation and its government became attuned to the sequence of perception of a need, followed by a royal commission or other investigation, followed by proposals for change, detailed discussion of these proposals, and ultimately some sort of legislation to impose the change. That the sphere of central government impinged on other spheres is undeniable; what may be debated are the rationale and priorities on which all sides based their negotiating standpoints. Scots became used to investigations and enquiries, and as the second millennium closes, developed a perhaps more sceptical view than was held by previous generations.

WOMEN AND PROFESSIONAL MEDICINE – THE FIRST FALTERING STEPS

In addition to women providing the focus of a number of medical advances as patients, initially in anaesthetics and antisepsis, this period also saw the initially fruitless attempts made by women themselves to enter the male-dominated sphere of qualified medicine. Assisting women to have children and survive in order to have more children was one thing; accepting that women could perform 'male' functions, particularly intellectual functions, was quite another. It is again a great irony that the appellation of hysteria to some emotional imbalances again makes the link to women's reproduction and reproductive organs.[59] The notion, highly current in this period, that gender differences necessitated separate spheres, was at the same time completely understandable and an almost insurmountable obstacle to the independent career progress of the 'other gender'.[60] Women had participated in the general sphere of medicine and medical care as long as men had, and indeed in some cultural areas more actively than men. The beginnings of the nursing profession heralded major change; the professionalisation of nurses and nursing has been ongoing ever since the later part of the nineteenth century. This perhaps met with rather less in the way of opposition than did the attempts made by Sophia Jex-Blake and others to enter the exclusive sphere of academic medicine. The gendering of roles in medicine and medical treatment, as in many other aspects of life, has become part of the historical and social account of progress. It seemed to be the case in the nineteenth century at least, that, whereas nursing was eventually deemed a suitable occupation for middle-class women, it was not thought acceptable for a woman to be in the position of having the right to dictate policy and treatment, particularly to male patients, and also having to be treated as equal to her male medical colleagues. It is from this period on that the gender distribution of medical roles has become more and more complex. For earlier periods it has been argued that physicians, although mostly of high social status, were regarded rather less highly than their colleagues in, say, the legal profession or the various shades of the cloth, because their role was seen to be towards the 'female' end of the professional spectrum. Physicians entered the homes of their patients as well as consulting in their own rooms or in hospital; they were allowed intimate contact with patients and were, therefore, perceived not to be as 'masculine' as other professionals. This may or may not be wholly the case; however, perhaps a reaction to this was the increasingly strong professional organisation of physicians and other medical professionals. However, at this time, women were not admitted to the other learned professions, so medicine was not unique in this respect. It may be that there was some sort of 'spectrum of maleness' in the professions, but it is more likely that attitudes to women rather than attitudes to the occupations themselves were the most significant factor.

In terms of gender mix, though, as nursing and the other paramedical occupations developed in the train of new technology and new thoughts on medical treatment, by the late twentieth century men have become increasingly involved in occupations which started off as exclusively female, and the reverse is also the case. There was a wide gulf between the roles of the nineteenth-century nurse, physician and surgeon. Nowadays there are not only female surgeons, physicians, paramedics and ambulance personnel, but there are also male physiotherapists, male nurses and male radiographers – occupations which were originally exclusively female. Nurse-practitioners carry out many of the tasks previously the province of junior doctors. The effect has been over time to create a gender mix of occupations just as much as gender inclusion or gender acceptance.

In terms of the introduction and integration of women into the formal sphere of orthodox medicine, there seem to have been two distinct paths, one of which was perhaps slightly easier underfoot than the other. It is difficult to avoid the accusation of gender bias on the part of those who controlled the official spheres and channels of medical training and practice. While the nursing profession evolved in the second half of the nineteenth century, enabled – though not wholly, or even mostly, due to – the work and influence of a few individuals such as Florence Nightingale, the wishes of women to become doctors in their own right were much harder to grant. A number of prejudices had to be overcome here. Firstly, this was the period of the 'separate spheres' in terms of the perceived roles which should be occupied by women, particularly middle-class women, from whom any professional group was likely to emerge. Women were generally regarded as being both physically and emotionally weaker than men, and, consequently, as not having the necessary strength of body or mind to cope with the rigours of the medical profession. As the nineteenth century wore on, and as more and more voluntary hospitals evolved, in which more and more patients died of hospitalism, it seemed that although Scotland was at the forefront of industry and empire building, medical and surgical outcomes remained relatively unchanged. This was a significant, if indirect, stimulus to the organisation and training of nurses and midwives.

The narrative of high-profile cases like that of Miss Jex-Blake serves both to highlight and perhaps distort the reality of the contemporary situation. Feminists and other historians of the modern period throw up their hands in horror at the apparently callous treatment meted out to women who wished to advance their intellectual situation. The resentment is well-founded, but care must be taken in making global assumptions about the wishes of women in general, and middle-class women in particular. It is perhaps the case that the cause of women was hindered to some extent by the emergence of the middle class, and that injustices of the sort highlighted by women who wished to become doctors were the result of the emergence of that particular class, which had very particular ideas about gender roles and the sort of activities which should be undertaken by women of this social and economic status.

Women who found themselves to be part of the working class did not experience occupational discrimination of this sort, or at least to the same extent. The effects of large-scale industrialisation may have prevented women from carrying out the heaviest of tasks, but industrialisation certainly did not remove women from the manual work force. The nature of the machinery or the limitations of their physical strength may have defined the particular tasks they carried out, but they were not constrained by the minutiae of etiquette or the full-blown ideology of separate spheres. Indeed, it is the contention of Whatley that women 'played a critical role' in the process of industrialisation in Scotland.[61] Similarly, women at the upper levels of society found that their lifestyles did not change markedly in spite of the rapid advancement of industrialisation and the beginnings of the transfer of financial power from the land to the factory or plant. Aristocratic women continued as they had done for centuries, and did not, on the whole, seek to 'work', either intellectually or otherwise, for financial gain.

It does seem that the women who did suffer most from the socio-economic realignment which was taking place in this period were middle-class women. They were increasingly separated off, particularly from the working class, and there quickly developed a complex and restrictive socio-ethical behavioural code which served to isolate many women, or confine their public activities to charitable works or perhaps a little genteel teaching. The misjudgement which is made by some historians, however, is the assumption that all, or most, of these women were unhappy with their lot and wished to break free from the restrictive bonds of middle-class mores. The cases of individuals like Sophia Jex-Blake and Florence Nightingale do serve to illustrate the problems faced by women who did wish to have careers; it is essential to remember, though, that they were a minority, and there is little in the way of direct evidence that there was a mass desire on the part of middle-class women to be liberated in this way.

This phase in the evolution of Scotland and its medicine did see the beginnings of the formalisation of nursing as a trained profession. It is undeniable that Florence Nightingale was of considerable importance; so was the much less heralded Mary Secole. But what seems to be rather more significant in the longer term was that by the mid- to late nineteenth century the same combination of factors which had necessitated the formalisation and standardisation of the medical profession had the effect of creating the need for trained nurses. In addition, there was the war factor, which affected Scotland just as much as anywhere. Traditionally, a large number of Scotsmen have served in the British armed forces, disproportionate in terms of population, but a historical phenomenon which still obtains today to some extent. The consequence was that for periods during which Britain was at war, considerable numbers of Scots were involved. In terms of the creation of opportunities for women rather than the medical consequences of the wounds of battle, it is easy enough to make the claim that the combination of industrialisation and the requirements and consequences of war meant that it was becoming perhaps easier for women of all classes to be allowed to take up employment deemed suitable for their circumstances. Whatever the case, it was clear that if the rapid progress which had been made in medicine, surgery, medical research, anaesthetics, antiseptics, medical training and, of course, the large voluntary hospitals was to have any significant or lasting effect, then structures would have to be put in place to ensure that patients were cared for to much higher standards in hospital than they had been in the past. The first nursing training school was established in Edinburgh in 1872 along the lines laid out by Nightingale, and from then on rapid progress was made in the field of nurse training, though it remained an exclusively female occupation well into the twentieth century.[62]

None the less, it is easy to see why the issue of women and medicine has been a very useful case-study for historians who purport to explain women's past in a new and more legitimate fashion. The feminist historians in particular have seized on it in an attempt to show the repression of women from the beginning of time. Some of their claims are of course legitimate, but the case of medicine is unique, in that women were attempting to enter a field which was not only intellectual but, of necessity practical. Nowadays, doctors of both sexes must form doctor/patient relationships with patients of both sexes; doctors of both sexes must *touch* patients of both sexes. Given the concurrence of factors in the Victorian period, such as the historic legal and practical subordination of women in Scotland and elsewhere; the hybrid nature of medicine (brain and hands); the artificial reticence and prescriptive code of middle-class behaviour, there is no surprise in the discovery that women found it more than difficult to gain a foothold in the medical profession. Indeed, the practical nature of medicine meant that many men found it an unsuitable occupation, even for the proverbial third or fourth son.

In assessing the role and status of women in medicine in Scotland it is less than helpful for historians at the extremes of the feminist spectrum to make statements like: 'The medical profession ... is not just another institution which happens to discriminate against us: it is a fortress designed and erected to exclude us ... It is deep-rooted, institutional sexism'.[63] This may be true in the most general sense, but it is not the whole explanation, or even an adequate explanation for a very complex situation. So, while there is little doubt that women who wished to become doctors faced very real problems, it is important to remember that they were at the beginning a minority, and a minority which often fought against the prejudices of women as much as of men.

Even within the ranks of the would-be medical women themselves, there was some dispute as to whether women should be educated separately or alongside men. Many of the continental and American institutions provided separate training for women, or were completely separate medical schools. While Jex-Blake would be forced eventually to set up a women's medical school herself, she and others saw this as a stopgap move which would help to tide things over until circumstances had changed to allow co-education to take place. So, again, the objections did not only come from male doctors or medical students, though they were certainly heavily involved.

In the same way that Scotland had pioneered medical training methods and improvements in the latter part of the eighteenth century, so it is perhaps appropriate that one of the most famous examples of the period had its main focus in Edinburgh. Events described as the 'Battle of Edinburgh'[64] took place in the 1870s. This was part of a more general campaign to open the universities to female students in many subjects, not just in medicine or science. The few women such as Elizabeth Garrett, who had managed to qualify in medicine, had been forced to do so abroad, but the redoubtable Miss Jex-Blake was prepared to take on the Scottish educational establishment. She applied for admission to the University of Edinburgh in 1869, and was helped initially by no less a figure than James Young Simpson. She was granted temporary admission, but this was reversed because it was felt that an exception should not be made in a single case. However, four other ladies quickly presented themselves, and the group was admitted, on condition that segregated teaching took place. The women had also to pay for this separate tuition. However, opposition was raising its head and profile in important quarters, centred on the current principal, Robert Christison who, ex-officio, sat on all of the relevant governing bodies of the University. The first obstacle came when one of the group, Elizabeth Pechey, outscored all of the male students in an examination, and part of the prize was her free access to a chemical laboratory. The tutor was persuaded to award the prize instead to a male student, on the dubious grounds that the women had not been part of the 'normal' (male) class. The ensuing battle of words occupied the front pages of the local press and caused a great deal of bitterness on all sides.

The next obstacle came when the managers of the Royal Infirmary, the major teaching hospital, were persuaded by the male medical students to deny the women access to the wards. Of course this meant that they could not complete their studies, as practical clinical training was by that time an integral and required part of the curriculum. A subsequent violent protest took place outside the anatomical dissecting room. Eventually the matter reached the Scottish law courts. Initially the verdict was in the women's favour, but, perhaps not surprisingly, reversed on appeal. Jex-Blake gave up the unequal struggle, qualified elsewhere and set up a separate school of medicine for women in London and subsequently in Edinburgh, although the latter was a short-lived affair.

As with many of these high-profile events, emotions cooled fairly quickly and it was left once again to a small band of dedicated women to try to continue the conflict. Even when higher education for women was accepted in Scotland in 1889, the Edinburgh Medical School contrived to prevent the introduction of co-educational teaching until the First World War, an event which perhaps did more to further the cause of female acceptance than many decades of protest beforehand. In all phases of Scottish history, war has had the effect of removing, at least temporarily, occupational gender demarcations.

Despite the eventual opening up of career pathways for medical women in Scotland, some confirmation of the assertion that the desire for advancement was confined to the minority comes from statistics on the uptake of places by women at medical schools. Ultimately, women were openly admitted to universities in 1892. However, in Aberdeen only one female joined the medical school; six took up the opportunity at St Andrews in 1989. Women in Edinburgh still faced a battle, as they were not allowed into the wards of the Infirmary until 1892, and fewer than ten women faced the challenge in the years leading up to the turn of the century. This is one area where it may have to be conceded that Edinburgh was less than pioneering in its efforts.

The situation did improve, though, and a recent and detailed study of the first women to study medicine in Glasgow indicates that, although the women were forced to study separately (and would do so for longer than elsewhere) in the Queen Margaret College, from the early 1890s, once medical training was available, it was taken up and many of the women who graduated as doctors had long and significant medical careers. In 1894 there were four female graduates out of a total of 84 (4.4 per cent), but by 1900 over 11 per cent were women. In terms of matriculated medical students, between 1892 and 1914 the female students comprised around 10–11 per cent.[65] It is also clear from this study that married women were able to continue their careers as doctors.

WHAT ABOUT THE ORDINARY PEOPLE?

While rapid advances in education, hospitals, towns and medical reform characterised this period, for much of the rural, remote population their medical care changed little. Many of the old superstitions persisted, and it was often not possible to reach orthodox medical care without incurring severe difficulties. Access to a qualified practitioner in the outer isles or remotest corners of the south-west continued to be much more difficult than in the urban areas, although there were difficulties there too. Many of the long-held ideas, superstitions and traditions continued, and folk medicine survived, often little altered for centuries. Evidence from the writings of David Rorie, who investigated lay medical practice in the north and east of Scotland, confirms this. For example, in Fife in the 1890s, it was considered that whooping cough could be cured by giving the patient roasted mouse dust; while among the cures for warts were rubbing with a piece of stolen meat (as the meat decayed, so would the warts), or tying knots in a string to represent the warts, and then burying the string.[66] This is all redolent of the disease transfer beliefs of much earlier periods.

CONCLUSION

The later Victorian period and early Edwardian era seems to show Scotland, Scots and their health, work and social conditions as markedly changed from the situation when Victoria ascended her several thrones. It is clear that in this period as in most others, it is impossible to disentangle completely the medical aspects from the general social, economic and political background. Victoria started her lengthy reign at a time when the full spectre of urban squalor was just beginning to be apparent; civic pride and civic government were solidly established but not yet entirely effective; Scotland was in the throes of empire-building but also of cholera and other devastating diseases; hospitals were more numerous but no more able to cure than they had been for half a century; doctors and surgeons still trained in a piecemeal and badly regulated fashion; operations were performed without anaesthetic and post-operative shock and infection claimed many lives; the Napoleonic wars were within living memory; and the economic situation was not propitious.

At the end of Victoria's occupancy of the throne many things had changed, some almost out of all recognition, though other things had not. Large towns were much larger; the problems in large towns were also greater but in some areas had been dealt with; anaesthetics and antiseptics played an important part in increasing the possibility of survival; civic pride and civic government had achieved much, whether or not by a coercive, authoritarian approach; medical education was rather more standardised and better organised; hospitals were staffed increasingly by trained nurses; women were at last able to attend university and eventually qualify as doctors; Scotland was perhaps at the height of its industrial and imperial importance; and, unfortunately, war was still a pressing problem and would be even more so in the next century. The Edwardian era saw the first of the devastating world wars, in which many Scots took part, and in which many Scots died or suffered severe physical or mental consequences. All of these elements would, in turn, help considerably to shape medicine in the first half of the twentieth century. Although the war was fought on foreign shores, Scottish medical practitioners were able to bring back new knowledge and skills.

In terms of assessment of interacting spheres, the main influences here would seem to be the increasing and increasingly complex inter-relationships between national government, local government and the medical institutions. The next period would see national policy on health taken to different levels, with mixed results. It would also see the rapid decline of Empire, the entry of party politics rather than the more complex politics of individual patronage into the politics of medicine, and attempts to regain some of the distinctive Scottishness which some believe was submerged within Great Britain. The identity of the Scot was now, however temporarily, inextricably linked with that of Britain and Empire. North Britain was now part of something much greater.

NOTES

1. *Reports on the Sanitary Condition of the Labouring Population of Scotland* (ed.) Laurie, W. L. (Greenock, 1842), 250–1.

2. Ibid., 266.

3. Jenkinson, Moss and Russell, *The Royal*, 50–3.

4. Patterson, S., 'Cholera, the great sanitary reformer?', *Proc. Roy. Coll. Phys. Ed.*, 22 (2) (1992), 238–53, argues that, in rural areas at least, cholera was not the main driving force behind any moves towards the imposition of measures to improve public health.

5. Robertson, E., *Glasgow's Doctor. James Burn Russell 1837–1904* (East Linton, 1998).

6. Quoted in ibid., 83.

7. Ibid., 99–100.

8. RCOSEd, Letter Books, 21 February 1890.

9. Finlayson, G., *Citizen, State, and Social Welfare in Britain 1839–1990* (Oxford, 1994) offers a comprehensive view on the relationships between citizen and state in terms of compulsion, co-operation, enabling and voluntaryism.

10. Thane, P., 'Government and society in England and Wales, 1750–1914', in Thompson, F. M. L. (ed.), *The Cambridge Social History of Britain 1750–1950* (Cambridge, 1990), 61.

11. Dupree, M., 'The provision of social services', in Daunton, M. (ed.), *The Cambridge Urban History of Britain. Volume III, 1840–1950* (Cambridge, 2000), 3.

12. Crowther, M. A., 'Poverty health and welfare', in Fraser, W. H. (ed.), *People and Society in Scotland. Vol. II 1830–1914* (Edinburgh, 1990), 265–87.

13. For a recent detailed account of the roots of the 1845 reforms, see Mitchison, R., *The Old Poor Law in Scotland* (Edinburgh, 2000), chs 7 and 8.

14. Full and detailed assessment of the workings of the Board in Blackden, S., 'The Board of Supervision and the Scottish Parochial Medical Service 1845–95', *Med. Hist.* 30 (1986), 145–72.

15. Ibid., 159.

16. Levitt, I., *Poverty and Welfare in Scotland 1890–1948* (Edinburgh, 1988), 89–90.

17. See analysis in Pennington, C. I., 'Mortality and medical care in nineteenth-century Glasgow', *Med. Hist.* 23 (1979), 442–50.

18. Dupree, M., 'Family care and hospital care: the "Sick Poor" in nineteenth-century Glasgow', *Soc. Hist. Med.* (1993), 195–211, assesses the admission of fever patients to the Glasgow Royal Infirmary in 1871 as a case study.

19. Gorsky, M., Johan, J. and Powell, M., 'British voluntary hospitals, 1871–1938: the

geography of provision and utilisation', *Journal of Historical Geography* 25 (4) (1999), 469, Table 2.

20. Medical societies were growing in range and number, and offered a focus for debate on medical matters and also medical politics. Full account and list of societies in Jenkinson, J. L. M., *Scottish Medical Societies 1731–1939* (Edinburgh, 1993).

21. Geissler, P. R., *The Royal Odonto-chirurgical Society of Scotland* (Edinburgh, 1997), 6; Jenkinson, *Scottish Medical Societies*, 185–6.

22. Geissler, *Royal Odonto-chirurgical Society*, 29.

23. Porter, *Greatest Benefit*, 381.

24. Hamilton, *Healers*, 213–4; Porter, *Greatest Benefit*, 386–8.

25. Jacyna, L. S., 'The laboratory and the clinic: the impact of pathology on surgical diagnosis in the Glasgow Western Infirmary, 1875–1910', *Bull. Hist. Med.* 62 (1968), 384–406; Porter, *Greatest Benefit*, 346–7.

26. Textbooks of surgery still describe the procedure, as in Rintoul, R. F. (ed.), *Farquharson's Textbook of Operative Surgery, Eighth Edition* (Edinburgh, 1995), 233, where it is described as 'the classical amputation in the region of the ankle'.

27. Masson, A. H. B., 'Edinburgh medicine in the time of Simpson', *Proc. Roy. Coll. Phys. Ed.* 27 (1997), 568–74.

28. Winter, A., *Mesmerised. Powers of Mind in Victorian Britain* (Chicago, 1998), 163–186.

29. The controversy is dealt with in detail in Baillie, T. W., *From Boston to Dumfries. The First Surgical Use of Anaesthetic Ether in the Old World* (Dumfries, 1969).

30. *Dumfries and Galloway Courier*, 2 March 1847.

31. Youngson, A., *The Scientific Revolution in Victorian Medicine* (London, 1979).

32. See Loudon, I., *The Tragedy of Childbed Fever* (Oxford, 2000).

33. Porter, *Greatest Benefit*, 369–70.

34. See Hamilton, *Healers*, 224, Table 6.1.

35. See also Cheyne, W., *Lister and his Achievement* (London, 1925).

36. For full discussion on these aspects, see Granshaw, '"Upon this principle I have based a practice": The development and reception of antisepsis in Britain, 1867–1900', in Pickstone, J. V. (ed.), *Medical Innovations in Historical Perspective* (Basingstoke, 1992), 17–46; Lawrence, C. and Dixey, A., 'Practising on principle: Joseph Lister and the germ theories of disease', in Lawrence, C. (ed.), *Medical Theory, Surgical Practice: Studies in the History of Surgery* (London, 1992), 153–215; Warboys, M., *Spreading Germs. Disease Theories and Medical Practice in Britain 1865–1900* (Cambridge, 2000).

37. Hamilton, D., 'The nineteenth-century surgical revolution – antisepsis or better nutrition', *Bull. Hist. Med.*, 56 (1982), 30–40.

38. Doody, G. A., Beveridge, A. and Johnstone, E. C., 'Poor and mad: a study of patients admitted to the Fife and Kinross District Asylum between 1874 and 1899', *Psychological Medicine* 26 (1996), 887–97.

39. Report of the Royal Edinburgh Asylum in 1885, quoted in Beveridge, A., 'Madness in Victorian Edinburgh: A study of patients admitted to the Royal Edinburgh Asylum under Thomas Clouston, 1873–1908', Part II, *History of Psychiatry* vi (1995), 144.

40. See Scull, A., 'Museums of madness revisited', *Soc. Hist. Med.* 6 (1) (1993), 3–24, which surveys recent opinion.

41. Beveridge, 'Madness in Victorian Edinburgh', II, 145.

42. See Sturdy, H., 'Boarding out the insane, 1857–1913. A study of the Scottish system' (unpublished Ph.D. thesis, University of Glasgow, 1996).

43. Quoted in Comrie, *History*, ii, 507.

44. Blair, J. S. G., *The Royal Army Medical Corps 1898–1991: Reflections of One Hundred Years of Service* (RAMC, 1998).

45. Blair, J. S. G, 'The Scots and Military Medicine', 26.

46. Crofton, E., *The Women of Royaumont. A Scottish Women's Hospital on the Western Front* (East Linton, 1997); Leneman, L., *In the Service of Life. The Story of Elsie Inglis and the Scottish Women's Hospitals* (Edinburgh, 1994); Ross, I. B., *Little Grey Partridge. First World War Diary of Ishobel Ross Who Served with the Scottish Women's Hospital in Serbia* (Aberdeen, 1998).

47. Porter, *Greatest Benefit*, 420.

48. Geyer-Kordesch and Macdonald, *Physicians and Surgeons in Glasgow*, 371.

49. The situation in St Andrews is well documented in Blair, *History of Medicine in St Andrews University*, chs 3 and 4.

50. Loudon, I., 'Medical Education and Medical Reform', in Nutton, V. and Porter, R. (eds), *The History of Medical Education in Britain* (Amsterdam, 1995), 231–4.

51. See Jenkinson, *Scottish Medical Societies*.

52. Creswell, *Royal College of Surgeons of Edinburgh*, 294.

53. Full account of the origins and development of the General Medical Council in Stacey, M., *Regulating British Medicine. The General Medical Council* (Chichester, 1992), especially ch. 3.

54. Detailed analysis of a sizeable body of medical students and their educational preferences in Bradley, J., Crowther, A. and Dupree, M., 'Mobility and selection in Scottish university medical education, 1858–1886', *Med. Hist.* 40 (1994), 1–24.

55. It is claimed that between 1836 and 1862 almost 2,000 postal degrees were awarded. Hamilton, *Healers*, 157.

56. For Aberdeen, see Pennington, C., *The Modernisation of Medical Teaching at Aberdeen in the Nineteenth Century* (Aberdeen, 1994); for St Andrews, see Blair, *History of Medicine at the University of St Andrews*.

57. RCOSEd, Minute Books, 21 October 1857.

58. Analysis of situation in Scottish universities in Bradley, Crowther and Dupree, 'Mobility and selection'.

59. Risse, G., 'Hysteria at the Edinburgh Infirmary'; Veith, I., *Hysteria. The History of a Disease* (Chicago, 1995).

60. Vickery, A., 'Golden age to separate spheres? A review of the categories and chronology of English women's history', in Shoemaker, R. and Vincent, M. (eds), *Gender and History in Western Europe*, London, 1998), 197–228.

61. Whatley, C. A., 'Women and the economic transformation of Scotland', 35.

62. See Baly, M., *Florence Nightingale and the Nursing Legacy* (London, 1988).

63. Ehrenreich, B. and English, D., *Witches, Midwives and Nurses. A History of Women Healers* (New York, 1972), 41.

64. Bonner, T., *To the Ends of the Earth. Women's Search for Education in Medicine* (Massachusetts, 1992).

65. Alexander, W., *First Ladies of Medicine. The Origins, Education and Destination of the Early Women Medical Graduates of Glasgow University* (Wellcome Trust Unit for the History of Medicine, Glasgow, 1987) 10–11. See also Geyer-Kordesch, J., *Blue Stockings, Black Gowns, White Coats. A Brief History of Women Entering Higher Education and the Medical Profession in Scotland in Celebration of One Hundred Years of Women Graduates at the University of Glasgow* (Glasgow, 1994).

66. Buchan, *Folk Tradition and Folk Medicine*, 243.

CHAPTER 9

MODERN MEDICINE IN MODERN SCOTLAND

INTRODUCTION

The twentieth century has seen the most far-reaching and, at times, almost incredible developments and changes in all areas of medicine in Scotland. This book has been completed at a time when technology seems to be threatening to overshadow the 'caring ethos'. It is very difficult to achieve a balance among the important aspects of the medical nation – knowledge, possibility, application and receipt of care. The medical student at the beginning of the new millennium shares (or, at least, should share) the ideals and ethos of his (and increasingly her) predecessors who signed up for an extra-mural anatomy class at Edinburgh or Glasgow University or took the tortuous journey to Leiden to sit at the feet of Boerhaave. What he or she is taught, however, is very different. The challenge for those who administer medicine in all its forms, from training to organisation and delivery, is to achieve high standards of all of these things, but not to lose sight of the idealism or altruism which seems to have been a core element of medicine through the ages, whether religious, secular, amateur or professional. Now that medicine is practised in a global context, and consultations can be made between doctor and patient separated by thousands of miles, the world of medicine is now locally-global as well as globally-local. Scotland is part of this macro- and micro-medical context, and it may still be claimed with some justification that the contributions made by such a small nation greatly exceed any geographical pro rata.

Among the major developments in the last century of the second millennium in terms of medicine in Scotland have been considerable advances in public health medicine, preventative medicine and technological medicine. The origins of large-scale municipal government lay in the nineteenth century; the twentieth century saw even larger-scale medicine, chiefly in terms of the advent of the National Health Service (NHS) and its great benefits and increasing problems. After the end of the First World War many measures were introduced gradually, particularly in areas such as health insurance, dental care and general practice. The idea of the Welfare State may not have been articulated directly, but ideas of 'Improving the Commonweal' certainly were, if not always from the purest of motives. The advent of the NHS and its increasing problems is a key theme in this final chapter. Attitudes to public welfare and universally available treatment shaped modern medicine, and produced recipients of medical care very different from those who were treated in previous times. Nowadays also, Scotland within Britain is, however reluctantly, a member of the European Union. This membership has considerable implications, particularly on the continent-wide regulation of medicine and medical practitioners and the ability to work freely in many countries despite often major problems of language and communication. Scots had practised medicine abroad for centuries, in foreign armies and in the various locations of the Empire, but the modern freedom of movement may be more problematic.

Some aspects of health and disease remain, of course, but often in somewhat changed forms. Bubonic plague has gone, cholera epidemics no longer wreak havoc on Scotland (though they undoubtedly do elsewhere), the more recent plagues of poliomyelitis and tuberculosis were thought to have been eliminated, though the latter is re-emerging for many of the same socio-economic reasons as before. New problems have appeared, though, particularly those related to HIV and to the consequences of various forms of substance addiction. In addition, the possibilities offered by transplantation, genetic engineering, a plethora of surgical specialties, and developments in assisted conception have brought in much anxiety as well as excitement, and stimulated heated debate as to the ethics of such procedures. The refining of techniques for early in utero diagnosis of malformation and disease in the fetus has allowed decisions to be made as to elective termination of the pregnancy. This is controversial for some, and viewed as interfering with nature (very much in line with attitudes to inoculation or pain relief in previous periods) or denigrating the value and potential contribution to society of those born with some disability. The sphere of nature has long played a part in medicine in Scotland and elsewhere, and in Christian-dominated areas in particular, the will of God was equated with, and seen through, the actions of 'nature'. Plagues and natural disasters were the result of God's anger; anaesthetics used in childbirth were denounced as contrary to nature; nowadays nature itself can be manipulated in many ways, and despite much greater knowledge of science and the much diluted influence of Christianity in Scotland, the nature card is still played by those who see medical technology as going too far. It is all very well to assist a woman to become pregnant; allowing her to choose the sex, physical appearance or characteristics of her offspring is quite another. Another important element is that, although there remain significant gender imbalances in a number of areas of medicine and surgery, women now play a much more equal role in professional medicine in all its aspects, not just in the areas thought previously to be within the sphere of women, such as the paramedical professions and nursing.

In the Victorian period the focus on public health was in line with the general context and trends towards the enforcement or enabling of measures which might build up the health of the nation as a whole, not just its medical health. Large-scale plans for vaccination, or provision of water supplies and detailed civic regulations were set out with a common purpose. That purpose was mainly twofold. Firstly, the aim was, as discussed, to improve the general health of the people so that they could in turn help to improve the general health of the nation. The second aim was to use these and other measures to build up the image and impor tance of the nation as part of an expanding British Empire. Civic pride was often the motive force behind prophylactic and improving measures, but civic pride influenced and directed by national and local aims and priorities. A boost to civic pride was also a boost to national pride.

By the early decades of the twentieth century things were changing a little. Politics had always played some part in the shaping of medicine in Scotland; twentieth-century politics were rather different, but still important. The effects of war on the subsequent progress of any nation are considerable; this was no less so at the end of the Great War, and would be even more the case following the Second World War. Rather than health being an issue of national concern, almost a non-political aspect of politics, the defining feature of twentieth-century public health and its policies seems to be that in some senses health has become the means rather than the end of political conflict. That is not to deny that a number of significant and effective initiatives have been taken during this time, or that there has always been a political aspect to most areas of medicine in Scotland from earliest times. However, since the end of the Second World War, health and medical issues have become focus points for particular political groupings, which use health and welfare politics as a means to gain more support for their general political standpoints. At times this has been to the benefit of the general public; at times it seems not to have been quite so beneficial.

This chapter will deal with modern spheres, looking at the effects of war, the advent of the NHS, the role of women in the medical and paramedical professions; the technology of medicine; and the increasing politicisation of medicine as a tool for politicians of all parties. It ends in a period of uncertainty as well as of huge potential. It also ends with

devolution, but rather too early to assess fully whether the Scottishness
of medicine will be reinforced, reactivated or recast. What is interesting
in a visual as well as historical context is that in the later chapters of this
book the number of sub-headed sections has proliferated. This is not just
a desire on the part of the author to make individual topics clear; it is
more an acknowledgement and demonstration of the fragmentation and
specialisation of health care, and the consequent, multi-faceted experience
of the patient. The many meta-narratives of the period combine to
influence the construction of modern medicine in modern Scotland. The
initial consultation with the general practitioner remains the entry point
to the diversity of specialist services on offer, but the sheer range of
specialties, sub-specialties and areas of medical, scientific and political
interest serves to ensure that, within orthodox medicine at least, it is no
longer possible for patient and practitioner to interact within a single,
general sphere of influence. The situation in Britain, though, still allows
for rather more of this sort of personal contact than, say, in the United
States, where there is no direct equivalent of the general practitioner.

POST-FIRST WORLD WAR INITIATIVES – RECOGNISING THE NEED FOR CHANGE

The origins of the NHS must be sought well before Beveridge, and can
be seen as part of the longer-term drive from Victorian times towards
increasing the levels of health in the general population, in terms more of
its economic potential than with particular or primary concern for the
state of health or otherwise of individual members of the public. To go
against the postmodernist reluctance to see any sort of continuity, it is
possible to do just that for Scottish health, or, perhaps better, the politics
of Scottish health. Once the realisation dawned in the first half of the
nineteenth century that a common approach had to be made in all
aspects of health, public and private, and in local government, and the
training and monitoring of the medical profession, the mentality of
legislation and standardisation became gradually inculcated into the
general population and its political and social leaders. It was clear by the
turn of the twentieth century that ad hoc, reactive or individualistic
measures could not ensure the minimum acceptable level of public
health and social comfort, and it was thenceforth somewhat easier to
legislate on these matters. It would not, however, be until the election of
a Labour administration after the Second World War that the concept of
free health care provision for all could be contemplated, let alone
accepted and enshrined in law. In addition, local government by the
1930s was faced by financial and organisational problems, which meant

that the 'bottom tier' of government was poorly equipped to deal with the increasing demands of national government. Local authorities were required to act as the tacksmen of the welfare state, to use a useful term from earlier times, and this would prove difficult.[1]

The NHS came into being in a period of optimism after the rigours and devastation of the Second World War, and as the pinnacle of the social conscience of the new Labour administration. The plan was ambitious and comprehensive, and its creators could not, perhaps, have foreseen that their grand design would, in only half a century, find itself under increasing iatrogenic strain. It is rather ironic that many of the current difficulties and problems facing the provision of a comprehensive, free medical service have arisen as a result of the very success of the service in enabling people to live for much longer periods and in allowing a variety of previously untreatable conditions to be treated successfully. The tripartite national, regional and local structure of the system was itself inherently problematic, and in addition, the forward vision of the 1940s was not one of increasingly sophisticated technology in medicine. The burgeoning technical aspects of modern medicine serve to compound all of these problems. Technology is expensive, but it can diagnose early and cure many, so that once again rates and numbers of survival are increased. In contrast, the general wealth levels of the country have not always increased apace, and it is now apparent that even in the currency of those who hold the legacy of 1940s Labour in their political hands, a fully comprehensive service at the point of need is no longer affordable, and, significantly in the view of some, perhaps not even desirable, although the latter is a political issue which will remain controversial. The difficulties faced by governments that wish to keep tax levels down mean that even the most universally approved government provision cannot be given free rein or unlimited amounts of extra money. The effects of progress and success are, indeed, at times difficult and complex.

As with many aspects of Scottish medicine in the modern period, there was a somewhat eclectic mix of features common to all areas and aspects unique to the circumstances of North Britain. In 1885 a major change in the way Scotland was governed had come about with the establishment of a Parliamentary Office for the Scottish Secretary of State. Prior to this, administration had been among the responsibilities of the Lord Advocate, thus under legal rather than political control. The new office meant that the Secretary of State and his responsibilities came within the political sphere, and the sphere of health politics. From that point a number of attempts were made to bring about parochial reform, and by 1918 the need for change was becoming more pressing. The

Local Government Board for Scotland, set up in 1894, had responsibility for the oversight of Public Health and Poor Law issues, but perhaps more significant was the Scottish Board of Health, established in January 1919.

This new body subsumed several groups already in existence, and one of the most important of these was the Highlands and Islands Medical Service (HIMS), established in 1913 to cater for the specific needs of people remote from centres of medical care. This scheme is generally seen as an important influence on the subsequent gestation of the NHS. As had been the case throughout many centuries, the highland areas were problematic, and had exercised the minds of successive kings and governments, generally with the focus on centralisation and political control. In terms of the enabling of health provision, the area was remote, it was difficult to find medical staff – who had to rely mainly on private income – and the National Health Insurance Scheme could not be applied to the highlands. In the normal scheme of things a commission was set up to investigate the situation. The Dewar Committee reported in 1912, and the proposals it made did to a large extent prefigure the national scheme.

Among the major proposals were for salaried medical practitioners, payment of doctors' travel costs, expansion of nursing services and the provision of a range of hospitals to provide basic health care. The scheme was implemented, but almost immediately faced considerable financial problems, so that ten years after its introduction many of the plans had not yet been put into operation. Some services were disrupted or suspended periodically thereafter. However, despite these problems, by the end of its life in 1948 the HIMS had achieved much, particularly in terms of improvements and extensions to remote hospitals and the provision of suitable consultants.[2] This is one of the areas where it may be claimed that the Scottish approach was distinctive. The combination of geographical problems and the apparent willingness of remote localities to submit to central control made for a well-planned scheme. It was not altogether successful, but did demonstrate clear possibilities, and paved the way for the fuller integration of remote medicine into the general compass of Scottish medicine under the NHS.

Other institutions which came within the remit of the Board of Health were the Scottish Insurance Commissioners and the Board of Local Government for Scotland. The Scottish Board of Health had a difficult birth and complicated infancy, but was influential in the formation and passage of the 1929 Local Government Act, the major aim of which was to rationalise public health provision in order to make it more efficient at local level.[3]

By 1929 the Board had been reborn as the Department of Health for Scotland. In terms of approach, the major feature of the twentieth century would seem to be the gradual move away from the 'sanitation' ethos – the attempt to improve health by removing nuisance – towards a more measured, scientific and condition-specific approach to individuals and their health, with particular focus on mothers and children. The aim appeared by that stage to be to prevent as well as to cure diseases.

The focus on children is illustrated by the note in the Local Government Board report in 1905 that:

> Scarcity of milk, its inferiority, and want of proper storage, free of contamination and cool, especially in our towns, promotes the notoriously high infant mortality and that mainly by infantile diarrhoea, which amounts to a summer plague. In fact through this and tuberculosis, milk may be said to be one of the main factors in the morbidity and mortality of children.

In terms of trying to put the intention into practice, steps were taken locally, and in 1903 the first health visitor was operating in Aberdeen, and by the time of the Board's annual report in 1907, health visitors were at work in Dundee and Greenock – a small start, but an important element in the individual rather than global approach to the problems of child health and welfare. It was important not just to cure diseases but also to improve general health, and the measures seemed to be working, as by 1912, infant mortality had dropped from 129 per thousand live births to 106.[4]

One area that seems to have been at the core of the drive to not only maintain health levels but also to enhance them, for whatever reason, was that of mothers and children, and the inter-war period saw considerable strides being made in that area. Despite the Victorian sanitary initiatives, by the turn of the twentieth century maternal and infant death rates were still unacceptably high. From that point progress in all areas relative to the health of mothers and young children was directed by a sequence familiar to other aspects of medicine covered in the foregoing chapters. A survey or royal commission defined a need; legislation was shaped to deal with the need; and universities or other validating institutions introduced training courses to educate those who would put the law into practice. For this sort of approach to work, it required some measure of co-operation among all the agencies involved – medical, educational and political – and perhaps it may be claimed that in Scotland the historical process had long been characterised by just that sort of interaction, and to a less troubled extent than south of the border.

There is no space here to elaborate on each piece of legislation and its effects,[5] but among the milestone measures were the Notification of

Births Act (1907), the Children's Act (1908), the Midwives (Scotland) Act (1915), the Nurses (Scotland) Act (1919) and the Maternity Services (Scotland) Act (1937). These acts promoted measures in a number of key areas. The three acts relating to nurses and midwives helped to regulate and standardise nurse and midwife training and, together with the important role of health visitors, laid the foundations for the professionalisation of maternal and child welfare services. Local government reorganisation in the 1930s resulted in larger units of supervision at a county level, while the Cathcart Report of 1936 encouraged progress in this area. With the coming of the NHS the focus shifted from cure to prevention and education and, to this end, the University of Edinburgh introduced the first Scottish course in Child Development in 1968, by which time the general thrust of NHS thinking was towards primary care in the community. The first comprehensive health centre in Scotland opened its doors in the Edinburgh suburb of Sighthill in 1953, followed by a similar enterprise in Stranraer in 1955. Nowadays the large, multi-service health centre is the norm in urban settlements of any size.

Although the focus was very much towards the locality, the home, school and community, one trend in the opposite direction was that of hospital births. Statistics from the post-war period show that in 1975, almost 99 per cent of births took place in hospital, and although there is a desire for home births on the part of many women nowadays, the trend is still the same. Whether the result of the hospitalisation of birth or of the more general measures taken to screen, supervise and sustain health, or the effects of the introduction of sulphonamides, followed by antibiotics, maternal mortality fell from over 4 per 1000 in the 1940s to 2.8 by 1975, and in 1982 there was a total of only 6 maternal deaths for the whole of Scotland.[6]

The campaign for immunisation against measles and rubella faced difficulties, but by 1975 over 80 per cent of 11 to 14-year-old girls were accepting the vaccine.[7]

The aim of improving the health of school-age children was also a priority and the School Health Service (SHS) did much sterling work, not just related to physical examination of children and the compilation of statistics, but also in areas such as school meals and employment of school-age children, not to mention the visits of the 'nit nurse' to primary schools. The re-organisation of the NHS in 1974 saw the end of a separate service, the functions of the SHS being subsumed within the more global, community care remit of the wider NHS itself. While in general terms the health of Scottish mothers and children has improved to a considerable extent, those who have the remit to promote health are faced with new problems, partly political and partly social, such as the greatly reduced time given to physical education in schools, the ongoing problems of social deprivation, incidence of cot death, and also, importantly, provision for children who in former times would not have survived because of severe disability or malfunction.

In addition to the measures put in place gradually to try to improve child health, some attempt was made to deal with some of the most pressing early twentieth-century plagues such as tuberculosis. This disease had been present among Scots for many centuries, variously described as scrofula, the King's Evil, or consumption. Many thousands had died, but it was not until the work of Robert Koch (1843–1910), who published his seminal work on the tubercle bacillus in 1882 and proved finally that the disease was infectious, that measures could be taken to combat it effectively. In Scotland the main credit for initiating steps to combat the disease must go to Sir Robert Philip, whose work was crucial to the organisation of measures to deal with and try to prevent the disease which was claiming the lives of many, not least the workers necessary to keep the wheels of industry turning, not to mention the problems of tuberculosis in the armed forces, which contributed to the deplorable state of fitness of many recruits. In 1908 the scheme which had been set up in Edinburgh, known as the Co-ordinated Edinburgh Scheme for the Control of Tuberculosis was implemented throughout Scotland, and a concerted drive to eradicate the disease would occupy at least the next half-century.

Sir Robert Philip, who had had first-hand sight of Koch's work, was a prime mover in the setting up of the Victoria Dispensary for Consumption in Edinburgh in 1887, and by 1894 the Victoria Hospital opened its doors to offer in-patient treatment to sufferers. As with a number of health initiatives, steps were taken at local level in Scotland often in advance of the situation in England, and before legislation was enacted to enforce such provisions. Once again it does seem that the powerful coincidence of circumstance, progress in scientific knowledge and the drive of key individuals were the major factors which brought about change. At an administrative level, the equally powerful combination of local health authority, voluntary groups and individual benefactors provided the necessary catalyst. Establishments appeared at Bridge of Weir and Glasgow, and by 1910 a dispensary service was available in Glasgow. The medical profession, under the drive of Philip took what was by now a common and logical step – it formed a medical society to disseminate knowledge and formulate medial policies. The Tuberculosis Society, which would later become the Scottish Thoracic Society, was founded in 1921. The Society still exists but, of course, with a much broader remit and compass.

In terms of the public administration and control of cases, compulsory notification was accepted in the first decade of the century, and by 1914 it was also necessary to notify cases of non-respiratory disease. The National Insurance Act of 1911 also made statutory provisions for the care of sufferers and their dependants. The result of these measures was that by 1914 the death rate was 162 per 100,000 of the population, as compared with 308 per 100,000 in 1887; a considerable improvement under the circumstances, before full implementation of measures nationally.[8] Although progress was much more limited during the First World War, the general measures of isolation, rest and fresh air continued to improve the statistics, but it would not be until the advent of antibiotics and the facilities for mass screening in the late 1940s that real progress would be made. Ultimately the BCG vaccination, as its ancestor the smallpox vaccine had done, would take control, at least until the end of the century, when the disease appears to be returning under many of the same causal circumstances as a century before.

In the present context, the fight against the 'white death' illustrates many of the 'Scottish' aspects. Measures were taken early, at local level, and were adopted gradually as a national policy, finally enforced by legislation. It has been claimed that Scotland in the modern period was easier to control in terms of health and medical administration. This may well be the case, and the reasons are complex and difficult to determine. It is not clear whether it is something specific in the Scottish consciousness, or merely that areas and regions are small and can be controlled with less effort than south of the border. It may be sheer luck that consensus between key medical men and key local politicians and charitable benefactors could be obtained. Whatever the case, the Scottish model was the best that could be conceived at that particular point, although there is a view that the sanatoria themselves were not particularly effective in controlling the disease, and were certainly not particularly cost-effective.[9]

There is no room here to rehearse in detail what was happening in all areas of health and disease, but some progress was made in dealing with syphilis, and the inevitable royal commission and its findings led to local authorities being required by 1917 to institute measures to deal with venereal disease. Unlike tuberculosis, the area of sexually transmitted disease was burdened with the heavy cloak of morality and this was reflected in the language of the debate. Given the nature of the disease it is perhaps unsurprising that many patients defaulted from treatment (as many as 43 per cent in Edinburgh in the 1920s), but this trend 'ran counter to the moral objectives of the social hygiene movement in Scotland, with its stress on self-control and discipline'.[10]

Many areas of medical treatment were influenced by the major strides in drug treatments of many sorts, which were developed in the middle decades of the last century. The release of penicillin for general use in 1945 was the beginning of what has been described as a 'therapeutic revolution', which would see the advent of steroids, betablockers and many other chemical agents, not to mention Valium (which produced severe problems of addiction), Prozac and Viagra. All of this produced genuine possibilities of treatment, but also a rising 'confidence in the powers of modern medicine'.[11]

The main obstacles in the way of full health care for all were also geographical and financial. In particular, care and treatment of the mentally ill and mentally handicapped, though under the aegis of the Board of Commissioners in Lunacy for Scotland, was less than adequate. The Mental Deficiency and Lunacy (Scotland) Act of 1913 replaced the Board and attempted to offer a more suitable service. The large institution was still the favoured option, and it was not until the very end of the century that the approach changed radically, so that individuals with mental problems are now mostly housed and cared for within local communities.

MEDICAL EDUCATION IN WARTIME AND PEACETIME

The treatment of the many thousands of casualties from the Great War served to confirm that in time of conflict careful and special arrangements had to be made. The particular conditions under which the Great War was conducted meant that a large proportion of the casualties suffered from mental trauma and the effects of gas rather than from gunshot or other wounds. Between the end of this war and the outbreak of the next, some progress was made in the provision of adequate numbers of hospital beds in suitable locations. There was not long to wait for the next conflict, and the 1930s can be seen as a decade of phoney war and preparation for medical war. When war did come, a major difference faced by the Scots was the large number of civilian casualties. The Great War happened abroad and the suffering of Scottish civilians lay in bereavement and the problems of caring in the long term for the effects of shell shock and other intractable conditions. The Second World War involved the whole nation as never before, and as a result, the medicine and surgery of war were applied to the entire population, not just those in uniform. Treatment of large numbers of casualties resulted in the development of surgical techniques which would be further developed in peace time, particularly in the area of plastic and reconstructive surgery.[12]

Another difference here was that the period before the war broke out was characterised by a general push towards improving the 'commonweal' and health of the nation as a whole. Medical insurance schemes provided some comfort, and the general background, unlike the period before the outbreak of the Great War, was one of forward planning to a greater extent than had been seen beforehand. The result was that the nation was perhaps a little better prepared for war in terms of hospitals and numbers of beds and, in turn, this preparation and organisation formed a template for at least part of the post-war push towards a national system of health care. The number of available beds in Scotland was greatly enhanced by the Emergency Medical Scheme (see below).

In terms of Scottish medical education and the role of the universities, a major effect was that both students and staff within the required age limits and levels of fitness were drafted into the armed services, leaving medical schools to be run by teaching staff who had retired or were unfit for service. After the war, a fast-track for demobilised medical students was instituted in order to boost the numbers of qualified practitioners in the years following the conflict. During the war, though, one development unique to Edinburgh was the establishment of the Polish Medical School at the University. Scots had enjoyed contacts with Poland for centuries, particularly in relation to trade. Scottish merchants had lived in Poland and doctors had practised in Poland, or at least the territory which included what is now Poland. Now, Poles were fighting for the Allies, and Polish medical students were able to train in Edinburgh. After the defeat of Poland, the Polish Army sought to regroup and reorganise, first in France, and then in Scotland. The circumstances were such that in February 1941 an agreement was concluded between the Polish Government and Edinburgh University, which resulted in a unique and symbolic enterprise.[13] The close connections between Scotland and Poland were thus reinforced, and in a very significant way. The Polish Medical School was the last of the extra-mural establishments in Scotland, and after the publication of the Goodenough Report in 1944, which opposed these outside routes to qualification, they gradually ceased to have any significant input into the primary production of doctors.

In more general ways, although medical education in Scotland retained a measure of distinctiveness, these days were numbered. One of the major advantages which had been enjoyed by Scottish medical schools was that they experienced rather better relations with the teaching hospitals and with the local authorities than was the case south of the border. The reasons for this are historical and have been alluded to in earlier chapters. Scottish universities before the Second World War period had still been pioneering, with, for example, the first full-time clinical professor being appointed at the University of Aberdeen as early as 1930. The trend towards salaried, full-time clinical medical teachers was one which was embraced fairly quickly by most of the Scottish universities, and after 1945 this became the norm, with clear benefits to the medical students and to their future patients.

After 1945 the Scottish Medical Schools enjoyed something of a revival in energy and reputation, and this was enabled by the historically close links between teaching hospitals and universities, and under the NHS in Scotland these hospitals came under the remit of the regional health authorities. Again, the benefits of a long history of educational co-operation, relatively small scale and a common purpose helped to ensure that Scottish medical schools were able to remain coherent and cohesive, for the time being at least. Although it may not be possible, or desirable, to claim any overarching trends, there is at least evidence that the consequences of previous groups of influences produced the circumstances in which new developments could be built.[14]

The teaching available within the medical schools, though, was perhaps not at the cutting edge of innovation or as yet in line with scientific progress or the burgeoning 'new ideas' about how teachers should teach and how students should learn. New areas had to be taught, such as general practice as a speciality rather than the basic general qualification of the previous century. To that end, the first Chair of General Practice in a Scottish university was established in Edinburgh in the early 1960s, at which time also the curriculum at several medical schools was altered to allow students to take an intercalated science degree during the period of their medical studies. Since then curricula have continued to evolve and change, so that nowadays the approach is much more systems-based, rather than concentrating on individual areas of the basic sciences before the period of clinical attachments begins. From the historian's point of view, what is clear, though, is that the 'apprenticeship' is still at the root of clinical training. Medical students still spend lengthy periods of attachment to a variety of hospital departments, general practices and other relevant institutions. The difference is precisely in this variety.

Students are also encouraged nowadays to participate in active learning, and the role of the patient is perhaps returning a little of the way towards what it had been many centuries ago, when the relationship between patient and practitioner was much more equal in terms of influence on diagnosis and treatment. One example comes from the Glasgow University Medical School, where students participated in group projects aimed at elucidation of the background social, economic and demographic context to the medical problems experienced by the patients.[15]

Most medical schools have continued to revise their curricula, not only
in line with developments in the medical field, but also in the
burgeoning area of educational theory. Medical students are encouraged
to look rather more holistically at their patients and their general circumstances – exactly the sort of approach advocated by Hippocrates. The
context and discourse of the modern period are of course vastly different,
but the sort of 'consultation' advocated by the ancients does seem once
again to be at the core of medical practice, or at least that is the aim.
Following the guidelines published by the GMC in 1996 under the title
Tomorrow's Doctors, the medical curriculum at Glasgow University was
restructured on a thematic basis. The previous clear distinction between
pre-clinical and clinical study was removed, and emphasis was placed on
an integrated, scientific and clinical approach. Ethics, gender issues and
palliative care are also covered. The current prospectus of the Medical
Faculty at Edinburgh University states that 'the curriculum is closely
aligned to changes in community and hospital care. It underpins the
nature of the Edinburgh medical graduate as a student who becomes
clinically competent in a research-rich environment'. It could be said
that this was exactly what it had sought to do in the later eighteenth
century; the language may have been different, but it can be claimed
with some justification that this is exactly what was happening in the age
of Cullen and Monro *Secundus*. The modern context is by nature rather
more impersonal, technological and high-speed than two millennia ago,
but the basic unit of medical practice, the consultation, cannot be
eclipsed, whether or not robots perform surgery or patients try to find
computer-aided diagnosis or surf the internet for the latest available
opinion or technique.

What the medical schools had produced at the beginning of the
twentieth century was, in effect, general practitioners who then proceeded
to practise in a variety of situations, including hospitals, institutions, the
armed forces, industry and asylums.[16] As the century progressed and
particularly once the extra-mural initial portals of entry closed and the
university provided initial training for all, the educational trend, as it has
been in many areas, was and is towards higher training as a basic
requirement for specialisation in a multiplicity of medical, surgical and
technological fields. By the time of the NHS reforms in the 1970s, it was
recognised by the colleges that 'Britain is the odd man out in not having
some form of examination to test qualifications in the major medical and
surgical specialities'.[17] The medical and surgical colleges in Glasgow and
Edinburgh offer higher qualifications and are increasingly providing
appropriate training courses and supervising the practical aspects, so that
fellowships and diplomas are available in all of the major specialities and

also in new areas such as Medical Informatics and Pre-hospital Care. The major problem facing the Scottish colleges at the beginning of the third millennium is that of whether a distinctive Scottish qualification should be maintained, or whether national higher medical and surgical qualifications should be the norm, as they already are in some specialist areas. There are intercollegiate fellowships in some of the major areas, such as cardiothoracic surgery, but developments in this area are problematic and influenced just as much by medical politics as by priorities in medical education or the 'Scottishness' factor.

The whole sphere of medical education has broadened in the twentieth century to include the training and validation of a wide range of nursing and paramedical disciplines. Nurse training has been subject to the same sorts of social, technological and educational influences as medical training, and has come a long way from the days of the 'boarding school' ethos of the nurses' home. Nursing training is now largely degree-based, and discipline-based. In the past, nurses undertook a general training before specialising in, for example, children's or mental health nursing. Nowadays, following the schemes outlined in Project 2000, nurses train to degree level in adult, child or mental health nursing.[18] Following this, should a nurse wish to work in a more specialised area, such as intensive care, further certificated training is necessary. Trends in nursing training do seem to mirror trends in medical education and in theories of education for occupations which combine theoretical and practical study.

As well as nursing, a proliferation of paramedical disciplines has evolved, including radiography, physiotherapy, podiatry, occupational therapy, and many others. Until the last decades of the twentieth century, training for most of these callings comprised practical and theoretical training, based in a teaching hospital. For example, radiography training at Edinburgh was centred at the Royal Infirmary until 1992, when it became part of the Department of Health Sciences at Queen Margaret University College, and is now a four-year honours degree. Most of the other paramedical disciplines have followed the same pattern, and the approach and opportunities would appear to be similar to those in other parts of the United Kingdom. The major trend has been the change from a mainly vocational orientation with added theory, to not quite the reverse, but a situation with a much more heavily academic bias.

THE COMING OF THE NHS

Returning to the 1940s, against a complex background and as a result of the work of consultative committees, boards, individuals and local initiatives, some progress had been made along the road towards the creation of a more comprehensive health care service. The next and potentially key milestone, or staging post, along the road to state-funded comprehensive health care services came in the form of the Cathcart Report, which appeared in 1936. The key to the proposals was a co-ordinated and integrated system of health and social welfare provision, but the plans did not meet with the wholehearted approval of the medical profession, which feared for its professional and clinical autonomy under such a scheme. The report was not adopted, apart from that part relating to maternity services, which shaped the Maternity Services (Scotland) Act of 1937, but it 'helped lay the groundwork for the operation of a distinctive health service suited to Scotland's specific health needs post-1948'.[19] Special attention to maternity care was necessary because of the significantly higher incidence of maternal and infant mortality and morbidity in Scotland as compared to the rest of the United Kingdom.

It has been claimed on occasion that 'a good war' tends to go much of the way towards dealing with mounting social or economic problems of one sort or another. This can be said about the Second World War in a number of ways. Not least of these were the giant strides which would be taken in surgery and the treatment of the victims of the conflict. However, what Scotland was forced to do in order to cope with the social effects of war would also help to shape the health of the peace. Fearing that the scattered and patchy provision of hospitals would be wholly inadequate to cope with the many thousands of expected wounded civilians, not to mention repatriated wounded soldiers (and prisoners of war), surveys were carried out and emergency legislation passed to facilitate the organisation of a national hospital service. The nightmare scenario did not materialise, but the Emergency Medical Service laid the groundwork for a national grid of hospital beds which would be utilised in many forms after the end of the war. The Civil Defence Act of 1939 allowed for the Emergency Hospital Scheme to be implemented throughout Britain, and over 16,000 additional hospital beds were made available in Scotland as a result.

Among the buildings and institutions pressed into service as an emergency hospital was Peel House in the Scottish borders. The house had been acquired in 1938 by Lady Craigmyle, who immediately offered it to the government for use as a convalescent home. The prevailing threat of renewed conflict, though, brought about its adoption as an emergency hospital under the control of Edinburgh Corporation. Huts were constructed to receive casualties, but even during the war attempts were made to involve the hospital in the treatment of crippled children, and after the war the hospital functioned as the only general hospital in the area until it was replaced by the new Borders General Hospital, which opened in 1988.[20] Several other hospitals around the country had similar origins.

What was in place at that point, then, was a devolved government department (Department of Health for Scotland), a comprehensive survey of the possibilities for corporate health provision, and the will on the part of at least some to ensure that health care would be supplied on a more comprehensive basis after the end of the war. What was needed in order to complete the 'package' of formative influence was an individual, or individuals, with the drive, insight and political will to ensure that ideals would eventually be translated into reality. In the case of Scotland, one such individual was Tom Johnston (1881–1965). Johnston occupied the post of Scottish Secretary during part of the war and in this capacity was closely involved in the co-ordination of medical arrangements and provisions. Perhaps his major achievement in this field was to secure an agreement whereby patients from the overcrowded and often inadequate voluntary hospitals could be treated at the wartime hospitals, and by the end of the war over 30,000 patients had been treated in this way. Johnston also managed to retain control of the EMS hospitals in the hands of the Scottish Office after the war.

Most large-scale schemes these days are tested initially by small-scale pilot projects. Such a test took place in the west of Scotland, and this became known as the Clyde Basin Experiment. It was probably not the case that those who set up the scheme knew that this was what they were doing. As late as the middle of the twentieth century, forward planning was not really at the heart of any rationale for change. As had been the case throughout the troubled and complex genesis of Scottish medicine, the fortuitous was often more significant than the planned. In any case, under the steerage of Johnston, some of the redundant military hospitals and the full panoply of specialist, and by now centrally controlled, medical services would be made available to the industrial workers in the crucible of Scottish industry. Under the more grandiose title of the Supplementary Medical Scheme, all of the facilities for treatment were co-ordinated and, importantly, the notion of preventative health care measures was a fully integrated part of the overall scheme.

The scheme started off on a relatively tentative footing, and was confined to the younger age groups, but was extended gradually to include most workers in most age groups in most parts of the country. Evidence of the workings and results of the scheme was transmitted to the government's Committee on Social and Allied Services (more widely known as the Beveridge Committee) during 1942, and by the end of that year the Beveridge Report had been compiled. At its core was the notion of the provision of a single, integrated scheme for the administration of social security nationwide, and also, crucially, the concept of free medical care for the entire population, free, in the famous phrase 'at the point of need'. The Beveridge plan did face considerable opposition from some quarters, though, both politically and medically. The wartime coalition government itself was not wholly in agreement with every detail of the proposed scheme. However, the mere existence of the proposal engendered its own momentum, and the individual on whom the subsequent clamour for action centred was Sir William Beveridge (1879–1963). Initial proposals were enshrined in a white paper, described as 'diffuse and confusing',[21] issued for discussion early in 1944, while the wartime consensus was holding together but with increasing difficulty.

In the optimistic days of early post-war Britain, perhaps one of the most abiding memories is that of Beveridge, on grainy black and white newsreel, speaking in the stilted tones of his time, about the aims and purpose of the new National Health Service, which was to be provided free to all at the point of need. This was to be made available by a new system of employer and employee contributions. No longer would primary care depend on whether the harassed mother of a large brood could afford the few shillings necessary to consult the local doctor. The implications were many. Conditions could be treated early, thus enabling the workforce to be more productive; children would be healthier; doctors and hospitals would be better organised; and all of this would mean that Scotland and Britain would continue to progress and be globally influential. However, the nature of the system meant that patients, most of whom had experienced wholly private (or partly subsidised) medicine hitherto, would have less freedom of choice – though in reality this may well have been restricted by socio-economic and geographical factors anyway.

A recent political history of the NHS, though largely focusing on England and Wales, emphasises the point that the NHS was not a 'spontaneous creation'.[22] It was realised, with increasing degrees of alarm, that the health care situation in most parts of Great Britain was much worse than in many other developed nations, including the 'white dominions', and that for political reasons, let alone health reasons, something had to be done to improve the situation. It was not the case, though, that this unanimity of sentiment brought about unanimity of aims and purpose to the political or medical nations. It was clear that the growing number of publicly funded health service provisions in Britain would have to be rationalised and standardised under a nationally directed scheme. What was certainly not clear, until the last possible moment, was the final shape that the new national service would take. Surprisingly also, it seems that the Scottish Labour Party had not put health at the top of its agenda in the lead-up to the 1945 General Election.[23]

A major sticking point in gaining acceptance of the scheme by the medical profession was the proposal that general practitioners should be given salaries by the local authorities and would, thus, be under their control. This measure was opposed strongly, particularly by older members of the profession, who guarded their clinical independence jealously and could not envisage their exclusive sphere of operation being controlled or influenced by non-medical individuals. Part of the background to the opposition was the enduring concept of professional fees as being the acceptable means of gaining remuneration, rather than a standard salary coming from a central body. The British Medical Association (BMA) shared these reservations. Matters came to a head after the 1945 election in the white heat of landslide Labour enthusiasm, when there was an increasing degree of polarisation between the medical profession and the government, during the period of Aneurin Bevan's negotiations with all parties. Bevan was also staunchly opposed to the idea of separate legislation for Scotland, although this was common and had been the case with many medical acts and Poor Law provisions in the past.

Negotiations progressed, and Bevan succeeded in dividing the opposition by gaining, to a certain extent, the support of a proportion of the hospital doctors for his plans and, consequently, ending the unanimity within the BMA.[24] Figures for voting patterns among medical practitioners indicate that at the final vote the Scottish medical profession voted relatively narrowly for the proposals, England and Wales substantially against, but the BMA did not consider that it would be able to wring further concessions out of the government, and gave tacit support. The general practitioners gained the status of independent contractors, although this was a mixed blessing in terms of the conditions of service they were able to achieve in the early decades of the NHS in operation. Final proposals were published in the National Health Service Bill in March 1946, and entered the statute book in November of that year. The parallel Scottish act took only a few months longer to achieve.

In Scotland there had, therefore, been at least three important strands of influence and initiative. Firstly, the industrial importance of Scotland had been recognised early, and measures taken to treat civilian casualties of the war, and thus keep the nation's war effort going. This had been made much easier by the fact that there were not the many thousands of expected military casualties to take up the beds in the emergency hospitals. Secondly, the Clyde Basin Scheme had proved a useful model for a more general scheme post-war, in line with what government assessed to be the feeling of the nation on 'free' schemes. Thirdly, the

success of the Clyde Basin Scheme was made known to central government at a time when it was considering what measures should be taken
to provide full health care, including preventative measures. Finally, the
general context seemed to require the specific or individual as the driving
force; this was present in Scotland in the person of Tom Johnston and
other like-minded individuals.

Following the sea-change in politics caused by the landslide Labour
victory in 1945, the political face of the proposed comprehensive health
care provision was changed, and was couched more in terms of a
nationalised industry than a standardisation of provision already existing
and organised at local level. None the less, the scheme that eventually
came into being in terms of the National Health Service (Scotland) Act
(1947) contained significant hints of what had taken place in Scotland
during the war, although some of the health care services which had
been provided by local authorities were removed. What the Scottish Act
provided was a higher profile for the hospital managers, and less of a
central role for the general practitioner, and the whole service was under
the remit of the Scottish Secretary. The new service would be responsible
for hospitals, which would be transferred to the remit of the Secretary of
State, from the various voluntary and other institutions, together with
health centres, research, ambulances, bacteriological services and blood
transfusion. Local health authorities would assume responsibility for
such matters as care of mothers and children and vaccination. The Act
stated grandly and comprehensively that:

> It shall be the duty of the Secretary of State for Scotland to promote the
> establishment in Scotland of a comprehensive health service designed to secure
> improvement in the physical and mental health of the people of Scotland and the
> prevention, diagnosis and treatment of illness and for that purpose to provide and
> secure the effective provision of services in accordance with the following
> provisions of the act.[25]

Once all the details had been agreed to the greatest extent possible, and
the act came into effect, its measures were ordained to begin on the
symbolic Appointed Day of 5 July 1948, a day chosen to coincide with
the implementation of other Labour-driven social reforms. It seems that,
despite the enormity of the concept and the difficulties in bringing about
agreement on the terms and conditions under which the scheme would
be introduced, the Appointed Day came and went with relatively little
trouble or difficulty. This was for several reasons, including the detailed
advance planning involved, and the fact that there were few completely
new medical services on offer. What patients experienced was free treatment and more comprehensive access to a range of services which
already existed, but which had been confined previously to certain

groups rather than society as a whole. The patient-practitioner relationship had changed, not perhaps in the medical sense, but in the
payment sense. The days of the GP being paid in kind – perhaps with a
succulent but questionably legal salmon or other practical remuneration
– were numbered.

What the NHS created within its own sphere was the third largest
organisation in Great Britain outside the military services (the list being
headed by the British Transport Commission and the National Coal
Board). This vast organisation, which represented some sort of medical
utopia in the minds of the population and of its progenitors, began
immediately to create the sort of overwhelming demand which would,
from the start, signal serious problems in the decades ahead. This was
not realised at the time, though, as there was little concept of the almost
incredible progress which would be made in medical and surgical
knowledge and technology, as well as the problems created by success in
preventative medicine in allowing life-span to increase substantially,
which would engender new and increasingly difficult problems.

The NHS was not as comprehensive as it might have been, and its
effects in the short term are difficult to assess. For example, the scheme
did not include direct provision for industrial or occupational health care
schemes or preventative measures, with the result that 'the historic
separation of work from health was now institutionalised' – a little ironic,
given the very real influence of industrial necessity on health care
improvements for the previous century.[26] Scottish medical history, as
indeed the history of the nation itself, is full of paradoxes. This, according to some historians, meant that crucial matters concerning occupational
health were much more difficult to control and deal with, a case in point
being the serious problems and high mortality caused by the widespread
use of asbestos in all aspects of industry and construction. Figures from the
Health and Safety Executive indicate that 183 deaths from mesothelioma
occurred among a surveyed group of industrial workers between 1900
and 1991, and it is claimed that the failure to include occupational health
within the compass of the NHS was a significant factor in delaying
measures to deal with the problem.

NEW SOLUTIONS BRING NEW PROBLEMS

Once the NHS was fully established, and once the older generation of
medical practitioners had been replaced by doctors who had not experienced the pre-NHS system, health care provisions under the terms of
the Act were, in most respects, adequate for their purpose. It was not too
long, though, before it became very clear that modifications and changes

would have to be made to the system in order to cope with the increasingly varied demands of post-war Britain, a Britain which, wide-eyed with hope and expectation, demanded more and more of its nationalised services, services which, it was often claimed, had been fought for during the war, a war fought to achieve 'a better future', whatever was meant by the term 'better'. By the early 1960s it was apparent that changes would have to be made and the service would have to be reorganised and streamlined, but it would take another decade before these reforms were achieved. Efforts were made to try to ensure that the existing system could be made to work better, and in Scotland the major figure to emerge during this period was Sir John Brotherston (1915–85), the Chief Medical Officer for Scotland. During the decade a number of trends were coming together, which would effectively render the NHS inadequate. These included a central drive to consolidate social work services under the aegis of local authorities; moves towards improvements in medical training, which would require teaching hospitals in England to be integrated as they were in Scotland; and a concurrent review of the organisation of local government itself.[27] At the core of all of these elements was the realisation that the administration of the various systems was too fragmented and thus difficult to control. As had been the case in the period of negotiation leading up to the inception of the NHS, the medical profession – in Scotland as in England and Wales – was very wary of the prospect of its being placed under the control of local authorities, in particular the Medical Officers of Health.

By the end of the 1960s the government was making serious efforts to come up with suitable plans for reorganisation which would result in a more integrated and rational service. The original tripartite structure of regional boards, local executive councils and hospital services had the major disadvantage that it was difficult for patients to cross the boundaries and receive treatment from more than one agency at the same time. There is something of an analogy here with the more recent problems of the so-called 'postcode lottery'. It was agreed that the prevailing situation did not 'enable us to make the most effective use of our preventative and curative resources', and, crucially, 'the difficulties of this administrative division are being *intensified by the advance of medicine*' [my italics].[28] This brings in a crucial theme which would both characterise and cause yet further problems for restructuring of the health services. The advance of medicine meant that more people could be cured rather than being merely cared for; more would live longer; developing treatments would mean that technology would become more complex; and everything would be increasingly expensive. A royal commission, set up in 1968 to look at the future of medical education concluded that 'the doctor of the future must therefore be educated not so much for the future as now we see it, but for a world in which everything – the content of medicine, the organisation of medical care, the doctor's relationship with his colleagues and the community, and indeed every feature of his professional life and work is now on the move'.[29] These aspects of Scottish medicine in the second half of the twentieth century drove change and brought about more and more difficulties in maintaining the comprehensive nature of medical provision which had been at the heart of Beveridge's grand design. Within twenty years the scheme was creaking at the seams; a further forty years would see it barely holding together. Barely ten years after the foundation of the NHS in Scotland, however, it was claimed that significant effects could be seen in the medical statistics. For example, in 1959 infant mortality had been reduced from 44.7 to 27.7 per 1,000 live births; while the death rate for respiratory tuberculosis was 12 as compared to 66 per 100,000; and the general death rate had reduced from 13.02 to 11.87 per 1,000, though it must be acknowledged that these trends were in place before 1948 and the effects may have been those of accelerating a process that was already taking place rather than a new development.[30]

The situation in Scotland was in some respects easier to control than in England. The major proposal was that health care should not be devolved to local authorities, but rather to some eighteen health boards, most of which would encompass the geographical areas of several smaller local authorities. Things did not run altogether smoothly, though, and it was not until July 1971 that a White Paper concerning Scottish health care was published, and the next National Health Service (Scotland) Act was passed in August 1972, a year earlier than the corresponding measures for England and Wales. Given the relatively weaker state of Scottish local government, and the realisation that individual local authorities would be unable to cope, particularly the smaller ones, it was not difficult to persuade all concerned that the concept of health boards would be the most suitable solution to the problems.

The price to be paid for agreement at grass roots level was the disappearance of the five regional health authorities. Again, Scotland perhaps had the advantage of its small size. The nation was small enough to be catered for by a combination of the eighteen area boards under the umbrella of the central Scottish Home and Health Department. Two further central bodies were set up under the Act: the Common Services Agency and the Scottish Health Service Planning Council. The cumulative effect of all these changes was to streamline Scottish health care provision to around 45 centres of organisation, as compared with some 160 before the reorganisation. Remaining problems concerned the political composition of the new boards, and ensuring that the patient's voice could still be heard above the administrative clamour. In most respects, though, Scotland's system was reorganised rather less painfully and more quickly than south of the border. Why this was the case may not be wholly the result of compact size. It may be that there was more of a corporate will and consensus among Scots as to how their health services should be organised. The Scottishness factor may be defined in terms of a distinct Scottish view on management strategies and the ability to realise that some degree of centralisation and standardisation was necessary, despite the political ascendancy of the Conservative Party at the time – a party which favours less, not more, in the way of centralisation of government and administration. This consensus was achieved in part, perhaps in large part, because on the whole the Scottish arm of the BMA was generally in favour of the principles involved, though not always of the precise details of their application.

Although Scotland was apparently somewhat simpler to deal with in terms of reorganisation, what seems to have happened after 1974 in Britain as a whole, was that medical provision became highly politicised in a manner in which it had not been previously. The advent of the Thatcher era brought in new attitudes towards the public services, and none was more public or potentially problematic than health and its provision and maintenance. As at no other time, cost and economics became the overriding engine of change and reform. The NHS came into being in a period when the country was in a severely impoverished state after the war, but the driving force was the new vision for a better future for Britain and the cost, although spiralling from early on, was a problem to be dealt with rather than a motive force for change. By the 1980s, as technology developed and as the population lived longer and required more and more medical services, it would be the financial aspects which would occupy the minds of politicians and planners closeted in think-tanks and various other advisory groups. A number of plans were put forward and possibilities discussed, including the difficult proposal for involvement of the private sector in mainstream medicine, and also the beginnings of charges for certain services which had been provided free of charge, such as eye examinations. Prescription charges also began to rise and have continued to increase over the years. Individuals were encouraged to take out private medical insurance, and organisations such as BUPA and PPP saw a great opportunity both to influence medicine and profit from it. The privatisation factor is becoming ever more politically sensitive.

The next major phase of reforms belongs to the very recent past. By the late 1980s the government was once again trying to refocus and reorganise health provision. The White Paper, *Working for Patients*, led to many changes in organisation and responsibility, and ushered in the age of the trusts and the directorates. The rationale behind most of these changes was couched in the often jargon-ridden terminology of management rather than medicine. Provision would now be expressed in terms of contracts between purchasers and providers, not patients and practitioners, whether larger area health boards or local primary care trusts. The terminology of business is of necessity impersonal and to a great extent inflexible, and change could not be implemented without a great deal of controversy and debate. One area which affected doctors directly was that they were obliged to involve themselves in the problems of management as well as in the clinical field. There has been an uneasy relationship between practitioners and managers, and, apparently, clinicians have been very slow to offer their services in management, although managers have acknowledged that success would be 'judged largely on the basis of clinical output', and thus is closely dependent on the actions and involvement of clinicians.[31] Suspicion on all sides will not be eliminated easily, given the very political nature of health care provision at the end of the second millennium, even more so now that the Scottish Parliament must seek to prove itself in one of the most sensitive and closely monitored areas of its remit.

As the 1990s wore on, the trusts, boards and directorates were accepted, if gradually, but with the ending of a lengthy period of Conservative political dominance and the beginning of New Labour, the Health Service again served as a major focus of political output. In 1997 yet more proposals were put forward in a new White Paper, *Designed to Care* (the Scottish equivalent of the 1997 NHS White Paper for England). This once again ushered in reforms and further attempts at restructuring. It is claimed that the proposals for Scotland were both simpler and more flexible than those put forward for England, and that there would be much less prescription and central control than south of the border. The proposals were for a three-tier system, headed by the Area Health Boards, then the Primary Care Trusts and Local Health Care Co-operatives. The terms 'purchaser' and 'provider' were still there, but the new words were 'localisation' and 'partnership'. Localisation implies a degree of regional autonomy and again this is claimed to be more of a feature in Scotland than elsewhere. The new structures have been in operation only since 1999, so it is very difficult to assess the extent to which they have succeeded or failed. However, one development that seems to have taken place within the ranks of the general practitioners, who are key to the success of primary care (but who were not guaranteed automatic representation on the executives), is that these once fully independent practitioners have undergone a 'micro-level shift from individualism to collegiality', that is, acting as groups to defend their status and bring about reforms as a body.[32] The discourse of general practice is nowadays that of the group practice or health centre. The days of the single-handed GP in the comfortable role of a Dr Finlay have long gone. So, it is natural that doctors who practise in partnership will speak with much more of a common or communal voice than they did in the past. If the practicalities of general practice are shared, the discourse will be to an extent modified, or sharpened and politicised, according to the group rather than the individual. The division is now more likely to be between the majority of GPs who operate in partnership and the fewer, single-handed practitioners who have to be offered financial inducements to take on remote practices – a sort of London Allowance in reverse.[33] Another factor which has proved controversial and less widely accepted in Scotland is the introduction of GP fundholding arrangements, which devolved financial control of practices to the partners themselves. While the trend towards primary care and care in the community continues, there is the apparent dichotomy between the legitimate needs of the 'scientific' side of medicine and of the primary care practitioners. The problem in Scotland would appear to be no less severe than elsewhere; although newspaper headlines such as, 'Almost half burnt-out GPs plan to retire early'[34] may be an exaggeration, it remains to be seen whether the 'enforcement of community health' will be a success. A recent, comprehensive survey of general practice in the lifetime of the NHS has highlighted these difficulties, but also claims a revival in the fortunes and status of general practice in Britain.[35]

There have been reports in the recent press, strongly denied, that the Scottish Executive is actively considering the possibility of discontinuing the trusts and replacing them with a more streamlined, larger-unit system. Whether or not this is the case, the very suggestion that the matter is under consideration yet again, would seem to indicate that there is significant concern that the present variation of NHS organisation is no less problematic than its several predecessors.

The 1990s was also the age of corporate privatism in medicine. Large companies began to offer private medical insurance to their employees as part of the salary package. Companies had in the past been closely involved in medical care, but in a rather different way. In the days of the white heat of industrialisation and the rapid development of hospitals in the middle part of the nineteenth century, it had become commonplace for industrialists to subscribe to hospitals in order that they could secure the admission of their workers suffering from industrial injury or disease, thus forcing the hospitals to change their policies and admit accident cases, which they had generally not done prior to this point. This was not a wholly altruistic step; the main priority was to keep the workers fit to work. Their descendants in the late twentieth century clearly wished this too, but there were extra dimensions. The private sector operates on behalf of both patient and practitioner, as well as in the broader health-care sphere, although it may be noted that when the current consultant contract providing for private practice was mooted, Scotland's consultants voted against it.

MODERN HEALTH PROBLEMS IN MODERN SCOTLAND, STRATEGIES FOR THE ENCOURAGEMENT OF HEALTH

As with most other ages and periods, modern Scotland, despite two millennia of social construction and interaction of spheres of influence, is still afflicted by serious health and environmental difficulties. The particular circumstances of each age produce particular diseases and conditions, brought about by various degrees of lack of medical knowledge and the socio-economic, demographic and political profile of the country at the time. In the medieval period, for example, plague and the scourges of famine and dearth, coupled with the political and religious influences of the Roman church, characterised the health problems of the Scots. Nineteenth-century Scotland saw the devastating effects of diseases propagated by the built environment of urban squalor. General living circumstances are relatively better in the present period, but pressing medical and social problems remain, particularly in the area of mental health.

Nowadays, once key problems are identified and defined, government policy towards dealing with these problems often takes the form of intimating medium- to long-term targets it hopes to achieve. The hope is to reduce problems exponentially, meaning that they may perhaps never be solved entirely but may be diminished greatly in their effects on individuals and on society as a whole. The Scottish Executive has identified cancer, heart disease and mental health problems as the major health issues for Scotland, and the official document *Our National Health: A Plan for Action, A Plan for Change* was published in 2000, outlining proposed strategies and statistical targets. The document sets out plans for new, unitary health boards and a policy of 'patient-centred' care. Like 'child-centred education', these phrases belie the difficulties in their implementation, and it remains to be seen whether any or all of the targets set by the Scottish Executive can be reached. With regard to cancer, for example, the aim is to reduce mortality in those under seventy-five by 20 per cent by 2010. It is also hoped to reduce adult smoking by a third in the same period, and to implement enhanced and new screening programmes for breast, colorectal and other cancers.

Similar aims have been outlined to try to lift Scotland from the bottom of the European heart disease table. There are currently over 12,000 deaths per annum from coronary heart disease, and around 500,000 people are estimated to suffer from the condition to a greater or lesser extent.[36] The solution of this particular problem, though, lies not just in medical or surgical advance, but in major change in society itself, its attitudes and priorities. The archetypal 'West of Scotland' heart disease patients may take a great deal of persuasion to abandon the 'West of Scotland' diet and dispose of their frying pans. There are, of course, broader issues here concerning social and economic deprivation, often relating to urban poverty.

The third priority identified by the Scottish Executive is that of mental health. Diseases and impairments of the mental faculties have always been a feature of the overall 'unhealth' profile of the country, but it was not until the late eighteenth century that attitudes towards the mentally ill and mentally handicapped began to change. The treatment and care of these patients was influenced by a combination of changing medical and social attitudes, as outlined in the previous chapter. By the end of the First World War – a conflict which brought into very sharp focus the considerable psychological problems of war – the so-called 'second psychiatric revolution' was underway, which encouraged an 'open doors' policy within the mental institutions. The Mental Deficiency and Lunacy (Scotland) Act of 1913 set out improved procedures for the voluntary admission of patients, and also established the General Board of Control for Scotland (the word 'control' perhaps having significance).

It was becoming the view among psychiatrists that a decrease in the use of enforced seclusion and physical restraint was necessary, and that other measures should be tested. The beginnings of group therapy had been introduced as early as the late nineteenth century by Dr W. Browne at Sunnyside Hospital, Montrose, but it would not be until the 1950s that open doors and group therapy were introduced throughout the Scottish mental health sphere (though the hospital at Dingleton near Melrose was opening its doors by 1949 and was one of the first hospitals in the world to do so).[37] In the early 1920s a new wing of the Royal Edinburgh Hospital had been built, connected to, but outside, the walls of the asylum itself, primarily to deal with psychologically damaged casualties from the Great War.

In line with most facets of the Scottish medical sphere, the shaping and implementation of mental health policy derived from a combination of central political initiatives coupled with gradual change in the medical practitioners' view of how these sorts of conditions should be dealt with. In addition, in the late nineteenth century it became clear that if medicine as a whole were to progress, then a human infrastructure in terms of trained nurses and medical ancillaries had to be provided. By the inter-war period it was equally clear that a similar infrastructure of trained mental nurses and psychiatric social workers was crucial, and consequently appropriate training was instituted in response to the need. This was assisted by the new practice of designating wards in ordinary hospitals to the care of the mentally ill, thus allowing better opportunities for clinical and nursing training, and observation. The academic aspect of the mental disorder sphere had started to establish itself somewhat earlier, with the foundation of a postgraduate Diploma in Psychiatry in 1912, and the creation of the first Chair of Psychiatry in Scotland in 1918. It is undeniable, though, that as in many other areas of medicine and society, the Great War was a considerable catalyst, and by the outbreak of the Second World War, mental health care had established itself firmly as a legitimate and important branch of the medical sphere. Policies were also shaped by social attitudes, and the definition of deviance or mental health problems was made in terms of social norms as articulated, directly or indirectly, at the time.

As with most other components of the medical sphere, the advent of the NHS brought change, but also greater opportunity for the development of new medical and rehabilitative techniques, in the areas of chemotherapy, insulin therapy, ECT and, occasionally, frontal lobotomy. Following the Mental Health (Scotland) Act of 1960, the trend has been towards voluntary admission to psychiatric beds rather than enforced treatment, and in the last few decades a number of psychiatric specialties have appeared, including child psychiatry, forensic psychiatry, the care of the elderly patient, and the increasingly prevalent problems caused by the misuse of toxic substances.

The trend over the last few decades has to some extent been directed by general government policy on the NHS in terms of the pursuit of moves towards a focus on community care, and a service centred on primary care facilities. This coincided to some extent with the 'third psychiatric revolution', which sought to reintegrate the mentally ill or mentally impaired into their communities – returning to the situation which existed many centuries previously, although in much altered form. Further legislation in 1984 encouraged this move, and also fostered the culture of self-help and the integration of the social work aspects of psychiatric care into the broad remit of social work as a whole. A further trend in this area has been the shift, as far as possible, from in-patient to out-patient treatment, so that while there were 109,308 out-patient attendances in Scotland in 1965, by 1983 the figure had risen to 227,994.[38] Most of the large institutions have now closed their doors, or are in the process of doing so, and in England, where there are many more institutions to deal with, the aim was to close almost all of the 120 establishments by 2000.[39]

In terms of the Scottishness or otherwise of the sphere of mental health, it would appear that although constrained and influenced to a greater extent by national policy, individual Scots in individual institutions continued to make a considerable contribution to new developments. It may be that at the end of the twentieth century some of the distinctiveness is in the nature of the mental illnesses and their causes, particularly those which are affected or engendered by poor socio-economic conditions. Just as Scots top the disease leagues for heart disease and lung cancer, so the incidence of suicide among young Scottish men has been increasing, from four per 100,000 of the population in 1975 to fifteen per 100,000 in 1999.[40] Much of this increase has been attributed to social and economic deprivation, to which must be added drug abuse and alcoholism, both of which severely affect the whole of Scotland, not just the western regions.

As with the other major components of health policy, the Scottish Executive has identified aims and objectives, outlined in the *Framework for Mental Health Services*, which was launched in 1997. These include particular focus on the relationships between primary care trusts, mental health services and social work provision. Work is in progress to lay down clinical standards in areas such as the treatment of schizophrenia, and eventually in all areas of mental health services. A further factor which now must be taken into consideration by governments, legislators and the medical profession is the all-encompassing nature of the Human Rights Act (2000).

The effectiveness of the strategies employed by the Scottish Executive, or the 'devolution factor', remains to be seen. Academic research is of necessity only just beginning in this area, but one view is that the differences among the component parts of the British Isles in terms of historical precedent, the precise nature of devolved government and the relationship between these, will inevitably produce policies and practices on health care which are diverse. In effect there will be four separate 'health services', rather than a single entity with local management.[41] What is not in doubt is that, whether politically driven or not, the devolved Scottish government appears to be making considerable efforts in the area of mental health as elsewhere. The Scottishness may now be measured in political rather than medical terms, and may indeed be overplayed by anyone who seeks to prove that Scotland is still distinctive, or is again becoming distinctive. The problem with a 300-year old phoenix is that its ashes cannot be reconstituted as they were at the time of its original demise.

THE TECHNOLOGY AND SPECIALISATION OF MEDICINE – THE STAMP OF THE MILLENNIUM?

As well as the major political, organisational and health changes which have affected the people and society of Scotland, perhaps the most rapid process in the last decades of the millennium has been the technologising and globalisation of medicine with the concomitant potential to revolutionise methods of treatment. The stage is apparently being reached at which robots will be used to carry out routine surgical procedures with a far greater level of consistency and accuracy than can be achieved by human operators. Indeed, a recent report in a medical journal describes a robotic operation performed on a patient in Strasbourg by a surgeon operating a computer in New York.[42] This is a far cry from the days of thirty-second amputations in a squalid room or rudimentary field hospital behind the lines of battle, but what does this do for the caring ethos? If the nation is its people; can robots or other computerised practitioners be said to be of the nation or moulded by the nation?

Among the many areas in which the technologising of medicine has proved to be more than useful are those of diagnosis and the shaping and focusing of technological treatments to treat only the affected part of the patient and not to damage otherwise healthy tissue or organs. Radiography and radiology are in the vanguard of these developments. The increasing sophistication of scanning apparatus means that diagnosis can be made without distressing and invasive procedures. Computerised treatment machines can deliver individually tailored and precisely calculated doses of complex chemicals and radiation. Drug therapy is progressing in an even more complex way, so that individual genes and cells can be targeted, whereas previously only roughly defined general areas of the body could be treated. All of this adds to long- and short-term survival rates from diseases and conditions which until relatively recently could only be given palliative treatment.

In relation to surgical treatment, one of the most well-known developments in the recent past has been minimal-access, or 'keyhole', surgery. This technique allows operations to be performed without the need for large incisions to be made. The resulting benefits are a more rapid recovery time and a reduced risk of infection entering the wound. Knock-on benefits relate also to reduced occupancy time for hospital beds, and, indeed shorter periods of absence from work to recover from

these procedures. Scottish surgeons have been at the forefront of developments here, the surgical colleges run training programmes and Scotland
has produced many experts in the technique.[43]

There is also the very important and still developing area of large-
scale screening programmes, enabled by continuing technological advances.
Once again, it is women and their gender-related conditions which have
been at the forefront of recent developments. In the 1950s and 1960s,
mass X-ray programmes to diagnose tuberculosis were the first major,
nationwide non-gendered activities in this area. The campaign was
aimed at eradicating the scourge of tuberculosis, which had been a
constant thread throughout many eras of Scottish history. More recently,
though, the major screening programmes have been aimed at the early
diagnosis of breast and cervical cancer. Further, more selective screening
can be obtained for the in utero diagnosis of a number of potentially
fatal, chronic, genetically transmitted and disabling conditions. This, of
course, brings in a further dilemma, that of taking a decision to terminate
a pregnancy or not. So, the rapid advances in medicine create often
insoluble moral, ethical and religious dilemmas.

It is interesting to note that many of these worthwhile and valuable
screening programmes are related to the specific needs of women. This
is not a gender issue per se, nor indeed an issue of nationality or
Scottishness; it is perhaps recognition that the health of women and their
offspring is crucial to the progress of any nation. It may be simply,
though, that the conditions which are screened are those for which
suitable and reliable techniques have been found. To redress the balance
somewhat, techniques are currently being developed for screening for
prostate and bowel cancer. Despite the best efforts of the medical profession, Scots are still in the regrettable position of world leaders in terms
of incidence of some of the major modern killer diseases, particularly
heart disease and lung cancer, and it will take a much more comprehensive change of attitude than the availability of a screening test to
change this situation.

In the so-called 'dark ages' of medicine, these decisions were not part
of the general experience and practice of medicine. What has emerged
seems to be a division between those who subscribe to or oppose the
view that medical science should have limits imposed, not necessarily
because of limitations of knowledge or capability, but limits imposed for
a number of interacting moral and ethical issues. It has been a contention
of this book that Scotland and its medicine were stifled in the medieval
period by the dominant language and discourse of the pre-Reformation
church. The present day pre-Reformation church still provides spiritual
sustenance for its members, and takes a very strong view on the question

of abortion. But modern problems are much more complex, and what has emerged in terms of medical ethics is a complexity of viewpoints put forward by both professional and lay individuals from many interest groups and opinions. The patient at the centre of all of these dilemmas is confronted with many difficulties. Because, say, a diagnosis of spina bifida or Down's syndrome can be made at a very early stage of gestation, does this mean that every such pregnancy should be terminated? There are many similar issues. The problems in Scotland are no less than elsewhere and are no less difficult to deal with. The interaction of spheres of influence is perhaps at its most complex at the beginning of the third millennium. The very success of scientific and technological advance has forced the topics of medical ethics and morals to the forefront of debate. Since much of this debate is now carried out in the very public sphere of the media, there are many forces at work on the shaping of ethical policy and guidelines.

Since at least the era of William Cullen and Joseph Black, Scottish scientists have been at the forefront of medical advance, and Scotland has played a crucial role in the increasingly difficult and ethically sensitive area of genetic manipulation. Dolly the sheep was created in Scotland; the first sheep to be produced by a cloning technique which could ultimately have important implications for medical science and, therefore, to future patients. Dolly may be blissfully unaware that she is at all different from her fellow sheep, but she has produced major controversy. Indeed, the controversy has deepened as it has been admitted recently that she is suffering from arthritis at a relatively young age – in sheep terms at least. The sphere of nature is still, perhaps, as important as it was in medieval Scotland. The great difference is that nature can now be manipulated more extensively than in the past, when the mere domestication of crops and animals could be seen as manipulation or distortion of the natural process.[44] It is mostly acceptable to the general public that experimentation and trials of new treatments are carried out with specific aims in view, particularly in relation to the potential treatment of life-threatening diseases such as cancer, and debilitating degenerative conditions such as multiple sclerosis. The problems faced by those who hold the ethical balance of medical research in their control are exacerbated by the results of the research and the continual pushing back of the horizons of scientific possibility. It was all very well to produce a Dolly, or a daughter or son of Dolly; it is quite another matter when the possibility arises that a human Dolly is coming within the realms of possibility.[45] The difficulties with genetic research are clear – and Scotland has been at the forefront of these developments – that while genetic explanations for cancer, genetic treatments of cystic fibrosis and genetic manipulation to screen out congenital malformations and conditions are welcomed, who is to say where the barrier is between that and the more morally unacceptable face of medicine – the cloning of a whole human being or the creation of 'designer babies'. These are problems which affect medical men and women all over the world, or at least in the developed world. Scotland is not an exception, and Scots have to face the same moral and ethical dilemmas as are faced elsewhere.

Another area in which Scotland in this period is challenged (as are most developed nations) is the politicisation of medicine to a degree perhaps not seen in previous eras. This is an era of litigation, power politics, management and government with, it seems, no real agreement as to how the nation's health provision should be organised. Now that Scottish health is a responsibility of the Scottish Parliament, there is perhaps a new opportunity to agree on and implement an integrated policy, provided that the political rivalries can be subordinated to the common good. We are, for example, confronted with the problems of whether hospitals should be built on the foundations of private finance, an apparently irreconcilable contradiction to the principle of a state-funded NHS, but a contradiction which is seen by some as the only possible means of providing hospitals in sufficient numbers and scope to cope with the many problems which have been created in part by the very success of the NHS.

The national press has reported considerable problems with new Scottish hospitals which have been enabled by private finance initiatives. For example, it was apparently the case at the new hospital in Wishaw that inadequate provision for the treatment of cancer patients had been made,[46] while the new Royal Infirmary of Edinburgh has been the subject of great controversy over matters such as parking and the number of beds it should have, almost since the project's conception a number of years ago.

Whatever the situation, and however patchy or inadequate is the provision of medical services, this is the framework which has to contain a plethora of medical and surgical specialties, each of which would claim priority in the hierarchy of fund allocation. A century ago there were surgeons and physicians. Nowadays there are general physicians, chest physicians, gastro-intestinal physicians, cardiologists, endocrine and renal physicians, not to mention psychiatrists, neurologists, rheumatologists and many others. In the surgical sphere there are general surgeons, ortho-paedic surgeons, plastic surgeons, transplant surgeons, cardio-thoracic surgeons, vascular surgeons, neurosurgeons and many others. This plethora of specialties reflects the huge increase in the technical possi-bilities of each specialty, so that it is now no longer possible for the generalist in any sphere to cover a wide spectrum. In addition, there are extensive laboratory facilities, pathologists, bacteriologists, medical physicists, radiologists, oncologists and haematologists. The infrastructure of early-modern medicine was no more than the patient's home and the apothecary's shop; the infrastructure of medicine in the Enlightenment period included rudimentary hospitals; that of the Victorian period required larger hospitals and rather more technical support, though decidedly primitive. What is required to support modern Scottish medicine and surgery is almost incalculable in comparison. A Scottish patient in a modern Scottish hospital might expect to encounter a consultant, several other doctors, nurses, physiotherapists, radiographers, occupational therapists, laboratory technicians, operating theatre technicians, dieticians and social workers, not to mention those who provide the 'hotel' services. The experience of the modern patient is, therefore, constructed by multiple factors, influenced to a great extent by medical and surgical advances as much as to socio-economic factors. Roy Porter claims that the medical profession has reached a point where 'its finest hour is the dawn of its dilemmas'.[47] As a result of progress, expectations have grown to the extent that there is less and less prospect that they can be satisfied. There is much to ponder here.

ALTERNATIVE MEDICINES IN MODERN SCOTLAND – OLD SPHERES RETURNING?

Another important interaction of spheres of influence relates to the vast range of so-called 'alternative' medicines. This group of treatments encompasses everything from crystal therapy to colonic irrigation. All sorts of practitioners advertise their treatments and the stage appears to have been reached at the beginning of the twenty-first century where some of these alternative therapies are practised alongside conventional medicine and indeed patients are referred by their general practitioners for some of these therapies. Alternative therapies have been sought, offered and used throughout the history of the country and its medicine. Here, though, it may be that the national identity of alternative medicine has faded. Locality was crucially important in terms of the kinds of beliefs which abounded and the methods of treatment applied. So, whereas many peripheral therapies are accepted and practised widely, they perhaps do not have the local or national distinctiveness that they once had. Aromatherapy in Scotland, for example, does not differ greatly from aromatherapy in England, or France, or the USA. Three or four centuries ago alternative cures for a cough, a sore throat, or infertility would differ according to locality and tradition. This is, though, a sphere which does appear to have come full circle. In early times, alternative medicine *was* medicine; gradually, professionalisation separated the qualified from the unqualified; more recently, qualified orthodox medicine and qualified unorthodox medicine have been uneasy companions. What is different from previous periods is that the whole population has relatively easy access to orthodox, state-funded medicine, and the option to look elsewhere is a choice, rather than the only option, as in earlier times. The world of alternative medicine contains areas which are very close to orthodox medicine. The chiropractor performs manipulations similar to those carried out by physiotherapists. Chiropractors and other alternative therapists undergo rigorous training, take qualifying examinations and are supervised by corporate bodies. Does this not make them professional? Why then are they considered to be of little use, or even dangerous, by many?

Some alternative therapies have origins in the even more distant past than classical Western orthodox medicine. Interestingly, more recently, some acknowledgement of the potential benefits of alternative therapies has appeared in relation to the ancient Chinese art of acupuncture.[48] In some areas of medicine, a more holistic approach to the range of potential orthodox and alternative treatments is now well-established. Important here is the care of cancer patients who cannot be treated further with conventional approaches, or who choose to try a two-pronged approach to their treatment. In some ways, then, Scottish medicine has really returned to whence it came – in Roman, Celtic and even later times, there was no real distinction between what could be offered by qualified practitioners or by lay medical men or women.

The question raised is: just what has happened to the medical sphere and, indeed, the nation, during the last two thousand years? In terms of custody of the knowledge, it would seem that the grip of the orthodox professional is slipping once again and that the beginnings of a return to something approaching a previous situation are becoming apparent. Patients can really no longer be described as 'paradigmatically passive' in terms of their acceptance of treatments offered by orthodox professionals. While it is still the case that orthodox treatments are regarded at least as the first line of action by most patients, it seems that nowadays Scottish patients are no different from patients anywhere else in the developed world, and are turning increasingly to the periphery to supplement orthodox treatment. It may be that at some point in the future the orthodoxy needs to be redefined. For the moment, though, the fact that Scottish doctors practise acupuncture or hypnosis as part of their overall package of services does not mean that the medical profession itself is being weakened.

HOSPICES AND HOLISTIC CARE CENTRES

In Scotland, as in other parts of Britain, respite and palliative care given outwith the general hospital setting has become an integral part of the services offered to patients suffering from cancer and other terminal illnesses, including children. Here, in terms of interacting spheres, matters have to some extent come full circle. In earlier ages, indeed until the nation's health could be maintained by measures other than repentance or prayer, death was an inescapable part of life at all ages, not just at the end of the allotted biblical span. The nineteenth-century image of the dead baby put in a drawer on the kitchen table to await a pauper's funeral gave way to the other extreme: death became a forbidden subject and something to be feared, rather than accepted as the natural end of life, whether or not individuals held any belief in some sort of future existence, in whatever form. Nowadays, though, death has once again been brought back to life. Patients are encouraged to talk about it and to make plans for the end of their lives, so that their final months or days can be spent, as far as possible, in the manner which they themselves would most like.

One of the most significant and visible parts of this process has been the emergence of the hospice movement. Hospices, which now exist in many parts of Scotland (such as St Columba's in Edinburgh, or Strathcarron in the central belt) provide a service which caters for respite care and death. Hospices are not hospitals; they resemble hospitals in some physical aspects, but the aim is to provide a more home-like environment and to control pain and distress in a manner which makes it possible for patients to live their lives to the fullest extent possible. The ethos of these places is, of necessity, care rather than cure – a situation which obtained in medicine in general until the early Victorian period because the possibilities of cure were often remote. Although slow to evolve, hospices are now a crucial part of the holistic care given to these patients. The major question now is whether these charitably funded institutions can continue without receiving some sort of guaranteed NHS status in terms of financial provision.[49] The time is past, largely, when doctors and other health care professionals were suspicious about hospices and other such institutions, perhaps fearing that their role as controllers and directors of medical care would be compromised. Nowadays the important role of supporting agencies of all sorts is well recognised.[50]

One of the earliest hospices to pioneer this aspect of medicine in Scotland was set up in Edinburgh,[51] and was given the name St Columba's, perhaps as a conscious link back through many centuries of healing in the Christian tradition. This hospice, together with the Marie Curie Centre at Fairmilehead, has served the terminally ill patients of the district for a number of years. It is in these centres that pioneering methods of pain control can be applied, and patients are treated in a very different atmosphere from that which pervades 'normal' hospitals, where the prime concern is to return patients to as near a state of full health as possible. The hospice movement is able to confront the fact that patients in its care will not return to health but are approaching the end of their lives. The situation in the hospices can in some ways be compared with what happened in medieval hospitals. There, as in the present hospices, the patients were given holistic care, both religious and secular, and there was less sense of an urgent need to treat the condition, however hopeless the situation. The well-known axiom 'Thou shalt not kill, but needst not strive officiously to keep alive' is one which is appropriate to the modern day medical and caring professions as well as to their ancestors. A religious ethos may not pervade the hospices, but in many other ways they are very similar, at least in intent, to the medieval hospitals.

The ills of the nation are likened by some to biblical plagues. AIDS and the results of alcohol abuse affect large numbers of people and are viewed by some as the consequences of particular lifestyles. It was believed that biblical plagues could not be eliminated other than by repentance and prayer. Late twentieth-century plagues can be treated and their effects can be reduced by less mystical means, but modern diseases in the modern world produce tensions no less difficult to assess than in previous centuries. The more that medicine becomes capable of intervention, the heavier are the burdens of 'morality' that are placed on those who have control of it. The problem facing the third-millennium doctor is not his or her inability to cure, but rather the increasing ability to intervene in all sorts of situations.

In recent years, while some diseases have been eradicated, other difficult afflictions have taken their place. AIDS and HIV have proved to be two of the major epidemic problems of the late twentieth century, and a branch of the hospice movement has developed specifically to take care of such patients. Scottish scientists have carried out major research on AIDS and possible measures to treat and prevent the condition. A milestone in the care of AIDS victims, aptly named Milestone House, was one of the earliest AIDS hospices to be opened, and it is situated in the grounds of an Edinburgh hospital.[52] Its future is now uncertain but it was certainly a pioneer in its field. Although some hospices south of the border achieved greater fame because of the high profile of royal patrons, the less publicised but no less important services provided in Scotland have continued the tradition of endeavouring to offer care to those suffering from all manner of diseases. The AIDS hospice in Edinburgh is situated on the outskirts of the city, but this does not have quite the same implications as the banishment of lepers to Liberton, another suburb, in earlier times.

Once wholly funded by voluntary means, and outwith the central core of medicine and the NHS, since the mid-1990s the hospice movement has been financed to a much greater degree from central funds. Since the era of NHS contracts dawned in 1991, the then Scottish Office undertook to meet 50 per cent of the normal running costs of the hospices. This commitment means, though, that detailed accountability is now much more of a priority, and in some ways much more problematic, given the holistic nature of hospice care, which makes it difficult to apply artificial boundaries between costs of different treatments. It was thought that this could, in some cases, result in the closure of particular centres, but it seems that at present the hospices have been able to weather this storm and are managing to keep their doors open, at least in the short term.[53]

Under the umbrella of alternative medicine, but an area perhaps of much less controversy, is the increasing development of holistic centres situated close to major treatment centres for cancer and other terminal illnesses. A typical such institution is Maggie's Centre in Edinburgh, which started in a very small way in a building in the grounds of the Western General Hospital. Its aim was to provide for the non-medical needs of cancer patients and their relatives. Here, many sorts of activities and alternative care are on offer, but the primary benefit lies in the social and communication aspects of the service. It is being accepted increasingly that environmental factors and the patient's general attitudes and reactions are important in improving quality of life, if not lifespan itself. These centres care for the families of sufferers, as well as the patients themselves, and help to prepare them for life after the death of their relative. What is most important, though, is that this sort of approach is now being accepted increasingly by the orthodox medical profession as a legitimate part of treatment in its widest sense. The medieval hospital with its holistic view is a not an inappropriate image or comparison here, although, of course, the ethos and discourse are rather more secular in nature.

A CATALOGUE OF CONFLICTS – PROBLEMS
FACED BY PRACTITIONERS AND PROVIDERS AT
THE END OF THE SECOND MILLENNIUM

Given the seemingly bipolar aspects of the universe and its inhabitants, and the apparent significance or at least inevitability of opposites (day/night; hot/cold; good/evil; orthodox/unorthodox) it should perhaps be expected that the unavoidable consequence of two millennia of – mostly – positive progress for both the nation, and its health and health care, could only produce difficulties, problems, frustrations and political difficulties. At the end of the twentieth century most Scots are in many ways healthier, they live longer, eat better and can assume a reasonably high level of medical care and attention. However, it is also unfortunately the case that in some areas of the country, Scots still top the world league tables in areas such as heart disease and lung cancer, not to mention the largely inappropriate 'West of Scotland diet'.

The effects of the NHS have been discussed already, and the major trends in Scottish politics outlined briefly. This final section will provide a note of caution in the assessment or prediction of future trends in Scotland and Scottish medicine. It would seem that as this book closes there appears to be little real cause for optimism, and the major factor seems to be the overt and growing politicisation of medicine and its exacerbating financial problems, not so much created by the profession itself as by politicians who see health care as a very suitable and opportune bandwagon. There is room for only a few examples to illustrate this claim.

Firstly, Scotland's general practitioners seem to be approaching crisis point very rapidly. At the beginning of the NHS, the family doctor was literally that; a *family* doctor. He, and increasingly, she, worked alone, usually at home, and was able to cater for most of the needs of the patients. At the time of the golden anniversary of the state medical system, the average GP works in a large health centre, often has too many patients yet too few colleagues, is obliged to undertake endless amounts of paperwork, is expected to have up-to-date knowledge of the latest developments in a myriad of branches of medicine, is expected to offer a 'cure' for everything, and is confronted with the social consequences of life in modern Scotland. On the other hand, there are the considerable advantages of modern communications, computers, practice nurses, ancillary staff and all sorts of added extras which were not there in 1948. If Scotland is to improve the general health of its people, it is not only necessary to improve the environment in the broadest sense, but also to take steps to recruit many more doctors to general practice, which has to compete against the more fashionable and glamorous hospital specialties. In order to do this, the government must be bold enough to take steps to depoliticise medicine, and the professional managers must achieve a suitable balance between managing and allowing clinical judgement to play an equal part. This is, of course, not to claim that doctors should be unaccountable, as they used to be. It is clearly necessary for there to be a balance between management and clinical freedom; it seems that at present the balance has yet to be reached or maintained.

Hospital medicine is another area where success has at times bred disaster or created major problems. The technology of medicine has advanced beyond all recognition, and with that advance the demand for technological services has increased. Scots live longer, but they also expect to be treated in the most up-to-date way, in the shortest possible time, with the best of equipment and the most advanced of techniques. This expectation is almost impossible to achieve. To give one example, in the field of cardiology, it is now possible, by means of laser treatment to cure cardiac arrhythmias and obviate the need for patients to be on drugs for life (itself a drain on NHS funds).[54] However, the technology is complex, the machinery expensive, and each procedure can take several hours to complete – and herein lies the dichotomy. It has been reported on a number of occasions recently in the press that Scottish hospitals have been unable to accept donations of expensive magnetic resonance imaging and other equipment, because there were no funds available to run the equipment or provide the necessary staff.

Now that management is apparently the key to progress, and given that review and assessment are essential aspects of the nature and accountability of medical practice, the process of medical and surgical audit is becoming increasingly important; particularly with regard to assessment of morbidity and mortality statistics. Medical and surgical audit can provide guidance and illustrate areas of practice which need to be improved. For example, the 1998 *Scottish Audit of Surgical Mortality*[55] reported the need for increased numbers of high-dependency beds as a means of reducing post-operative mortality in Scottish Hospitals. Audits are ongoing on many aspects of medicine and surgery, aided by the increasing sophistication of computing equipment, and this is one area where technology provides the means to supervise techniques and survey results. Mortality statistics published in early eighteenth-century newspapers pointed out disturbing trends and epidemics; modern statistics can do much more. Medical statistics and informatics are now specialties in their own right.

CONCLUSION

The consequences of good advice have often brought problems in their wake. The eradication of crippling diseases like poliomyelitis has reduced the burden of that type of care on the health services. Indeed, hospitals created in Scotland specifically to care for 'crippled children' are being closed.[56] This development has, though, been more than counterbalanced by modern afflictions such as AIDS or the consequences of individuals who choose to smoke, to consume a seriously unsuitable diet or to start on the dangerous path of experimentation with drugs and other noxious substances.

In their own turn, though, the great achievements of the NHS have, increasingly, generated even greater problems, so that the concept of medical care 'free to all at the point of need', is almost impossible to sustain. This book ends with the NHS apparently in terminal crisis and about to disintegrate because of the sheer burden placed on limited financial resources. As mentioned, the very success of the NHS has created a situation in which it is almost impossible to continue to supply the full aims of the original Act. In the latter part of the twentieth century, the NHS underwent several revisions and attempted reorganisations, dividing the country into fewer, larger areas and introducing NHS trusts and other management systems, by which it was hoped that the requirements of patients and practitioners in an age of almost limitless, medical possibilities could be covered.

The relatively short period covered by this final chapter has witnessed some of the most important developments, not only in medicine and surgery themselves, but, importantly, also in the areas of government policy, general attitudes towards health care, the promotion of healthy lifestyles as well as regaining health after disease or injury, and the considerable technological advances which have taken place. In terms of the discourse of medicine and the public perceptions of practitioners and the rights and role of the patients, the overwhelming impression is one of politicisation and the dominance of both medical and national politics over organisational progress. All of the major trends identified in previous chapters are there; their relative importance and emphasis may be different, and new factors added, but at the core is still the presence of disease, the need to treat it and the need for new knowledge to be gained and applied in a suitable manner. Modern medical discourse is about organisation and management systems, about manipulation of the NHS to try to control the problems it has itself created, and which have been created by the changing socio-economic and political profile of society in general. The nature of the consultation process may be different, but medicine has not yet progressed to the extent where face-to-face consultation is no longer necessary. The sphere of medicine has expanded greatly over the two millennia. It contains many and increasingly complicated elements, and is still influenced to a great extent by politics. The politics of the nation are as important as ever, and as complex as ever. The Scottish Parliament has yet to make a full impact on Scottish life as well as medicine. Critical analysis of Scottish medicine under devolved government is a topic for a future historian of medicine in Scotland.

NOTES

1. See Davis, J., 'Central government and the towns', in Daunton, M. (ed.), *The Cambridge Urban History of Britain. Volume III*, 260–86.

2. Blackden, S., 'From physicians' enquiry to Dewar Report: a survey of medical services in the west highlands and islands of Scotland, 1852–1912', Parts I and II, *Proc. Roy. Coll. Phys. Ed. 28* (1998), 51–66; 207–17; Hamilton, *Healers*, 247–52.

3. The work of the Scottish Board of Health is described in detail in Jenkinson, J. L. M., 'Scottish Health Policy 1918–1938', in Nottingham, C. (ed.), *The NHS in Scotland. The Legacy of the Past and the Prospect of the Future* (Aldershot, 2000), 1–20.

4. Quoted in *Health in Scotland 2000*, Scottish Executive Health Department, 2. Jenkinson's forthcoming book on health policy will add considerably to the historiography of this area. Jenkinson, J. L. M., *Scotland's Health 1919–1948* (Oxford, forthcoming).

5. Detailed summary in Tait, H., 'Maternity and Child Welfare', in McLachlan, G. (ed.), *Improving the Commonweal. Aspects of Scottish Health Services, 1900–1984* (Edinburgh, 1987), 414–38.

6. Ibid., 420.

7. Wilson, S., 'The public health services', in McLachlan (ed.), *Improving the Common Weal*, 307.

8. Clayson, C., 'Tuberculosis', in McLachlan, (ed.), *Improving the Common Weal*, 393.

9. McFarlane, N., 'Hospitals, housing and tuberculosis in Glasgow, 1911–1951', *Soc. Hist. Med. 2* (1989), 59–85.

10. Davidson, R., 'Measuring "the social evil": the incidence of venereal disease in inter-war Scotland', *Medical History 37* (1993), 185.

11. Hardy, A., *Health and Medicine in Britain Since 1860* (Basingstoke, 2001), 155. See also pp. 139–72, the 'Golden Age', which details developments in treatments for many diseases and conditions.

12. Porter, *Greatest Benefit*, 618–9.

13. Full account in Tomaszewski, W. (ed.), *The University of Edinburgh and Poland* (Edinburgh, 1969), 41–52. See also Wojcik, W. A., 'Time in context – the Polish School of Medicine and Paderewski Polish Hospital in Edinburgh 1941 to 1949', *Proc. Roy. Coll. Phys. Ed. 31* (2001), 69–76.

14. For factual information on the major Scottish medical schools, see Blair, *History of Medicine at the University of St Andrews;* Comrie, *History*, vol. ii; Pennington, *Modernisation of Medical Teaching at Aberdeen*.

15. Davison, H., Capewell, S., MacNaughton, J., Murray, S., Hanlon, P. and McEwen, J., 'Community-oriented medical education in Glasgow: developing a community diagnosis exercise', *Medical Education 33* (1999), 55–62.

16. Dupree, M. and Crowther, M. A., 'A profile of the medical profession in Scotland in the early twentieth century: the *Medical Directory* as a historical source', *Bull. Hist. Med.* 65 (1991), 209–33.

17. Hull, A. and Geyer-Kordesch, J., *The Shaping of the Medical Profession. The History of the Royal College of Physicians and Surgeons of Glasgow, 1858–1999* (Oxford, 1999), 226, quote from T. Gibson, November 1977.

18. See Bradshaw, A., *The Project 2000 Nurse: The Remaking of British General Nursing, 1978–2000* (London, 2001).

19. Jenkinson, 'Scottish Health Policy', 7.

20. Full account of the origins and development of the hospital in Austin, T., *The Story of Peel Hospital, Galashiels* (Selkirk, 1996).

21. Webster, C., *The National Health Service. A Political History* (Oxford, 1998), 2.

22. Webster, *National Health Service*, 10.

23. Hutchison, I. G. C., *Scottish Politics in the Twentieth Century* , 92.

24. Fuller account of these negotiations in Hamilton, *Healers*, 259–62.

25. National Health Service (Scotland) Act, 10 & 11 Geo VI, Cap 27.

26. Johnston, R. and McIvor, A., 'Whatever happened to the occupational health service? The NHS, the OHS and the asbestos tragedy on Clydeside', in Nottingham (ed.), *NHS in Scotland*, 84.

27. Webster, *National Health Service*, 87–93.

28. *Reasons for Restructuring. Administrative Reorganisation of the Scottish Health Services* (HMSO, Edinburgh, 1968), 7.

29. *Report of the Royal Commission on Medical Education* (HMSO, London, 1968), 56.

30. *The National Health Service in Scotland* (Department of Health for Scotland, 1959).

31. Bruce, A. and Hill, S., 'Relationships between doctors and managers: the Scottish experience' *Journal of Management in Medicine*, 8 (5) (1994), 51.

32. Hudson, B. and Hardy, B., 'Localisation and partnership in the "New National Health Service": England and Scotland compared', *Public Administration* 79 (2) (2001), 330.

33. Green, J., 'Time and space revisited: the creation of community in single-handed British General Practice', *Health and Place* 2 (2) (1996), 85–94.

34. *The Times*, 18 October 2001.

35. Loudon, K., Horder, J. and Webster, C. (eds), *General Practice Under the National Health Service 1948–1997* (London, 1998).

36. Full details and statistics of health policies can be found in *Health in Scotland 2000*.

37. Hunter, T. D., 'Mental Health', in McLachlan, G. (ed.), *Improving the Common Weal. Aspects of Scottish Health Services 1900–1984* (Edinburgh, 1987), 341.

38. Ibid., 346.

39. Lane, J., *A Social History of Medicine. Health, Healing and Disease in England, 1750–1950* (London, 2001), 113.

40. *Health in Scotland 2000, Part 3, Mental Health*, 1.

41. Exworthy, M., 'Primary care in the UK: understanding the dynamics of devolution', *Health and Social Care in the Community* 9 (5) (2001), 266–78.

42. Marescaux, J., Leroy, J., Rubino, F., Smith, M., et al., 'Transcontinental robot-assisted remote telesurgery: feasibility and potential applications', *Annals of Surgery* 235 (4) (2002), 487–92.

43. The Royal College of Surgeons of Edinburgh, and other institutions, run regular basic and advanced courses on the techniques of minimal access surgery.

44. Wilmut, I., *The Second Creation. Dolly and the Art of Biological Control by the Scientists who Cloned Dolly* (London, 2000).

45. It was reported recently that American scientists had developed the technology for human cloning. *The Herald*, 26 November 2001.

46. As reported in the *Glasgow Evening Times* (3 September 2001), 'Furious staff blast health minister at crisis hospital'.

47. Porter, *Greatest Benefit*, 718.

48. See, for example, *The Times*, 26 June 2000, which carried the headline 'BMA calls for acupuncture on the NHS'.

49. Sims, M. T., 'Can the hospices survive the market? A financial analysis of palliative care provision in Scotland', *Journal of Management in Medicine* 9 (4) (1995) 6–16.

50. Macdonald, E. T. and Macdonald, J. B., 'How do local doctors react to a hospice?', *Health Bulletin Edinburgh*, 50 (5) (1992), 351–5.

51. For an account of St Columba's, see Bostock, Y., *Letting Go and Living: the Story of St Columba's Hospice* (Edinburgh, 1991).

52. Murie, J., 'A milestone in AIDS care', *Nursing Times* 88 (42) (1992), 24–7.

53. Sims, M. T. R., 'Can the hospices survive the market? A financial analysis of palliative care provision in Scotland', *Journal of Management in Medicine*, 9 (4) (1995), 4–16.

54. Grubb, N. R. and Furniss, S., 'Science, medicine and the future: radiofrequency ablation for atrial fibrillation', *British Medical Journal*, 322 (7289) (2001), 777–80.

55. *Scottish Audit of Surgical Mortality* (Glasgow, 1998), 3.

56. Hospitals such as the Princess Margaret Rose Orthopaedic Hospital in Edinburgh, which was founded to care for children crippled by poliomyelitis, and then congenital dislocation of the hip – a condition which because of early diagnosis and treatment nowadays does not require lengthy hospitalisation and surgery in all cases.

CONCLUSION

Whither Scottish medicine now? The changing needs of an ever more demanding population, set against ever diminishing finance, mean that the ills of the nation are very much bound up with the progress, problems and successes of the nation itself, as much as with the influence of any individual or institution. Policies on nations and their health are matters of government and politics and finance. The noble aims of the National Health Service were enunciated in a time when life expectancy was shorter and fewer individuals were expected to live long enough to become a major economic drain on medical resources. The technology of medicine was much more primitive, and the possibilities and financial implications of sophisticated diagnostic and therapeutic machinery were unknown and, therefore unconsidered, in the bold promise of free treatment for all 'at the point of need'. In many ways the very distinction of Scottish medical men and women has, ironically, produced problems which appear to be almost insoluble. The means to cure diseases and to prolong life have brought the nation's medical services to crisis point, a situation which Beveridge and his political allies could never have anticipated. Britain as a whole spends much less per capita on health care than most other European countries (and in a recent survey came a poor eighteenth out of the top twenty nations in Europe), and it seems that economics have served to make British – and, therefore, Scottish – medicine much more dependent on finance and management rather than political ideals, altruistic intent or medical genius. It remains to be seen whether the devolved Scottish Parliament can do anything to remedy these problems, and while it has been claimed that the Scottish Executive has already met its spending targets on health for 2005, Scots still suffer worse health than in many parts of the developed world. Locality has been crucial in all aspects of history, not least in the evolution of the Scottish nation, the British state and the transient period of Empire. Historians have perhaps rather neglected the localities; even in these days of postmodernism, where nothing apparently derives from anything else, it is beneficial to consider them.

Spheres of medical influence have come almost full circle. Nowadays patients have once again rather more influence on their treatments (should they wish to have), or, at least, access to knowledge about their conditions. These influences, though, are rather different from the doctor-patient relationships in previous eras and in differently related spheres. Scotland may be about to be 'a nation again' but medicine will probably not regain a separate Scottishness, and indeed the nation can never be the same 'nation again'. There is no doubt, however, that British medicine and the medicine of much of the developed world bear, however faintly now, the mark of Scotland's medical history and, indirectly, Scotland's national history and defining characteristics.

Scots are still to be found at the head of national medical and surgical institutions; Scots doctors and surgeons are, however, no less fallible than their counterparts elsewhere, as witnessed by several high-profile cases in the recent past. When he wrote his famous treatise on surgery four centuries ago, and included a detailed account of how to amputate a leg, Peter Lowe can scarcely have conceived of the possibility of a surgeon amputating a perfectly healthy limb because of a patient's disturbed body image. However, on closer consideration, is this very much different from the widespread use of trepanning to let out evil spirits in earlier times? If each activity is judged according to the belief systems, attitudes and practices of the time, it is possible to see yet again that mind and body and their care bring up different questions of ethics and practice in any age. What seems outrageous to the allegedly rational modern mind may not have appeared in the least extraordinary in the Dark Ages, when the only way to rid the body of evil was to force it out by whatever means deemed necessary.

But what of the distinctive nationality of Scottish medicine? This account ends at a time of considerable flux and, perhaps, even excitement, in the history of Scotland and her relations with her contiguous territories and global partners. Many individual Scots are prominent in medicine, medical organisations and medical advances; for example, in research into Creutzfeldt-Jakob Disease and its effects, but is there anything left that can be cited truly as Scottish medicine rather than medicine in Scotland? This is very much the same sort of debate as the historiographical controversies over the Enlightenment, a period in which Scotland and Scots were not only prominent, but were world leaders, particularly in medicine and scientific matters. Historians agonise over whether there was a Scottish Enlightenment, or the Enlightenment in Scotland; the same debate may be entered into with regard to medicine at the start of, for at least that part of the population of Scotland which adheres to the Christian calendar (if not religion), the third millennium. Early-modern Scottish medicine was distinctive because of its close contacts with Europe, the acceptance of individuals from lower social ranks as medical equals, the evolution of the universities, and the relatively small size of the nation, which meant that in some senses 'Scottish' medicine was 'local' medicine. Scotland's population is heterogeneous today; but it has always been so. The peoples who inhabited Scotland before the start of the first millennium were members of a number of disparate tribes and peoples. The mixture was spiced up by the addition of Romans, Normans, Saxons, Angles and many others over the centuries, so, although Scotland may perhaps be heading towards a period of greater political independence, her people are no more homogeneous than they have ever been. The current mixture of ethnic groups in Scotland may be rather different from what it was many centuries ago, but there has always been such a mix. Wallace and Bruce may have fought for the freedom of Scotland and the Scots, but the people on whose behalf they fought were not a uniform people of uniform origins, and indeed Bruce's own ancestors were French.

In that case, can Scottish medicine, or medicine in Scotland, be claimed ever to have been distinctive or even unique? Certainly, the characteristics of the Scottish nation include a historic recognition of the importance of education. The 'school in every parish' may have been a pipe dream in the days of John Knox, and the 'lad o' pairts' no more than the expression of an ideal rather than a description of specific or real individuals, but education is one factor which seems to have played a part in making Scotland different. The very high regard in which early-modern Scottish surgeons were held in comparison to their English counterparts was due at least in part to the general willingness of Scots and Scotland to accept individuals with a combination of lower social status and higher-level education, the former not necessarily precluding the latter as it did in many other areas of Britain and the world. A competent Scottish surgeon of relatively low social rank could still find acceptance as surgeon to the king. A key influence here was the early, strong and continuing favour of Scots medical men by nobles and royalty. Patronage was everything in the medieval and early-modern periods. It is still important, but perhaps clothed in a more subtle disguise.

Future historians of medicine in Scotland will, no doubt, have much more to say on the subject of the nationality of medicine and medical practice. For the moment, it is perhaps sufficient to re-emphasise the very significant contributions made by Scots and Scotland in a field which is growing ever more complex and global in its manifestations.

Scotland, as a nation of people suffering ills of all sorts, progressed through a complex network of interacting spheres of influence and levels of potential. Patients in the middle ages demanded different things from their medical attendants than patients in the early-modern period, the Victorian period, in wartime, in natural or unnatural disasters, or in the late twentieth century, when many body parts can be replaced, done without, reconstructed or otherwise manipulated. Whether or not Scottish medicine is better than it ever was, is quite another matter. The state of the nation is perhaps even more problematic. It is rather too early in the new scheme of things to give judgement on how a devolved Scotland is working for the nation or for its medicine. There are indications that the state of the NHS in Scotland is not quite so parlous or dangerous as its counterpart south of the border. This situation is due to a number of factors, such as different patterns of population concentration, and differences in the composition and functions of the urban setting. There is, though, no guarantee that the situation will not deteriorate. Recently, it has been claimed that a substantial majority of the general practitioners in Scotland have indicated their willingness to resign en masse from the NHS in protest at perceived mismanagement and severe underfunding as negotiations for a new contract continue. There is little doubt that British medicine is in a period of crisis; it remains to be seen whether Scotland can weather that crisis more easily than the rest of the UK.

If some sort of human analogy is needed, in terms of the evolution of medicine, the diseases of mind and body became very separate spheres of causation and treatment, at least by the end of the eighteenth century. On the fringes of orthodox medicine at least, a more holistic view is now being taken of the body and all its functions, including those of the mind. The Scottish nation itself started as a series of mutating and changing parts; by the beginning of the fourteenth century the 'body' became more or less fixed in scope, though not in terms of 'peace of mind'; by the beginning of the seventeenth century, Scotland was part of a much bigger body; in turn, the British body became the core of an empire in a larger and globally disparate body; by the end of the second millennium, the British body had shrunk and the Scottish part had threatened to detach itself once more. What this means for Scotland and Scottish medicine is, at present, enigmatic and difficult to assess.

This book ends at a crossroads, for both the nation and its medicine and medical health. Scotland has come through two turbulent millennia and is, in some ways, a little uncertain as to her real identity. This has been an ongoing issue for two thousand years. When the early tribes melded themselves from Picts, Scots, Angles and others into Alba, what was created was no nearer to being a unified identity or entity. The corporate aspects of Scotland related to groups of domination and opposition to other groups which desired a greater measure of territorial power. What shaped the destiny of the Scots in at least the first millennium was leadership and the influence of regional kings and groups of nobles who were able to use their leadership skills, power bases and at times sheer luck, in order to take the nation part of the way along the long road to consolidation. Once consolidated under a single dynastic progression, the destiny of Scotland was bound up inextricably with the fate and actions of other nations and other influential leaders. It has been claimed that a nation that loses its identity tries to construct a history, perhaps not always founded on facts. The origin-legends of Scotland are a case in point. In many ways this is true of second-millennium Scotland, particularly post-eighteenth-century Scotland. The myth and legend of the Scot have become linked symbolically with the myth and legend of the highlander. The 'tartanisation' of Scotland has been a very mixed blessing – positive for the tourist industry but rather less effective in portraying the complexities and core of the nation or of its medicine.

How did all of this help to shape the destiny and fate of medicine and its practitioners in Scotland? In some ways medicine and society developed hand in hand, each dependent on progress in the other aspect. In other ways, though, what happened in terms of health care provision was increasingly taken out of the sphere of the specific nation. It seems from the foregoing chapters that in most of the periods under discussion, a combination, often a complex combination, of interacting influences shaped the nation, its medical practitioners and, importantly, its patients. In addition, the combination and interaction of influences was not standard across the whole country, particularly in earlier times. Geography, demographic change, urbanisation and communication all played their part in influencing exactly who was where in Scotland, and who received what kind of medical training or treatment.

At the end of two millennia some things have changed out of all recognition, while other things seem to have changed hardly at all. At the beginning of the first millennium Scotland did not exist. At the turn of the second millennium Scotland almost existed but not quite, although its main constituent groups of inhabitants were mostly in place. At the turn of the third millennium Scotland most certainly exists, and is possibly on the brink of breaking away from its southern, dominant partner. So there has never been an individual who could be described as the 'standard' Scot, and the territory known as Scotland has only been so for less than half of the period under review in this book.

PATIENTS, PRACTITIONERS AND POWER

One of the defining characteristics of medicine through the ages has been the nature of the relationship between patient and practitioner. The balance of power, and the factors influencing that relationship have changed considerably, and these changes have themselves helped to characterise the medical sphere of different periods. In very early times, power was wholly local, and any bias of power towards the healer probably related to acknowledgement that the healer had special gifts. There was no national concept of anything, let alone medicine. In medieval times the power base of medicine in Scotland was the Roman Catholic church, which dominated the nation, but Scotland was still a nation essentially of localities, linked together by the relationships between the centre of government and the local nobles. Feudal society was hierarchical, but feudal medicine was still local. One difference, though, was that high status patients held the balance of power in any relationship with a medical practitioner.

The early-modern period saw the beginnings of very different power structures. Two new factors here were, firstly, the acceleration in the urbanisation process, and, secondly, the emergence of institutions which trained the 'orthodox' practitioners and allowed them to claim power within the ranks of the practitioners as well as over the patients. At this point politics assumed a much greater degree of importance, as patronage of some sort was the key to maintenance of status or privilege. These general trends continued during the eighteenth century, which was characterised by new debates over both the nature of medical knowledge itself and the efforts by the practitioners to maintain custody of that knowledge in a sphere of wider access to knowledge of all sorts. The patronage of royalty, nobility and politicians continued to matter greatly. Perhaps by this time, in official medicine at least, the patient was becoming less powerful in the consultation and treatment situation.

In the Victorian period and the more modern era, the trends towards urbanisation, hospitals as the élite focus of medicine, new knowledge, new technology and new problems have continued. What is rather different, though, is the nature of political involvement. Politics continues to affect medical power, but the effects are twofold. Firstly, medicine in all its aspects has become increasingly controlled by legislation and the force of central government, whether or not the responsibility for implementation is devolved to the localities. Secondly, and a strong feature of the recent past, medicine has itself become a political tool for politicians to manipulate for the ends of political power rather than the health of the patients. The patient may have regained a little more power within the consultation situation, but medical politics is now an integral part of national politics for its own sake.

SOURCES

One very illuminating aspect of this study has been the consideration of the sources on which the book has been based. The very marked changes in the nature of these sources provide a useful indicator of how medicine and nation have changed. Assessment of medicine and surgery in the very early period was based largely on the evidence left from physical remains and artefacts. Archaeology rather than manuscript records provided most of the surviving evidence. Nowadays, the techniques of environmental history can lend their aid also to the historian of early medicine. The preponderance of fragmentary physical evidence gave way to the equally fragmentary and incomplete manuscript evidence for the Dark Age and medieval periods. The manuscripts themselves were derived from Hippocrates and Galen, but increasingly the evidence was religious and Roman Catholic in compass. The tale of medicine in medieval Scotland was that of religion. What was added to this tale in the early-modern period were the records of the emerging medical and surgical institutions, and also of town councils and of other secular bodies. The trend is clear, then, of the secularising and institutionalising process at work and this trend is reflected in the surviving evidence. The casebooks of a few Scottish practitioners add to the institutional records, while 'Poor Man's Guides' and other lay records confirm the continuing importance of that substantial facet of the medical sphere. As the Scots moved into the age of the Enlightenment, so the physical nature of the evidence began to change again. To hand now were not only the writings of individuals and institutional records, but also the new sphere of the medical journal, which contained the collected evidence of the latest trends and thoughts in medicine and surgery. These records confirm two further processes: the interaction between individual genius and the growing public; and the published sphere of information, discussion, debate and dissemination.

From this period onwards, there is an even more decisive change in the nature of the records. What the Victorian period produced in profusion was the records of officialdom and government intervention. Medicine and surgery became more and more affected and controlled by the process of large-scale national and municipal government. National legislation, royal commissions and local legislation provided a new legal framework for medical practice and also medical training. Historians of medicine are confronted by a much wider variety of source materials, reflecting the more complex nature of medicine itself. Government records are supplemented by hospital records, training records, the press and the medical press. The modern period, particularly post-1945, has offered even more illuminating illustration. There are now two very different strands. One of these strands is the large volumes of official sources from government and health institutions. However, there is also the burgeoning historiography of medicine, which itself is extremely significant. A glance through the secondary references for the chapter on the modern period very quickly reveals that for coverage of the very recent past, the historian has to look in journals of management rather than journals dealing with the general history of medicine and surgery. Information is also available in works coming out of the spheres of sociology, politics and technology. The fragmentation of the historiography reflects the fragmentation of medicine and surgery into specialisms and also the increasingly political and politicised nature of medicine and medical practice. The medical sphere has always relied on politics, but politics of an ever changing nature.

THEORIES AND CONCEPTS

As mentioned at the beginning of this book, any attempt to impose a sociological or other sort of theory on the evolution of the nation and its medicine is fraught with considerable difficulty. Habermas, Jordanova, or any other theorist, may be appropriate as a starting point, or as an initial method of harnessing thoughts and information. Consideration of the intermingling of spheres of interaction and influence is certainly useful in helping to portray the complexities of factors which brought about change but also maintained continuity throughout this very long period.

This type of survey or global history may be seen as a postmodernist's worst nightmare. There is no doubt that detailed local or specific studies are crucial to an understanding of the greater whole, but some attempt at an overall perspective may offer a useful framework on which to build the local, the detailed and the specific. Certain dominant themes and causal sequences have been highlighted unashamedly here, making the book susceptible to accusations of Whiggishness. It is certainly not intended to give a Whiggish political slant, far from it, but in terms of the demonstration of chains of interaction, planned or spontaneous, which led to a particular state or set of circumstances, it is possible to rebut the accusation and turn it into a positive feature. The aim is not Whiggish in the sense of trying to demonstrate that the state of either Scotland or its medicine in 2002 was the direct, or inevitable, consequence of what happened twenty centuries ago, or even ten. The aim in suggesting some sort of historical causality has been to point out the dialectic confluence of local, national and at times international circumstances which influenced the shape, scope and Scottishness of medicine.

It is also possible to apply many other theoretical perspectives. Those who subscribe to the views of Foucault on social control could certainly find ready evidence in some of the events and processes which have been described, particularly in relation to developments in the treatment of mental illness, or in the emergence of big government and national legislation on poor relief and public health in the nineteenth century. Those of a more Marxist persuasion might feel that Scottish medicine was shaped, in the industrial period at least, by the consequences of the class struggle and the emergence of different divisions among groups in society. Individuals who take a more conservative or Conservative perspective could, though with perhaps a little more difficulty than with some approaches, point to a more organic or osmotic process, through which Scotland and Scottish medicine progressed together over the centuries.

Another viewpoint, which does seem to have some merit in this case relates to the role of the individual. While the 'great doctors' or 'names and places' view of this history of medicine has been largely, and rightly, criticised as insufficient or old-fashioned, a more useful perspective might be to look at the role of the individual in combination with his or her contemporary circumstances. It is clear that many developments in medicine and surgery could not have been made without the input and influence of specific individuals, but these individuals could not have functioned in isolation. They were members of their own age, time and society, and imbued with the same influences as the rest of the population. So, the creative dialectic between crucial individual genius and general background trends seems to have been of some importance here.

Whatever the case, and whatever theory might be claimed to be the most plausible, there is no doubt that medicine, medical training, and the experiences of Scots as patients and practitioners has been influenced, to varying degrees at various times, by the 'outside world', as well as by the nation itself. A key factor may have been the disproportionate number of prominent individual Scots who practised in medicine and in other areas of intellectual prominence; it may have been the crucial involvement and support of those in power in society, particularly successive monarchs over the ages; it may have been the undefinable 'Scottishness' factor. Whatever the explanation, it can be claimed with some justification that there was something distinctive about Scottish medicine for at least part of the period. Medicine in Scotland, rather than Scottish medicine, is what is practised at the present time, but there is also no doubt that medicine as a whole, worldwide, has been touched by Scottish medicine, just as all corners of the globe have been touched by Scots of all sorts.

A FINAL WORD OF CAUTION

As stated clearly at the beginning of this book, a work such as this cannot do more than scratch at the surface. A project of this nature is open to all sorts of accusations and criticisms that this or that point was not made, or this or that aspect was not given full, in-depth treatment. It must be emphasised that the purpose was, and remains, to offer a general perspective as a basis for further, detailed research. Many scholarly monographs would be needed to cover two thousand years in depth. It is hoped that this book will at least give some suggestions as to possible directions for more detailed research in the future. No claim is made that definitive answers are given; the aim and intention has been to raise issues, highlight key themes and pose questions for discussion, research and elucidation in the future. The teaching of the history of medicine is a relatively new area, particularly so in Scotland, and more particularly in mainstream university history departments. This work is aimed also at serving this aspect of academic history as a basic sounding board. Many of the points made in these chapters have been influenced by discussions in honours classes in the history of medicine in Scotland at the universities of Stirling and Edinburgh; it is hoped that future works will be similarly influenced and stimulated.

FURTHER READING

Since the book covers a very long time scale and has been able only to hint at progress, controversy or historiography in many areas, the following list suggests further reading on the major topics covered and comprises material not referenced directly at any other point in the book. It has been necessary to be brief and selective, but the material mentioned here will act at least as a starting point to further, more detailed research. In many cases the bibliographies of the cited works will offer guidance for further reading. This listing is thematic, rather than chronological in composition, to indicate more easily items relating to topics rather than to specific time-periods. A separate 'Select Bibliography' contains a brief list of major works cited in this book.

HISTORICAL THEORY

Burrage, M. and Torstendahl, R. (eds), *Professions in Theory and History* (London, 1980).
Evans, R., *In Defence of History* (London, 1998).
Jordanova, L., *History in Practice* (London, 2000).
Marwick, A., *The Nature of History*, 3rd edn (Basingstoke, 1989).
Tosh, R., *The Pursuit of History*, 3rd edn (London, 2000).

SCOTTISH HISTORY

SCOTLAND FROM EARLY TIMES TO c. 1750

Armit, I., *Celtic Scotland* (London, 1997).
Ashmore, P. J., *Neolithic and Bronze Age Scotland* (London, 1996).
Bannerman, J., *Studies in the History of Dalriada* (Edinburgh, 1974).
Breeze, D., *Roman Scotland: Frontier Country* (London, 1996).
Brotherstone, T. and Ditchburn, D. (eds), *Freedom and Authority. Historical and Historiographical Essays presented to Grant G. Simpson* (East Linton, 2000).
Cowan, E. G. and Macdonald, R. A. (eds), *Alba. Celtic Scotland in the Medieval Era* (East Linton, 2000).
Crawford, B. E. (ed.), *Scotland in Dark Age Britain. The Proceedings of a Day Conference held on 18 February 1995* (Aberdeen, 1996).
Dingwall, H. M., *Late Seventeenth-Century Edinburgh: A Demographic Study* (Aldershot, 1994).

Ditchburn, D., *Scotland and Europe. The Medieval Kingdom and its Contacts with Christendom, 1214–1560* (East Linton, 2001).

Donaldson, G., *James V to James VII* (Edinburgh, 1965).

Ewan, E. and Meikle, M. (eds), *Women in Scotland c. 1100–c. 1750* (East Linton, 1999).

Ferguson, W., *Scotland's Relations with England. A Survey to 1707*, 2nd edn (Edinburgh, 1994).

Grant, A. and Stringer, K. L. (eds), *Medieval Scotland. Crown, Lordship and Community. Essays Presented to G. W. S. Barrow* (Edinburgh, 1998).

Lynch, M. (ed.), *The Early Modern Town in Scotland* (Edinburgh, 1987).

McCrone, D., *The Making of Scotland. Nation, Culture and Social Change* (Edinburgh, 1989).

Maxwell, G. S., *The Romans and Scotland* (Edinburgh, 1989).

Ritchie, G. J. N., *Scotland. Archaeology and Early History* (Edinburgh, 1991).

Whatley, C. A., *Bought and Sold for English Gold? Explaining the Union of 1707* (East Linton, 2001).

Withers, C. W. J., *Geography, Science and National Identity. Scotland Since 1520* (Cambridge, 2001).

Yeoman, P., *Pilgrimage in Medieval Scotland* (London, 1999).

MODERN SCOTLAND FROM c. 1750

Allan, D., *Scotland in the Eighteenth Century. Union and Enlightenment* (Harlow, 2002).

Breitenbach, E. and Gordon, E., *Out of Bounds. Women and Scottish Society 1800–1945* (Edinburgh, 1992).

Broadie, A., *The Scottish Enlightenment. The Historical Age of the Historical Nation* (Edinburgh, 2001).

Camic, C., *Experience and Enlightenment: Socialisation for Cultural Change in Eighteenth-century Scotland* (Edinburgh, 1983).

Campbell, R. H. and Skinner, A. (eds), *The Origins and Nature of the Enlightenment in Scotland* (Edinburgh, 1982).

Carter, J. and Pittock-Wesson, J. (eds), *Aberdeen and the Enlightenment* (Edinburgh, 1989).

Checkland, S. and Checkland, O., *Industry and Ethos. Scotland 1832–1914* (Edinburgh, 1984).

Devine, T. M. and Finlay, R. J. (eds), *Scotland in the Twentieth Century* (Edinburgh, 1996).

Devine, T. M. and Mitchison, R. (eds), *People and Society in Scotland Volume 1, 1760–1830* (Edinburgh, 1988).

Devine, T. M. and Young, J. D. (eds) *Eighteenth-century Scotland. New Perspectives* (East Linton, 1999).

Dickson, T. and Treble, J. H. (eds) *People and Society in Scotland Volume III: 1914 to the Present* (Edinburgh, 1992).

Dwyer, J. H., *Virtuous Discourse. Sensibility and Community in Late Eighteenth-century Scotland* (Edinburgh, 1987).

Dwyer, J. and Sher, R., *Sociability and Society in Eighteenth-century Scotland* (Edinburgh, 1993).

Finlay, R. J., *A Partnership for Good? Scottish Politics and the Union since 1880* (Edinburgh, 1997).

Fraser, W. H. (ed.), *People and Society in Scotland Volume II, 1830–1914* (Edinburgh, 1990).

Harvie, C., *No Gods and Precious Few Heroes. Scotland 1914–1980* (Edinburgh, 1981).

Hook, A. and Sher, R . B., *The Glasgow Enlightenment* (East Linton, 1995).

Houston, R. A., 'Literacy, education and the culture of print in Enlightenment Edinburgh', *History* 78 (1993), 373–92.

Lenman, B. P., *Integration and Enlightenment. Scotland 1746–1832* (London, 1981).

Murdoch, A., *British History 1660–1832. National Identity and Local Culture* (London, 1998).

Porter, R., *The Enlightenment* (Basingstoke, 2001).

Robbins, K., *Nineteenth-century Britain. England, Scotland and Wales: The Making of a Nation* (Oxford, 1988).

Smout, T. C., *A Century of the Scottish People, 1850–1950* (London, 1986).

Withrington, D. J., 'What was distinctive about the Scottish Enlightenment?', in *Aberdeen and the Enlightenment* (eds) Phillipson, N. T. and Mitchison, R., (Edinburgh, 1970), 169–99.

Youngson, A. J., *The Making of Classical Edinburgh, 1750–1840* (Edinburgh, 1966).

MEDICINE

GENERAL

Bynum, W. F. and Porter, R. (eds), *Companion Encyclopedia of the History of Medicine* (London, 1993).

Cartwright, F. F., *A Social History of Medicine* (London, 1977).

Grell, O. P. and Cunningham, A. (eds), *Medicine and the Reformation* (London, 1993).

Guthrie, D., *A History of Medicine* (London, 1960).

Guthrie, D. *Janus in the Doorway* (London, 1963).

Lawrence, C., *Medical Theory, Surgical Practice. Studies in the History of Surgery* (London, 1992).

Loudon, I., *Western Medicine. An Illustrated History* (Oxford, 1997).

Porter, R., *The Cambridge Illustrated History of Medicine* (Cambridge, 1996).

ALTERNATIVE MEDICINE

Bradley, J., Dupree, M. and Durie, A., 'Taking the Water Cure. The Hydropathic Movement in Scotland 1840–1940', *Business and Economic History* 26 (2) (1977), 426–37.

Complementary Medicine and the National Health Service: An Examination of Acupuncture, Homeopathy, Chiropractic and Osteopathy. A Report by the National Medical Advisory Committee (Scottish Office, Edinburgh, 1997).

Davidson, T., *Rowan Tree and Red Thread: A Scottish Witchcraft Miscellany of Tales, Legends and Ballads* (Edinburgh, 1949).

Davies, O., 'Healing charms in use in England and Wales 1700–1950', *Folklore* 197 (1996), 19–32.

Estes, L., 'The medical origins of the European witch craze – a hypothesis', *Journal of Social History* 17 (2) (1983), 271–84.

Kirkpatrick, E. M., *The Little Book of Scottish Grannies' Remedies* (London, 2001).

Porter, R., *Health for Sale. Quackery in England, 1650–1850* (Manchester, 1989).

Sharma, U., *Complementary Medicine Today. Practitioners and Patients* (London, 1992).

DENTISTRY

Forbes, E., 'The professionalisation of dentistry in the United Kingdom, *Med. Hist.* 29 (1985), 169–81.

Macdonald, A. G., 'John Henry Hill Lewellin: the first etherist in Glasgow', *British Journal of Anaesthesia* 70 (1993), 228–34.

Marlborough, H. S., 'The emergence of a graduate dental profession, 1858–1957' (unpublished Ph.D. thesis, University of Glasgow, 1995).

Menzies, C. J., *Dentistry Then and Now* (Glasgow, 1981).

Merrill, H. W., 'Thoughts on the history of dentistry in Scotland', *Dental History* 23 (1992), 15–24.

Meyer, R., M., 'The development of dentistry: A Scottish perspective c. 1800–1921' (unpublished Ph.D. thesis, University of Glasgow, 1994).

Noble, H. W., 'Dental practice in Glasgow, 1790–1799', *Dental History* 27 (1994), 1–7.

EDUCATION

Berry, D., 'Richard Bright (1789–1858): Student days in Edinburgh', *Proc. Roy. Coll. Phys. Ed.* 24 (3) (1994), 383–96.

Collins, K. E., 'Jewish medical students and graduates in Scotland, 1739–1862', *Jewish Historical Studies* 29 (1982), 75–96.

Dow, D. and Moss, M., 'The medical curriculum at Glasgow in the early Nineteenth Century', *History of Universities* 7 (1988), 227–57.

French, R., 'Medical teaching in Aberdeen from the foundation of the university to the middle of the seventeenth century', *History of Universities* 3 (1983), 127–57.

Geary, S., 'Australian medical students in 19th-century Scotland', *Proc. Roy. Coll. Phys. Ed.* 26 (3) (1996), 472–86.

Geyer-Kordesch, J., 'Comparative difficulties: Scottish medical education in the European Context (c. 1690–1830)', *Clio Medica* 30 (1995), 94–115.

Guthrie, D., *Extra-mural Medical Education in Edinburgh and the School of Medicine of the Royal Colleges* (Edinburgh, 1965).

Hoolihan, C., 'Thomas Young. M.D. (1726?–1783) and Obstetrical Education at Edinburgh', *Journal of the History of Medicine* 40 (1985), 327–45.

Innes-Smith, R. W., *English-speaking Students of Medicine at the University of Leiden* (Edinburgh, 1932).

Jacyna, S., 'Theory of medicine; science of life: The place of physiology in the Edinburgh Medical Curriculum, 1790–1870', *Clio Medica* 39 (1995), 141–52.

Kaufman, M. H., and Best, J. J. K., 'Monro secundus and Eighteenth-century lymphangiography', *Proc. Roy. Coll. Phys. Ed.* 26 (1) (1996), 75–90.

Lawrence, C., 'Alexander Monro *Primus* and the Edinburgh Manner of Anatomy', *Bull. Hist. Med.* 62 (1988), 193–214.

Lindeboom, G. A., *Herman Boerhaave: The Man and His Work* (London, 1968).

Risse, G. B., 'Clinical instruction in Hospitals: the Boerhaavian tradition in Leyden, Edinburgh, Vienna and Pavia', *Clio Medica* 21 (1987–88), 1–19.

Taylor, D. W., 'The manuscript lecture notes of Alexander Monro *primus* (1697–1767)', *Med. Hist.* 30 (1986), 444–67.

Turner, A. L. (ed.), *History of the University of Edinburgh, 1833–1933* (Edinburgh, 1933).

ENLIGHTENMENT (SCIENCE AND MEDICINE)

Broman, T., 'The Habermasian public sphere and 'science "in" the enlightenment', *History of Science,* 36 (2) (1998), 123–49.

Daiches, D., Jones, P. and Jones, J. (eds) *A Hotbed of Genius. The Scottish Enlightenment 1730–1790* (Edinburgh, 1986).

Doig, A., Ferguson, J. P. S., Milne, I. A. and Passmore, R. (eds.), *William Cullen and the Eighteenth-century Medical World* (Edinburgh, 1993).

Donovan, A. L., *Philosophical Chemistry in the Scottish Enlightenment: The Doctrines and Discoveries of William Cullen and Joseph Black* (Edinburgh, 1975).

Emerson, R. L., 'Sir Robert Sibbald, Kt, the Royal Society of Scotland and the Origins of the Scottish Enlightenment', *Annals of Science* 45 (1988), 41–72.

Emerson, R. L., 'The Philosophical Society of Edinburgh 1768–1783', *British Journal of the History of Science* 18 (1985), 255–303.

Golinski, J. V., 'Utility and audience in eighteenth-century chemistry: case studies of William Cullen and Joseph Priestley', *British Journal of the History of Science* 21 (1988), 1–31.

Guerrini, A., 'Archibald Pitcairne and Newtonian medicine', *Med. Hist.* 32 (1987), 70–83.

Hamilton, D., 'The Scottish Enlightenment and clinical medicine', in Dow, D. (ed.), *The Influence of Scottish Medicine* (London, 1988), 103–13.

Kaufman, M. H., 'Caesarean operations performed in Edinburgh during the eighteenth century', *British Journal of Obstetrics and Gynaecology* 102 (1995), 186–91.

Jones, P. (ed.), *Philosophy and Science in the Scottish Enlightenment* (Edinburgh, 1988).

Lawrence, C., 'Cullen, Brown and the Poverty of Essentialism', *Med. Hist.,* Supplement No. 8 (1988), 1–21.

Lawrence, C. and Shapin, S. (eds), *Science Incarnate. Historical Embodiments of Natural Knowledge* (Chicago, 1998).

Lowis, G. W., 'Epidemiology of puerperal fever: the contributions of Alexander Gordon', *Med. Hist.* 37 (1993), 399–410.

McGirr, E. M. and Stoddart, W., 'Changing theories in 18th-century medicine. The inheritance and legacy of William Cullen', *Scottish Medical Journal* 36 (1991), 23–6.

Porter, R., *Medicine in the Enlightenment* (Amsterdam, 1995).

Porter, R., *Spreading Medical Enlightenment: The Popularisation of Medicine in Georgian England* (London, 1992).

Stott, R., 'Health and Virtue: Or, how to keep out of harm's way. Lectures on pathology and therapeutics by William Cullen c. 1770', *Med. Hist.* 31 (1987), 123–42.

HOSPITALS (SELECTIVE LIST)

Austin, T., *The Story of Peel Hospital, Galashiels* (Selkirk, 1996).

Boyd, D. H. A., *Leith Hospital 1848–1988* (Edinburgh, 1990).

Campbell, D., *The Hospitals of Peterhead and District* (Aberdeen, 1994).

Catford, E. F., *The Royal Infirmary of Edinburgh 1929–1979* (Edinburgh, 1984).

Eastwood, M. and Jenkinson, A., *A History of the Western General Hospital, Edinburgh* (Edinburgh, 1995).

Gray, J. A., *The Edinburgh City Hospital* (East Linton, 1999).

Hendrie, W. F. and Macleod, D. A. D., *The Bangour Story. A History of Bangour Village and General Hospitals* (Aberdeen, 1991).

Levack, I. and Dudley, H., *Aberdeen Royal Infirmary. The People's Hospital of the North-east* (London, 1992).

Porter, I. A., *Epidemic Diseases in Aberdeen and the History of the City Hospital* (Aberdeen, 2001).

Poynter, F. N. L. (ed.), *The Evolution of Hospitals in Britain* (London, 1964).

Risse, G. B., 'Britannia rules the seas: The health of seamen, Edinburgh, 1791–1800', *Journal of the History of Medicine and Allied Sciences* 43 (1988), 426–446.

Turner, A. L., *Story of a Great Hospital; The Royal Infirmary of Edinburgh, 1729–1929* (Edinburgh, 1937).

Williams, M., *History of Crichton Royal Hospital 1839–1989* (Dumfries, 1989).

Willocks, J. and Calder, A. A., 'The Glasgow Royal Maternity Hospital, 1834–1984'. 150 years of service in a changing obstetric world', *Scottish Medical Journal* 30 (1985), 247–54.

Woodward, J., *To Do the Sick No Harm. A Study of the British Voluntary Hospital System to 1875* (London, 1974).

Yule, B., *Matrons, Medics and Maladies. Edinburgh Royal Infirmary in the 1840s* (East Linton, 1999).

INSTITUTIONS

Cant, R. G., *The University of St Andrews. A Short History* (Edinburgh, 1970).

Clark, G., *A History of the Royal College of Physicians of London, Vol 1* (London, 1964).

Cope, Z., *The History of the Royal College of Surgeons of England* (London, 1959).

Duncan, A., *Memorials of the Faculty of Physicians and Surgeons of Glasgow* (Glasgow, 1896).

Eccles, W., *An Historical Account of the Rights and Privileges of the Royal College of Physicians, and of the Incorporation of Chirurgions in Edinburgh* (Edinburgh, 1707).

Gairdner, J., *Historical Sketch of the Royal College of Surgeons of Edinburgh* (Edinburgh, 1860).

Gray, J., *History of the Royal Medical Society, 1737–1937* (Edinburgh, 1952).

Horn, D. B., *A Short History of the University of Edinburgh* (Edinburgh, 1967).

Mackie, J. D., *The University of Glasgow 1451–1951* (Glasgow, 1954).

O'Day, R., *The Professions in Early Modern* England (London, 2000).

Passmore, R. (ed.), *Proceedings of the Royal College of Physicians of Edinburgh. Tercentenary Congress 1981* (Cambridge, 1982).

Ritchie, P., *The Early Days of the Royall Colledge of Phisitians, Edinburgh* (Edinburgh, 1899).

MENTAL HEALTH

Jones, K., *Asylums and After. A Revised History of the Mental Health Services: From the Early 18th Century to the 1990s* (London, 1993).

Porter, R., *A Social History of Madness* (London, 1987).

Scull, A., *Madhouses, Mad-Doctors and Madmen: The Social History of Psychiatry in the Victorian Era* (London, 1981).

Scull, A., *The Most Solitary of Afflictions. Madness and Society in Britain, 1700–1900* (London, 1993).

Weir, R. I., 'An experimental course of lectures on moral treatment for mentally ill people', *Journal of Advanced Nursing* 17 (1992), 390–5.

MILITARY

Blair, J. S. G., *The Royal Army Medical Corps 1898–1998. Reflections of One Hundred Years of Service* (RAMC, 1998).

Cook, H. J., 'Practical medicine and the British armed forces after the "Glorious Revolution"', *Med. Hist.* 34 (1990), 1–26.

Kaufman, M. H., 'Clinical case histories and sketches of gun-shot injuries from the Carlist war', *Journal of the Royal College of Surgeons of Edinburgh* 46 (5) (2001), 279–89.

Kaufman, M. H., 'The gunner with silver mask: observations on the management of severe maxillo-facial lesions over the last 160 years', *Journal of the Royal College of Surgeons of Edinburgh* 42 (1997), 367–75.

Kaufman, M. H., *Surgeons at War. Medical Arrangements for the Treatment of the Sick and wounded in the British Army During the Late Eighteenth and Nineteenth Centuries* (London, 2001).

Kaufman, M. H., Purdue, B. N. and Carswell, A. L., 'Old wounds and distant battles: The Alcock-Ballingall collection of military surgery at the University of Edinburgh', *Journal of the Royal College of Surgeons of Edinburgh* 41 (1996), 339–50.

Lind, J., *An Essay on the Most Effectual Means of Preserving the Health of Seamen in the Royal Navy: And a Dissertation on Fevers and Infections: Together with Observations on the Jail Distemper and the Proper Means of Preventing and Stopping its Infections* (London, 1774).

Pringle, J., *Observations on the Diseases of the Army* (London, 1764).

PUBLIC AND NATIONAL HEALTH TOPICS

Allison, W. P., *Observations on the Management of the Poor in Scotland and its Effects on the Health of the Great Towns* (Edinburgh, 1840).

Berridge, V., *Health and Society in Britain Since 1939* (Cambridge, 1999).

Brotherston, J. H. F., *Observations on the Early Public Health Movement in Scotland* (London, 1952).

Brunton, D., 'Practitioners versus legislators: the shaping of the Scottish Vaccination Act', *Proc. Roy. Coll. Phys. Ed.* 23 (1993), 193–201.

Carstairs, V. and Russell, M., *Deprivation and Health in Scotland* (Aberdeen, 1991).

Checkland, O. (ed.), *Health Care as Social History. The Glasgow Case* (Aberdeen, 1982).

Davidson, R., *Dangerous Liaisons. A Social History of Venereal Disease in Twentieth-century Scotland* (Amsterdam, 2000).

Ilett, I., and Laughlin, S., 'Devolving health and building a healthy Scotland: from the Medical Social Model in the post-devolution environment', *Renewal* 9 (1) (2001), 26–35.

Jacyna, S., '"A host of experienced microscopists": the establishment of histology in nineteenth-century Edinburgh', *Bull. Hist. Med.* 75 (2) (2001), 225–53.

Loudon, I., *Medical Care and the General Practitioner 1750–1850* (Oxford, 1986).

Loudon, R., Horder, J. and Webster, C. (eds), *General Practice under the National Health Service 1948–1997* (Oxford, 1998).

Macdonald, F., 'Vaccination Policy of the Faculty of Physicians and Surgeons of Glasgow, 1801–1863', *Med. Hist.* 41 (1997), 291–321.

Macdonald, I. S., 'The Origins of the Government's Doctors in Scotland', *Health Bulletin* 49 (2) (1991), 118–35.

Mathieson, R., *The Survival of the Unfittest. The Highland Clearances and the End of Isolation* (Edinburgh, 2000).

Pelling, M., *The Common Lot. Sickness, Medical Occupations and the Urban Poor in Early Modern England* (London, 1998).

Porter, R., *Disease, Medicine and Society in England, 1550–1860* (Cambridge, 1993).

Rushman, G. B., *A Short History of Anaesthesia* (London, 1996)

Smith, R. G., 'The Development of Ethical Guidance for Medical Practitioners by the General Medical Council', *Med. Hist.* 37 (1993), 56–67.

Tait, H. P., *A Doctor and Two Policemen: The History of Edinburgh Health Department, 1862–1974* (Edinburgh, 1974).

WOMEN

Bashford, A., *Purity and Pollution. Gender, Embodiment and Victorian Medicine* (London, 2000).

Bonner, T. N., 'Medical woman abroad: a new dimension of women's push for opportunity in medicine, 1850–1914', *Bull. Hist. Med.* 62 (1988).

Dyhouse, C., *No Distinction of Sex? Women in British Universities 1870–1939* (London, 1995).

Gordon, W. M., 'The right of women to graduate in medicine – Scottish judicial attitudes in the nineteenth century', *Journal of Legal History* 52 (1984), 136–51.

Lutzker, E., *Women Gain a Place in Medicine* (London, 1969).

Roberts, S., *Sophia Jex-Blake. A Woman Pioneer in Nineteenth-century Medical Reform* (London, 1993).

SELECT BIBLIOGRAPHY

The following brief and highly selective bibliography lists some of the major works referred to in this book. It is by no means exhaustive, and does not include journal articles. Fuller bibliographical references may be found in the 'Further Reading' section, and in the notes for each chapter.

Allan, D., *Virtue, Learning and the Scottish Enlightenment* (Edinburgh, 1993).

Anderson, B. R. O., *Imagined Communities: Reflections on the Origins and Spread of Nationalism* (London, 1991).

Armit, I., *Scotland's Hidden History* (Stroud, 1999).

Bannerman, J., *The Beatons. A Medical Kindred in the Classical Gaelic Tradition* (Edinburgh, 1986).

Barrell, A. D. M, *Medieval Scotland* (Cambridge, 2000).

Beith, M., *Healing Threads. Traditional Medicine of the Highlands and Islands* (Edinburgh, 1995).

Blair, J. S. G., *History of Medicine in the University of St Andrews* (Edinburgh, 1987).

Bonner, T., *To the Ends of the Earth. Women's Search for Education in Medicine* (Massachusetts, 1992).

Brockliss, L. and Jones, C., *The Medical World of Early Modern France* (Oxford, 1997).

Broun, D., Finlay, R. and Lynch, M. (eds), *Image and Identity. The Making and Remaking of Scotland Through the Ages* (Edinburgh, 1998).

Brown, C., *Religion and Society in Scotland Since 1707* (Edinburgh, 1999).

Brown, K. M., *Kingdom or Province? Scotland and the Regal Union, 1603–1707* (London, 1992).

Buchan, D., *Folk Tradition and Folk Medicine in Scotland. The Writings of David Rorie* (Edinburgh, 1994).

Campbell, R. A. and Skinner, A. S. (eds), *The Origins and Nature of the Scottish Enlightenment* (Edinburgh, 1982).

Chitnis, A. C., *The Scottish Enlightenment. A Social History* (Edinburgh, 1976).

Colley, L., *Britons. Forging the Nation* (London, 1992).

Comrie, J. D., *History of Scottish Medicine*, 2 vols (Oxford, 1932).

Conrad, L. L. et al., *The Western Medical Tradition 800BC–1800AD* (Cambridge, 1995).

Craig, W. S., *History of the Royal College of Physicians of Edinburgh* (Oxford, 1976).

Creswell, C. H., *The Royal College of Surgeons of Edinburgh. Historical Notes from 1505–1905* (Edinburgh, 1926).

Cunningham, A. and French, R. A. (eds), *The Medical Enlightenment of the Eighteenth Century* (London, 1990).

Darwin, T., *The Scots Herbal. The Plant Lore of Scotland* (Edinburgh, 1996).

Daunton, M. (ed.), *The Cambridge Urban History of Britain. Volume III, 1840–1950* (Cambridge, 2000).

Devine, T. M., *The Scottish Nation 1700–2000* (Edinburgh, 1999).

Devine, T. M. and Jackson, G. (eds), *Glasgow Vol I. Beginnings to 1830* (Manchester, 1995).

Dingwall, H. M., *Physicians, Surgeons and Apothecaries. Medical Practice in Seventeenth-century Edinburgh* (East Linton, 1995).

Dow, D. (ed.), *The Influence of Scottish Medicine* (London, 1986).

Finlayson, G., *Citizen, State and Social Welfare in Britain 1839–1990* (Oxford, 1994).

Fraser, W. H. and Maver, I. (eds), *Glasgow Vol II. 1830–1912* (Manchester, 1996).

Gentilcore, D., *Healers and Healing in Early Modern Italy* (Manchester, 1998).

Gelfand, T., *Professionalising Modern Medicine. Paris Surgeons and Medical Science Institutions in the Eighteenth Century* (London, 1980).

Geyer-Kordesch, J. and Macdonald, F., *Physicians and Surgeons in Glasgow. The History of the Royal College of Physicians and Surgeons of Glasgow* (Oxford, 1999).

Grant, A., *Independence and Nationhood. Scotland 1306–1469* (Edinburgh, 1984).

Habermas, J., *The Structural Transformation of the Public Sphere. An Inquiry into a Category of Bourgeois Society*, trans. Burger, T. (Cambridge, 1989).

Hamilton, D., *The Healers. A History of Medicine in Scotland* (Edinburgh, 1981).

Hardy, A., *Health and Medicine in Britain Since 1860* (Basingstoke, 2001). (Basingstoke, 2001).

Henry, J., *The Scientific Revolution and the Origins of Modern Science* (Basingstoke, 1997).

Houston, R. A., *Madness and Society in Eighteenth-century Scotland* (Oxford, 2000).

Houston, R. A. and Whyte, I. D. (eds), *Scottish Society 1500–1800* (Cambridge, 1989).

Hull, A. and Geyer-Kordesch, J., *The Shaping of the Medical Profession. The History of the Royal College of Physicians and Surgeons of Glasgow, 1858–1999* (Oxford, 1999).

Hutchison, I. G. C., *Scottish Politics in the Twentieth Century* (Basingstoke, 2001).

Jacyna, S., *Philosophic Whigs. Medicine, Science and Citizenship in Edinburgh, 1789–1848* (London, 1994).

Jenkinson, J. L. M., *Scottish Medical Societies 1731–1939* (Edinburgh, 1993).

Jenkinson, J. L. M., Moss, M., and Russell, I. (eds) *The Royal. The History of Glasgow Royal Infirmary, 1794–1994* (Glasgow, 1994).

Lane, J., *A Social History of Medicine. Health, Healing and Disease in England, 1750–1950* (London, 2001).

Larner, C., *Enemies of God. The Witch Hunt in Scotland* (Edinburgh, 1983).

Lawrence, C., *Medicine in the Making of Modern Britain* (London, 1994).

Lenman, B. P., *An Economic History of Modern Scotland* (Edinburgh, 1977).

Levitt, I., *Poverty and Welfare in Scotland 1890–1948* (Edinburgh, 1998).

Lynch, M., *Scotland. A New History* (London, 1991).

MacQueen, J., *Humanism in Renaissance Scotland* (Edinburgh, 1990).

McLachlan, G. (ed.), *Improving the Common Weal. Aspects of Scottish Health Services, 1900–1984* (Edinburgh, 1987).

Martin, M., *A Description of the Western Highlands and Islands of Scotland Circa 1695* (Edinburgh, 1999).

Mitchison, R., *The Old Poor Law in Scotland* (Edinburgh, 2000).

Nottingham, C. (ed.), *The NHS in Scotland. The Legacy of the Past and the Prospect of the Future* (Aldershot, 2000).

Nutton, V. and Porter, R. (eds), *History of Medical Education in Britain* (Amsterdam, 1995).

Pennington, C., *The Modernisation of Medical Teaching at Aberdeen in the Nineteenth Century* (Aberdeen, 1994).

Phillipson, N. T. and Mitchison, R. (eds), *Scotland in the Age of Improvement* (Edinburgh, 1970).

Porter, R., *The Greatest Benefit to Mankind. A Medical History of Humanity from Antiquity to the Present* (London, 1997).

Porter, R. and Teich, M. (eds), *The Enlightenment in its National Context* (London, 1981).

Risse, G., *Hospital Life in Enlightenment Scotland. Care and Teaching at the Edinburgh Infirmary* (Cambridge, 1986).

Risse, G., *Mending Bodies. Saving Souls,. A History of Hospitals* (Oxford, 1999).

Robertson, E., *Glasgow's Doctor. James Burn Russell, 1837–1904* (East Linton, 1998).

Rosner, L., *Medical Education in the Age of Improvement* (Edinburgh, 1991).

Shaw, J. J., *The Politics of Eighteenth-century Scotland* (London, 1999).

Thomson, F. M. L. (ed.), *The Cambridge Social History of Britain. Volume III 1750–1950* (Cambridge, 1990).

Watson, F., *Scotland. A History* (Stroud, 2001).

Webster, B., *Medieval Scotland. The Making of an Identity* (London, 1997).

Webster, C., *The National Health Service. A Political History* (Oxford, 1998).

Whatley, C. A., *Scottish Society 1707–1830* (Manchester, 2000).

Whyte, I. D., *Scotland Before the Industrial Revolution* c. 1050–1750 (London, 1995).

Wood, P. (ed.), *The Scottish Enlightenment. Essays in Reinterpretation* (Rochester, 2000).

Young, S., *Annals of the Barber Surgeons of London* (London, 1980).

INDEX